Lecture Notes in Computer Science 5128

Commenced Publication in 1973
Founding and Former Series Editors:
Gerhard Goos, Juris Hartmanis, ~~and Jan van Leeuwen~~

Takeyoshi Dohi   Ichiro Sakuma
Hongen Liao (Eds.)

Medical Imaging and Augmented Reality

4th International Workshop
Tokyo, Japan, August 1-2, 2008
Proceedings

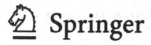
Springer

Volume Editors

Takeyoshi Dohi
The University of Tokyo
Department of Mechano-Informatics
Tokyo, Japan
E-mail: takdohi@i.u-tokyo.ac.jp

Ichiro Sakuma
The University of Tokyo
Department of Precision Engineering
Tokyo, Japan
E-mail: sakuma@bmpe.t.u-tokyo.ac.jp

Hongen Liao
The University of Tokyo
Department of Bioengineering
Tokyo, Japan
E-mail: liao@bmpe.t.u-tokyo.ac.jp

Library of Congress Control Number: 2008931096

CR Subject Classification (1998): I.5, I.4, I.3.5-8, I.2.9-10, J.3, I.6

LNCS Sublibrary: SL 6 – Image Processing, Computer Vision, Pattern Recognition, and Graphics

ISSN   0302-9743
ISBN-10   3-540-79981-8 Springer Berlin Heidelberg New York
ISBN-13   978-3-540-79981-8 Springer Berlin Heidelberg New York

Springer is a part of Springer Science+Business Media

springer.com

© Springer-Verlag Berlin Heidelberg 2008

Typesetting: Camera-ready by author, data conversion by Scientific Publishing Services, Chennai, India
Printed on acid-free paper   SPIN: 12446698   06/3180   5 4 3 2 1 0

Preface

The 4th International Workshop on Medical Imaging and Augmented Reality, MIAR 2008, was held at the University of Tokyo, Tokyo, Japan during August 1–2, 2008.

The goal of MIAR 2008 was to bring together researchers in medical imaging and intervention to present state-of-the-art developments in this ever-growing research area. Rapid technical advances in medical imaging, including its growing application in drug/gene therapy and invasive/interventional procedures, have attracted significant interest in the close integration of research in the life sciences, medicine, physical sciences, and engineering. Current research is also motivated by the fact that medical imaging is moving increasingly from a primarily diagnostic modality towards a therapeutic and interventional aid, driven by the streamlining of diagnostic and therapeutic processes for human diseases by means of imaging modalities and robotic-assisted surgery.

The impact of MIAR on these fields increases each year, and the quality of submitted papers this year was very impressive. We received 90 full submissions, which were subsequently reviewed by up to five reviewers. Reviewer affiliations were carefully checked against author affiliations to avoid conflicts of interest, and the review process was run as a double-blind process. A special procedure was also devised for papers from the universities of the organizers, upholding a double-blind review process for these papers. The MIAR 2008 Program Committee finally accepted 44 full papers. For this workshop, we also included three papers from the invited speakers covering registration and segmentation, virtual reality, and perceptual docking for robotic control. The meeting consisted of a single track of oral/poster presentations, with each session led by an invited lecture from our distinguished international faculty.

Running such a workshop requires dedication, and we appreciate the commitment of the MIAR 2008 Program Committee and reviewers who worked in putting together this workshop. We are grateful to everyone who participated in the review process; they donated a large amount of time and effort to make these volumes possible and insure a high level of quality. We thank the invited speakers Makoto Hashizume from Kyushu University, Japan, Koji Ikuta from Nagoya University, Japan, Nassir Navab from Technische Universität München (TUM), Germany, Terry Peters from the University of Western Ontario, Canada, Stephen Wong from Methodist Hospital-Weill Cornell Medical College, USA, and Guang-Zhong Yang from Imperial College, London, UK. A series of sponsors helped make the conference possible, and for this they are thanked.

It was our great pleasure to welcome this year's MIAR attendees to Tokyo, which is an ideal center for exploring history and culture, and for natural beauty as well as for shopping. Tokyo also boasts 240 art museums and galleries and more than 270 parks and gardens, drawing a large crowd of visitors. Tokyo is a multicultural metropolis with both modern and traditional Japanese features and we trust that the attendees took the opportunity to explore many different aspects of the city in addition to attending the workshop.

For those who were unable to attend, we hope this volume will act as a valuable reference to the MIAR disciplines, and we look forward to meeting you at future MIAR workshops.

August 2008

Takeyoshi Dohi
Ichiro Sakuma
Hongen Liao

Organization

Executive Committee

General Chair

Takeyoshi Dohi — Department of Mechano-Informatics, The University of Tokyo, Japan

Program Chair

Ichiro Sakuma — Department of Precision Engineering, The University of Tokyo, Japan

Organization Chair

Hongen Liao — Department of Bioengineering, The University of Tokyo, Japan

Program Committee

Nicholas Ayache — INRIA, France
Christian Barillot — IRISA, Rennes, France
Yiyu Cai — Nanyang Technological University, Singapore
Gary Egan — Howard Florey Institute, Australia
Gabor Fichtinger — Queen's University, Canada
David Firmin — Imperial College, UK
Masakatsu G. Fujie — Waseda University, Japan
James Gee — University of Pennsylvania, USA
Guido Gerig — University of North Carolina at Chapel Hill, USA
Lixu Gu — Shanghai Jiaotong University, China
Makoto Hashizume — Kyushu University, Japan
Karl Heinz Hoehne — University Medical Center Hamburg-Eppendorf, Germany
Xiaoping Hu — Emory University, USA
Koji Ikuta — Nagoya University, Japan
Horace Ip — City University of Hong Kong, China
Hiroshi Iseki — Tokyo Women's Medical University, Japan
Tianzi Jiang — NLPR, Institute of Automation, CAS, China
Ron Kikinis — Brigham & Women's Hospital, Harvard Medical School, USA
Young-Soo Kim — Hanyang University, Korea
Zhi-Pei Liang — University of Illinois at Urbana-Champaign, USA

Tianming Liu	Weill Medical College of Cornell University, USA
Anthony Maeder	CSIRO, Australia
Ken Masamune	The University of Tokyo, Japan
Yoichi Matsumoto	The University of Tokyo, Japan
Mamoru Mitsuishi	The University of Tokyo, Japan
Kensaku Mori	Nagoya University, Japan
Nassir Navab	Technische Universität/München, Germany
Xiaochuan Pan	University of Chicago, USA
Terry Peters	Robarts Research Institute, Canada
Stephen Riederer	Mayo Clinic, USA
Yoshinobu Sato	Osaka University, Japan
Dinggang Shen	University of Pennsylvania, USA
Pengcheng Shi	Hong Kong University of Science and Technology, China
Jin-Suck Suh	Yonsei University College of Medicine, Korea
Naoki Suzuki	Jikei University School of Medicine, Japan
Russell H. Taylor	Johns Hopkins University, USA
Max Viergever	University Medical Center Utrecht, The Netherlands
Yingxiao Wang	University of Illinois at Urbana-Champaign, USA
Stephen TC Wong	Methodist Hospital - Weill Cornell Medical College, USA
Chenyang Xu	Siemens Research, USA
Guang-Zhong Yang	Imperial College London, UK

Poster Coordination

Yasushi Yamauchi   Toyo University, Japan

Student Awards Coordination

Yoshitaka Masutani   The University of Tokyo, Japan

Sponsor and Exhibits Coordination

Etsuko Kobayashi   The University of Tokyo, Japan

Local Organizing Committee

Jaesung Hong	Kyushu University, Japan
Norihiro Koizumi	The University of Tokyo, Japan
Masahiko Nakamoto	Osaka University, Japan
Ryoichi Nakamura	Tokyo Women's Medical University, Japan
Hiromasa Yamashita	The University of Tokyo, Japan
Kiyoshi Yoshinaka	The University of Tokyo, Japan

Conference Secretariat

Nicholas Herlambang The University of Tokyo, Japan

Reviewers

Purang Abolmaesumi
Brian Avants
Suyash Awate
Yiyu Cai
Vassilis Charissis
Adrian Chung
Moo K. Chung
Philip Cook
Xiang Deng
Gary Egan
Gabor Fichtinger
Michael Figl
David Firmin
James Gee
Guido Gerig
Ali Gooya
Lixu Gu
Yujum Guo
Makoto Hashizume
Yong He
Nicholas Herlambang
Jaesung Hong
Xiaoping Hu
Ameet Jain
Tianzi Jiang
Jongmyon Kim
Sang-Youn Kim
Young-Soo Kim
Norihiro Koizumi
Nina Kozic
Susanne Kraemer
Jeongjin Lee
Yeon Soo Lee
Ming Li
Jianming Liang
Hongen Liao
Huafeng Liu
Tianming Liu

Zhentai Lu
Anthony Maeder
Ken Masamune
Ashraf Mohamed
Kensaku Mori
Ryoichi Nakamura
Hsiao Piau Ng
Marek Ogiela
Xiaochuan Pan
Terry Peters
Matthias Raspe
Mauricio Reyes
Stephen J. Riederer
Su Ruan
Yoshinobu Sato
Dinggang Shen
Pengcheng Shi
Danail Stoyanov
Hui Sun
Hotaka Takizawa
Xiaodong Tao
Russell H. Taylor
Thomas Tolxdorff
Joerg Traub
Nicholas Tustison
Tomaz Vrtovec
Lei Wang
Liansheng Wang
Linwei Wang
Yingxiao Wang
Changhua Wu
Hiromasa Yamashita
Faguo Yang
Guang-Zhong Yang
Paul Yushkevich
Heye Zhang
Guoyan Zheng
Chaozhe Zhu

Sponsors and Partners

Aloka Co., Ltd.
Fukuda Foundation for Medical Technology
Hoya Corporation (Pentax)
Inoue Foundation for Science
Japan Interaction in Science & Technology Forum
Japan Society of Computer Aided Surgery
NDI-Northern Digital Inc.
Olympus Corporation
Shinko Optical Co., Ltd.
Siemens Corporate Research
Terumo Corporation
The Precise Measurement Technique Promoting Foundation
The University of Tokyo
Totoku Electric Co., Ltd.
Translational Systems Biology and Medicine Initiative

Table of Contents

Invited Contributions

Towards a Medical Virtual Reality Environment for Minimally Invasive
Cardiac Surgery 1
  *Terry M. Peters, Cristian A. Linte, John Moore, Daniel Bainbridge,
  Douglas L. Jones, and Gérard M. Guiraudon*

Joint Registration and Segmentation of Serial Lung CT Images in
Microendoscopy Molecular Image-Guided Therapy 12
  Zhong Xue, Kelvin Wong, and Stephen Wong

Perceptual Docking for Robotic Control............................ 21
  *Guang-Zhong Yang, George P. Mylonas, Ka-Wai Kwok, and
  Adrian Chung*

Surgical Planning and Simulation

An Integration of Statistical Deformable Model and Finite Element
Method for Bone-Related Soft Tissue Prediction in Orthognathic
Surgery Planning 31
  Qizhen He, Jun Feng, Horace H.S. Ip, James Xia, and Xianbin Cao

Automated Preoperative Planning of Femoral Component for Total
Hip Arthroplasty (THA) from 3D CT Images........................ 40
  *Itaru Otomaru, Masahiko Nakamoto, Masaki Takao,
  Nobuhiko Sugano, Yoshiyuki Kagiyama, Hideki Yoshikawa,
  Yukio Tada, and Yoshinobu Sato*

Validation of Viscoelastic and Nonlinear Liver Model for Needle
Insertion from in Vivo Experiments 50
  *Yo Kobayashi, Akinori Onishi, Takeharu Hoshi, Kazuya Kawamura,
  Makoto Hashizume, and Masakatsu G. Fujie*

Simulation of Active Cardiac Electromechanical Dynamics 60
  *Ken C.L. Wong, Linwei Wang, Heye Zhang, Huafeng Liu, and
  Pengcheng Shi*

Wheelchair Propulsion Analysis System That Incorporates Human
Skeletal Muscular Model Analyses on the Flat Floor and Slope 70
  *Akihiko Hanafusa, Motoki Sugawara, Teruhiko Fuwa,
  Tomozumi Ikeda, Naoki Suzuki, and Asaki Hattori*

Medical Image Computing

Automatic Detection of Fiducial Marker Center Based on Shape Index
and Curvedness   81
   Manning Wang and Zhijian Song

Modality-Independent Determination of Vertebral Position and
Rotation in 3D   89
   Tomaž Vrtovec

Coupled Meshfree-BEM Platform for Electrocardiographic Simulation:
Modeling and Validations   98
   Linwei Wang, Heye Zhang, Ken C.L. Wong, and Pengcheng Shi

Source Localization of Subtopographies Decomposed by Radial Basis
Functions   108
   Adil Deniz Duru and Ahmet Ademoglu

Estimation of the Current Density in a Dynamic Heart Model and
Visualization of Its Propagation   116
   Liansheng Wang, Pheng Ann Heng, and Wong Tien Tsin

Image Analysis

Identification of Atrophy Patterns in Alzheimer's Disease Based on
SVM Feature Selection and Anatomical Parcellation   124
   Lilia Mesrob, Benoit Magnin, Olivier Colliot, Marie Sarazin,
   Valérie Hahn-Barma, Bruno Dubois, Patrick Gallinari,
   Stéphane Lehéricy, Serge Kinkingnéhun, and Habib Benali

A Surface-Based Fractal Information Dimension Method for Cortical
Complexity Analysis   133
   Yuanchao Zhang, Jiefeng Jiang, Lei Lin, Feng Shi, Yuan Zhou,
   Chunshui Yu, Kuncheng Li, and Tianzi Jiang

Wavelet-Based Compression and Segmentation of Hyperspectral Images
in Surgery   142
   Hamed Akbari, Yukio Kosugi, Kazuyuki Kojima, and
   Naofumi Tanaka

A Novel Level Set Based Shape Prior Method for Liver Segmentation
from MRI Images   150
   Kan Cheng, Lixu Gu, Jianghua Wu, Wei Li, and Jianrong Xu

Shape Modeling and Morphometry

Statistical Shape Space Analysis Based on Level Sets   160
   Nina Kozic, Miguel Á. González Ballester, Moritz Tannast,
   Lutz P. Nolte, and Mauricio Reyes

Statistical Piecewise Assembled Model (SPAM) for the Representation
of Highly Deformable Medical Organs 168
    Jun Feng, Peng Du, and Horace H.S. Ip

Amygdala Surface Modeling with Weighted Spherical Harmonics 177
    Moo K. Chung, Brendon M. Nacewicz, Shubing Wang,
    Kim M. Dalton, Seth Pollak, and Richard J. Davidson

Kalman Filtering for Frame-by-Frame CT to Ultrasound Rigid
Registration 185
    Haydar Talib, Matthias Peterhans, Jaime García,
    Martin Styner, and Miguel A. González Ballester

Cardiac PET Motion Correction Using Materially Constrained
Transform Models.. 193
    Adrian J. Chung, Paolo G. Camici, and Guang-Zhong Yang

Image-Guided Robotics

Image Guidance for Robotic Minimally Invasive Coronary Artery
Bypass 202
    Michael Figl, Daniel Rueckert, David Hawkes, Roberto Casula,
    Mingxing Hu, Ose Pedro, Dong Ping Zhang, Graeme Penney,
    Fernando Bello, and Philip Edwards

MRI-Compatible Rigid and Flexible Outer Sheath Device with
Pneumatic Locking Mechanism for Minimally Invasive Surgery......... 210
    Siyang Zuo, Noriaki Yamanaka, Ikuma Sato, Ken Masamune,
    Hongen Liao, Kiyoshi Matsumiya, and Takeyoshi Dohi

MR Compatible Tactile Sensing and Noise Analysis in a 1.5 Tesla MR
System 220
    Abbi Hamed, Zion Tsz Ho Tse, Ian Young, and Michael Lamperth

A Framework of the Non-invasive Ultrasound Theragnostic System 231
    Norihiro Koizumi, Deukhee Lee, Kohei Ota, Shin Yoshizawa,
    Kiyoshi Yoshinaka, Yoichiro Matsumoto, and Mamoru Mitsuishi

Image-Guided Intervention

In Vivo Evaluation of a Guidance System for Computer Assisted
Robotized Needle Insertion Devoted to Small Animals 241
    Stephane A. Nicolau, Luis Mendoza-Burgos, Luc Soler,
    Didier Mutter, and Jacques Marescaux

Composite-Type Optical Fiberscope for Laser Surgery for Twin-to-Twin
Transfusion Syndrome 251
    Kiyoshi Oka, Akihiro Naganawa, Hiromasa Yamashita,
    Tetsuya Nakamura, and Toshio Chiba

Surgical Manipulator with Balloon for Stabilizing Fetus in Utero under
Ultrasound Guidance 260
    Noriaki Yamanaka, Hiromasa Yamashita, Kiyoshi Matsumiya,
    Hongen Liao, Ken Masamune, Toshio Chiba, and Takeyoshi Dohi

Investigation of Partial Directed Coherence for Hand-Eye Coordination
in Laparoscopic Training 270
    Julian J.H. Leong, Louis Atallah, George P. Mylonas, Daniel R. Leff,
    Roger J. Emery, Ara W. Darzi, and Guang-Zhong Yang

A Virtual Reality Patient and Environments for Image Guided
Diagnosis 279
    Barnabas Takacs, David Hanak, and Kirby G. Voshburg

Interventional Imaging

A Navigation System for Brain Surgery Using Computer Vision
Technology 289
    Jiann-Der Lee, Chung-Wei Lin, Chung-Hsien Huang,
    Shin-Tseng Lee, and Chien-Tsai Wu

Computer-Aided Delivery of High-Intensity Focused Ultrasound
(HIFU) for Creation of an Atrial Septal Defect in Vivo 300
    Hiromasa Yamashita, Tetsuko Ishii, Akihiko Ishiyama,
    Noriyoshi Nakayama, Toshinobu Miyoshi, Yoshitaka Miyamoto,
    Gontaro Kitazumi, Yasumasa Katsuike, Makoto Okazaki,
    Takashi Azuma, Masayuki Fujisaki, Shinichi Takamoto, and
    Toshio Chiba

Basic Study on Real-Time Simulation Using Mass Spring System for
Robotic Surgery 311
    Kazuya Kawamura, Yo Kobayashi, and Masakatsu G. Fujie

A Precise Robotic Ablation and Division Mechanism for Liver
Resection 320
    Florence Leong, Liangjing Yang, Stephen Chang, Aun Neow Poo,
    Ichiro Sakuma, and Chee-Kong Chui

Image Registration

Fast Image Mapping of Endoscopic Image Mosaics with
Three-Dimensional Ultrasound Image for Intrauterine Treatment of
Twin-to-Twin Transfusion Syndrome 329
    Hongen Liao, Masayoshi Tsuzuki, Etsuko Kobayashi,
    Takeyoshi Dohi, Toshio Chiba, Takashi Mochizuki, and
    Ichiro Sakuma

Non-rigid 2D-3D Registration Based on Support Vector Regression
Estimated Similarity Metric   339
     Wenyuan Qi, Lixu Gu, and Jianrong Xu

Real-Time Autostereoscopic Visualization of Registration-Generated
4D MR Image of Beating Heart   349
     Nicholas Herlambang, Hongen Liao, Kiyoshi Matsumiya,
     Ken Masamune, and Takeyoshi Dohi

Augmented Reality

Realtime Organ Tracking for Endoscopic Augmented Reality
Visualization Using Miniature Wireless Magnetic Tracker   359
     Masahiko Nakamoto, Osamu Ukimura, Inderbir S. Gill,
     Arul Mahadevan, Tsuneharu Miki, Makoto Hashizume, and
     Yoshinobu Sato

Fusion of Laser Guidance and 3-D Autostereoscopic Image Overlay for
Precision-Guided Surgery   367
     Hongen Liao, Hirotaka Ishihara, Huy Hoang Tran, Ken Masamune,
     Ichiro Sakuma, and Takeyoshi Dohi

Augmented Display of Anatomical Names of Bronchial Branches for
Bronchoscopy Assistance   377
     Shunsuke Ota, Daisuke Deguchi, Takayuki Kitasaka, Kensaku Mori,
     Yasuhito Suenaga, Yoshinori Hasegawa, Kazuyoshi Imaizumi,
     Hirotsugu Takabatake, Masaki Mori, and Hiroshi Natori

Non-metal Slice Image Overlay Display System Used Inside the Open
Type MRI   385
     Ken Masamune, Ikuma Sato, Hongen Liao, and Takeyoshi Dohi

Image Segmentation

Extracting Curve Skeletons from Gray Value Images for Virtual
Endoscopy   393
     Christian Bauer and Horst Bischof

Automatic Hepatic Vessel Segmentation Using Graphics Hardware   403
     Marius Erdt, Matthias Raspe, and Michael Suehling

Learning Longitudinal Deformations for Adaptive Segmentation of
Lung Fields from Serial Chest Radiographs   413
     Yonghong Shi and Dinggang Shen

Automatic Extraction of Proximal Femur Contours from Calibrated
X-Ray Images Using 3D Statistical Models   421
     Xiao Dong and Guoyan Zheng

Anisotropic Haralick Edge Detection Scheme with Application to Vessel
Segmentation.. 430
    Ali Gooya, Takeyoshi Dohi, Ichiro Sakuma, and Hongen Liao

Author Index.. 439

Towards a Medical Virtual Reality Environment for Minimally Invasive Cardiac Surgery

Terry M. Peters[1,2,5], Cristian A. Linte[1,2], John Moore[1], Daniel Bainbridge[3], Douglas L. Jones[4,5], and Gérard M. Guiraudon[1,5]

[1] Imaging Research Laboratories, Robarts Research Institute,
[2] Biomedical Engineering Graduate Program, University of Western Ontario,
[3] Division of Anaesthesia, University of Western Ontario,
[4] Department of Physiology & Pharmacology, University of Western Ontario,
[5] Canadian Surgical Technologies and Advanced Robotics,
London, Ontario, Canada

Abstract. We have developed a visualization environment to assist surgeons with therapy delivery inside the beating heart, in absence of direct vision. This system employs virtual reality techniques to integrate pre-operative anatomical models, real-time intra-operative imaging, and models of magnetically-tracked surgical tools. Visualization is enhanced via 3D dynamic cardiac models constructed from high-resolution pre-operative MR or CT data and registered within the intra-operative imaging environment. In this paper, we report our experience with a feature-based registration technique to fuse the pre- and intra-operative data during an *in vivo* intracardiac procedure on a porcine subject. Good alignment of the pre- and intra-operative anatomy within the virtual reality environment is ensured through the registration of easily identifiable landmarks. We present our initial experience in translating this work into the operating room and employing this system to guide typical intracardiac interventions. Given its extensive capabilities in providing surgical guidance in the absence of direct vision, our virtual environment is an ideal candidate for performing off-pump intracardiac interventions.

Keywords: Minimally Invasive Surgery, Off-pump Cardiac Procedures, Intra-procedure Imaging, Organ Modeling, Virtual Augmented Reality.

1 Introduction

While recent technological advancements have enabled the use of less invasive approaches to reduce morbidity during surgical interventions, the translation of these enhancements to minimally invasive intracardiac therapy has been slow. Most complex procedures are hampered by inadequate access and visualization inside the beating heart. Consequently, such interventions are currently performed under direct target vision via a sternotomy or thoracotomy, and rely on the use of cardio-pulmonary bypass.

McVeigh et al [1] recently demonstrated that interventional MRI systems could provide the surgeon with comprehensive dynamic cardiac images for intra-procedure guidance. However, MRI is not readily available in the operating room

T. Dohi, I. Sakuma, and H. Liao (Eds.): MIAR 2008, LNCS 5128, pp. 1–11, 2008.

(OR), and its use as an interventional modality is limited due to the restricted surgical access, incompatibility with most standard OR equipment, and cost. "CT fluoroscopy"is a high-quality intra-procedure image guidance technique, and Lauritsch *et al.* [2] have investigated the feasibility of C-arm image guidance both in *in vitro* and *in vivo* pre-clinical studies. Nevertheless, neither CT nor fluoroscopy images possess the necessary contrast to identify various features in cardiac anatomy without contrast enhancement. On the other hand, ultrasound (US) imaging is an attractive modality for intra-procedure guidance, given its wide availability and compatibility with the OR environment. While real-time 2D US images have relatively high spatial and temporal resolution, it is often difficult to perceive the target in its appropriate surgical context. Accurate navigation of surgical tools is an essential component in the optimization of the surgical path, and unfortunately 2D images cannot appropriately portray the entire 3D scene, particularly when it includes both surgical instruments and anatomical targets.

We previously introduced a novel minimally-invasive image-guidance system and demonstrated its use for cardiac therapy inside the beating heart [3]. Our system relies on intra-procedure 2D trans-esophageal echocardiography (TEE) images augmented by a VR environment, with pre-operative information and a virtual representation of the surgical instruments tracked in real time using a magnetic tracking system [3,4]. As a result, the intra-procedure TEE information can be interpreted within its 3D anatomical context to enhance intra-procedure navigation. In the context of an *in vivo* porcine study, we show how intra-procedure images can be augmented with cardiac models to assist the surgeon during procedure guidance. All animal experiments were approved by the Animal Care and Use Committee of The University of Western Ontario and followed the guidelines of the Canadian Council on Animal Care.

2   Surgical Platform Components

2.1   Pre-operative Anatomical Models

Given their high spatial resolution and excellent capabilities for soft tissue characterization without contrast enhancement, MR images allow for a clear definition of various anatomical features and can be used to construct anatomical models. Pre-operative cardiac images of the pig were acquired on a 1.5 T MRI scanner (CVMR, General Electric, Milwaukee, USA), using the fast cine gradient echo pulse sequence. The image acquisition was gated to the R-wave of the animal's ECG and 20 images were reconstructed per slice, depicting the heart at different cardiac phases, resulting in a complete dataset comprising 50 sagittal images slices for each cardiac phase. To ensure that all slices were acquired at the same point in the respiratory cycle, and to minimize the image artifacts due to breathing, each slice was acquired while the pig's respiration was consistently suspended at end-expiration using the mechanical ventilator.

The dynamic MR image dataset was processed to generate the pre-procedural cardiac models of the pig's heart. These models require different levels of

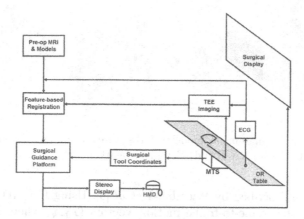

Fig. 1. Schematic representation of the operating room setup during a minimally invasive procedure conducted via virtual reality-enhanced ultrasound guidance

complexity, according to the clinical application under investigation. Our approach to cardiac modeling consists of first generating individual models for different cardiac components, and then assembling them according to the complexity of the procedure. The main features of interest include the left ventricle myocardium (LV), the left atrium (LA), and the right atrium and ventricle (RA/RV).

We extracted all anatomical features using manual segmentation of the mid-diastole (MD) image of the 4D dataset (Fig. 2) by outlining the region enclosed by the endocardial and epicardial contours [5]. The resulting binary image was then processed using the Marching Cubes algorithm [5] to generate a surface model of each organ component (Fig. 3).

To portray the dynamic behaviour of the heart, we employed a technique previously developed in the lab to reconstruct the heart motion throughout the cardiac cycle. A 3D free-form deformation field that describes the trajectories of all points in the surface model was extracted using image registration, according

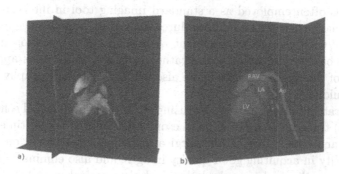

Fig. 2. a) Porcine heart image at MD; b) Porcine heart model at MD showing the left ventricle (LV), left atrium (LA) and right atrium & ventricle (RA/RV)

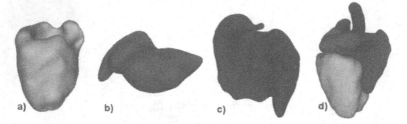

Fig. 3. Pre-operative anatomical models of the heart chambers all shown at mid-diastole: a) LV; b) LA; c) RA/RV; d) Complete heart model

to the technique described by Wierzbicki *et al* [6]. Using the MD heart image as a reference, the frame-to-frame motion vectors (T_{0-k}, where $k = 1\,\text{to}\,19$) were computed by non-rigidly registering the 3D MD image (corresponding to $k = 0$) to each of the remaining frames in the 4D dataset.Ultimately, the dynamic cardiac model was obtained by sequentially animating the static model at MD with the motion vectors previously estimated. Fig. 4 depicts the global heart model at different time points in the cardiac cycle.

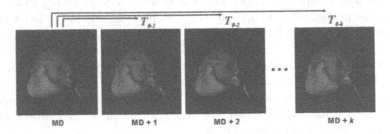

Fig. 4. Dynamic heart model displayed at different cardiac phases obtained by animating the static model with the motion extracted using non-rigid registration

2.2   Intra-operative Imaging

Ultrasound is often employed as a standard imaging tool in interventional radiology for many catheter-based procedures, due to its non-invasive nature and compatibility with the OR environment. Although our application in its current form is based on a direct access rather than a percutaneous approach to the interior of the cardiac chambers, we also employ echocardiography for intra-procedure guidance.

Intra-operative images are acquired using a 2D trans-esophageal echocardiography (TEE) transducer inserted in the esophagus, supplying real-time information on the anatomical targets and surgical instruments. In addition, 2D TEE offers flexibility in acquiring good-quality images, and also eliminates the interference between the probe manipulation and the surgical work-flow. However, the main disadvantage of the 2D US images is the inadequate representation of the anatomical targets and surgical tools required for intra-procedure guidance.

To address these limitations, we augment the 2D intra-procedure images with anatomical context supplied in the form of pre-operative cardiac models, as described in Section3.1.

2D TEE images were acquired using a Philips SONOS 7500 machine (Philips Ultrasound Division, Bothell, WA, USA). The images were encoded spatially using the tracking information provided by the NDI Aurora magnetic tracking system (MTS) (Northern Digital Inc., Waterloo, Ontario, Canada). A 6 degree-of-freedom (DOF) magnetic sensor coil was rigidly attached to the US probe and calibrated using a Z-string phantom [7] prior to its insertion in the esophagus. The image acquisition was gated to the R-wave of the ECG using a standard 3-lead configuration. All images were acquired during breath-holding, by shutting off the mechanical ventilator at end-expiration. A subset of 19 2D images were acquired at each cardiac phase, by rotating the TEE transducer about its normal axis at 10° angular increments.

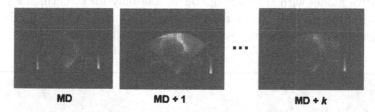

Fig. 5. Intra-operatively reconstructed 3D images of the intra-operative anatomy images at different cardiac phases

A pseudo 3D US image was reconstructed at each cardiac phase, by inserting each of the 2D US image frames into its appropriate location within a 3D image volume, according to its position and orientation information recorded by the magnetic tracking system, and its temporal information encoded by the ECG gating. This process ultimately led to a set of volumetric displays of the intra-operative anatomy reconstructed by assembling all angular frames acquired at each cardiac phase (Fig. 5). The main advantage of this 3D display is that it allows us to identify and select anatomical features that will be further used to drive the model-to-subject registration.

3 Virtual Reality Environment and Surgical Guidance

3.1 Model-to-Subject Registration

A feature-based registration algorithm was employed to augment the intra-operative VR environment with the pre-operative cardiac models. Easily identifiable targets — the mitral (MVA) and aortic (AVA) valve annuli — in both the pre- and intra-procedure image datasets, were chosen to drive the model-to-subject registration algorithm. The pre-operative annuli were segmented manually under the guidance of an experienced cardiologist, using a custom-developed spline-based segmentation tool similar to that available in the clinic within the TomTec 4D MV Assessment Software (Unterschleissheim, Germany). Similarly, the intra-operative annuli were also segmented manually by an echocardiographer, by sweeping the image fan of the magnetically tracked 2D TEE probe across each annulus and identifying the points of interest.

Image registration was achieved by aligning the AVA and MVA (Fig. 6b) defined in the model, with those identified intra-operatively (Fig. 6a). The algorithm first performed the translational component of the registration by aligning the centroids of the homologous pre- and intra-operative annuli, then performed the rotational component by aligning the unit normal vectors corresponding to the homologous structures. Ultimately, the registration was refined using an iterative closest point approach to ensure a good alignment of the pre- and intra-operative mitral and aortic annuli. This registration technique was assessed in a previous study involving 3D MR and US data of a healthy human subject as described by Linte *et al* [8]. We achieved a 4.8 mm average accuracy in aligning the pre-operative model with the intra-operative anatomy for structures located in the vicinity of the valvular valvular region (basal region of LV, LA and RA/RV), while larger misalignments were observed at remoter locations.

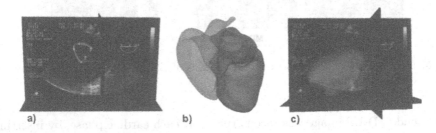

a)   b)   c)

Fig. 6. a) Intra-operatively reconstructed 3D US image showing the MVA and AVA; b) Pre-operative model displaying the MVA and AVA; c) Pre-operative model fused with the intra-operative US image after registration

This feature-based registration technique was used to augment the intra-operative imaging environment by overlaying the pre-operative 3D model onto the 2D TEE US image (Fig. 6c). This pre- to intra-procedure registration approach is suitable for cardiac interventions, as the selected valvular structures are easily identifiable in both the pre-operative and intra-operative images, and they also ensure a good alignment of the pre- and intra-operative surgical targets. Furthermore, given the location of the features used to drive the registration, we achieve a good anatomical alignment in the surrounding regions, enabling us to employ this technique for various image-guided interventions within the heart.

Fig. 7a shows an example of a 2D intra-procedure image used for guidance during a different experiment, displayed within the pre-operative anatomical context. Ultimately, the virtual environment is complemented with vitrual representations of the surgical instruments, enabling their tracking within the virtual surgical space (Fig. 7b).

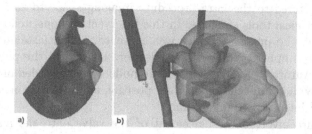

Fig. 7. a) Intra-operative 2D US image complemented by the pre-operative cardiac model; b) Complete augmented reality environment including pre-operative model, intra-operative US image, TEE transducer, and virtual models of the surgical tools

3.2 Applications in Procedure Guidance

In this section we describe our preliminary experience in the operating room in guiding some typical intracardiac procedures on the beating heart in porcine subjects, including a mitral valve implantation procedure, an ASD closure intervention, and an attempt to a radio-frequency ablation procedure.

Intracardiac access was achieved using the Universal Cardiac Introducer® (UCI) [9], a device used to gain access inside the chambers of the beating heart. The UCI comprises an attachment cuff and a versatile airlock introductory chamber. It attaches to the epicardial surface of the chamber of interest and allows the introduction of surgical instruments inside the beating heart through the designed access ports with minimal blood loss.

Mitral Valve Implantation. One of the most challenging interventions that we have attempted using our hybrid image-guidance system is the mitral valve implantation procedure. Following the success achieved during the *in vitro* studies in our laboratory in both a cardiac phantom [4], as well as in *ex vivo* porcine hearts [3], we attempted a preliminary translation of the work into the OR on porcine models.

A magnetically-tracked 2D trans-esophageal US transducer was employed for real-time intra-procedure image-guidance. Pre-operative models of the pig's

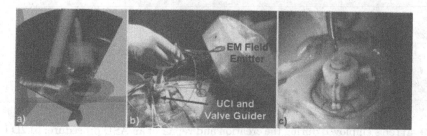

Fig. 8. a) Virtual models of the US probe, 2D image fan, and surgical instruments; b) Typical OR setup during a mitral valve implantation procedure; c) Post-procedure assessment showing the prosthesis attached with surgical clips to the native annulus

heart were registered to the intra-procedure imaging space to add anatomical context. The surgical tools employed in this intervention consisted of a guiding tool, onto which the prosthetic valve was attached, and a fastening tool — a laparoscopic clip applier. While these tools were tracked in the physical space using the NDI Aurora™ MTS, their virtual models were included in the VR environment, providing information on their position and orientation with respect to the pre- and intra-procedure anatomy.

The procedure involved the placement of the valve onto the native mitral annulus, followed by its attachment to the underlying tissue. The surgical instruments were navigated to the target under guidance provided by the virtual tool and organ models, followed by the correct positioning of the valve and proper application of the surgical fasteners, performed under US guidance (Fig. 8).

Atrial Septal Defect Repair. Any optimal minimally invasive ASD closure procedure should combine off-pump techniques with the effectiveness and versatility of the traditional open-heart approach. We report our experience in guiding an off-pump ASD closure in a porcine model. Our goal was to first create an atrial septal defect over the fossa ovale, and then close it by positioning a patch over its surface. The right atrium (RA) of the pig was exposed via a right lateral thoracotomy, and the UCI was attached to the free right atrial wall.

The septal defect was created using a custom made punch tool used to resect a circular region of tissue from the fossa ovale (FO) under real-time US guidance. A repair patch, attached to a guiding tool, and a fastening device were then introduced into the RA via the UCI. Using the pre-operative anatomical information and the virtual models of the surgical tools, the patch was guided to the target. One minor challenge arose due to the slightly oversized laparoscopic clip applier which collided with the patch guiding tool during navigation. Once on target, the surgeon relied on the US imaging to correctly position the patch onto the created ASD. The correct placement of the patch completely occluding the ASD orifice was also confirmed in the post-procedure assessment (Fig. 9). The off-pump ASD closure procedure was safe and the VR-enhanced US guidance provided significant assistance in both navigation and positioning. This study

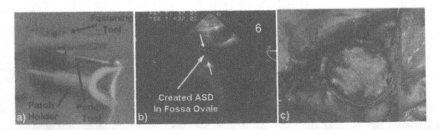

Fig. 9. a) Tools employed during the creation and repair of an ASD procedure; b) 2D US image showing a resected region in the fossa ovale; c) Image showing the repair patch covering the previously created septal defect and secured to the underlying tissue

also raised the need to improve the design of our guiding and fastening fastening tools to better suit the limited intracardiac space.

4   Discussion

Although two-dimensional TEE plays a significant role in our interventional system as it provides the operator with real-time intra-procedure information, the 2D images are of limited use when trying to identify the surgical tools and their positions and orientations with respect to the target. For our intracardiac therapy applications, we employ the pre-operative anatomical models to replace the traditional view of the surgical field with a virtual reality space, since the surgeon is no longer able to directly look inside the chambers while the heart is beating. This virtual space resembles the real surgical space and consists of images of the heart gathered both before and during the operation, as well as models of the instruments used in surgery. As such, the surgeon has access to a global 3D view of the heart from images taken prior to surgery, a detailed view of the surgical target from images acquired during surgery, as well as information on the position and information of the surgical instruments.

One of the benefits of employing anatomical models for intra-procedure guidance, as opposed to just using pre-operative images, consists of their capability to display the anatomy in a much clearer manner. Depending on the procedure performed and the location of the surgical target, only the required parts of the model can be displayed within the virtual reality environment, while the user controls the translucency level of each component. Furthermore, these models do not depend on the access route chosen to enter the heart, and are therefore feasible with either direct access through the atrial appendage or the ventricular apex, or even through one of the major blood vessels for catheter-driven procedures.

The quality of the pre-operatively acquired images may also impose certain limitations upon how much detail can be achieved when segmenting the anatomy of certain organs. For mitral valve applications, it is almost impossible to identify and segment the anatomy of the mitral apparatus from clinical quality, 6 mm slice-thickness MR images. Similar challenges may be encountered whenever the surgical targets consist of delicate anatomical structures that are not readily identifiable in the acquired images. This limitation points to the desirability of employing dynamic volume rendered images in the OR environment [10].

Our results show that the model-to-subject registration technique employed to augment the intra-procedure images with the pre-operative models ensures a $\sim$ 5 mm alignment accuracy for the cardiac structures located within 10 mm from the valvular region. From a surgical perspective the overall accuracy achieved in building and aligning the pre-operative cardiac models with the intra-procedure anatomical images is acceptable, recognizing that pre-operative models are used as aids for providing anatomical context during navigation, while real-time US imaging is employed for final target positioning.

The accuracy of the VR-enhanced US guidance system was assessed from the surgeon's point of view in our laboratory. Three surgical guidance modalities were tested: (i) 2D US image guidance only ("US only"); (ii) virtual reality guidance with tracked surgical tools ("VR only"); and (iii) 2D US image guidance augmented by virtual reality ("VR + US"). The user was asked to guide a probe tip onto a small target within a cardiac phantom. The only information available to the user was the US image, the VR interface, and the VR-augmented US interface for "US only", "VR only" and "VR + US" guidance modalities, respectively. The achieved localization accuracy, reduced to the single point root-mean-squared (RMS) statistic, was 5.42 mm, 1.02 mm and 1.47 mm for the "US only", "VR only" and "VR + US" guidance modalities, respectively [4].

Several approaches have been considered regarding the most appropriate means of delivering the virtual environment data to the physician: the image can be displayed on a simple computer monitor, on a stereoscopic screen that enables 3D visualization, or using head-mounted display which allow the surgeons to directly "navigate" within a virtual volume, as suggested by Sauer *et al.* [11] or Birkfellner [12]. However, the displays contain a great deal of information in a form unfamiliar to the surgeon, and we believe that further research must be performed to determine the optimal visualization paradigm.

5 Conclusions

We conclude that the use of the VR environment is a key element in enhancing the performance of off-pump beating heart intracardiac surgery. Augmented with both US imaging and virtual models of organs and surgical tools, this system provides extensive support for target visualization, planning optimal routes to the target, and guidance for directing therapeutic interventions. This initial work has demonstrated the potential of multi-modality imaging, combined with tracking of tools and real-time US, to enable both the guidance and assessment of surgical intervention in a manner that will ultimately provide an appropriate surrogate to direct vision.

Acknowledgments. The authors thank Dr. Marcin Wierzbicki, Dr. Usaf Aladl and Dr. David Gobbi for assistance with software development and Sheri VanLingen and Louis Estey for technical support. We also acknowledge funding for this work provided by the Natural Sciences and Engineering Research Council (Grant R3146A01), the Canadian Institutes of health Research (Grant MOP-74626), the Ontario Research and Development Challenge Fund, Ontario Innovation Trust, and the Canadian Foundation for Innovation.

References

1. McVeigh, E.R., Guttman, M.A., Kellman, P., Raval, A.A., Lederman, R.J.: Realtime, interactive MRI for cardiovascular interventions. Acad Radiol 12, 1221–1227 (2005)

2. Lauritsch, G., Boese, J., Wigström, L., Kemeth, H., Fahrig, R.: Towards cardiac C-arm computed tomography. IEEE Trans. Med. Imaging 25, 922–934 (2006)
3. Linte, C.A., Wiles, A.D., Hill, N., Moore, J., Wedlake, C., Guiraudon, G.M., Jones, D.L., Bainbridge, D., Peters, T.M.: An augmented reality environment for image-guidance of off-pump mitral valve implantation. In: Medical Imaging 2007: Visualization and Image-Guided Procedures. Proc. of SPIE, vol. 6509 (2007) 65090N–12
4. Wiles, A.D., Guiraudon, G.M., Moore, J., Wedlake, C., Linte, C.A., Jones, D.L., Bainbridge, D., Peters, T.M.: Navigation accuracy for an intracardiac procedure using virtual reality-enhanced ultrasound. In: Medical Imaging 2007: Visualization and Image-Guided Procedures. Proc. of SPIE, vol. 6509 (2007) 61410W–10
5. Wierzbicki, M., Drangova, M., Guiraudon, G.M., Peters, T.M.: Validation of dynamic heart models obtained using non-linear registration for virtual reality training, planning, and guidance of minimally invasive cardiac surgeries. Med. Image Anal. 8, 387–401 (2004)
6. Wierzbicki, M., Peters, T.M.: Determining epicardial surface motion using elastic registration: Towards virtual reality guidance of minimally-invasive cardiac interventions. In: Ellis, R.E., Peters, T.M. (eds.) MICCAI 2003. LNCS, vol. 2878, pp. 722–729. Springer, Heidelberg (2003)
7. Gobbi, D.G., Comeau, R.M., Peters, T.M.: Ultrasound probe tracking for real-time ultrasound/MRI overlay and visualization of brain shift. In: Taylor, C., Colchester, A. (eds.) MICCAI 1999. LNCS, vol. 1679, pp. 920–927. Springer, Heidelberg (1999)
8. Linte, C.A., Wierzbicki, M., Moore, J., Guiraudon, G.M., Jones, D.L., Peters, T.M.: On enhancing planning and navigation of beating-heart mitral valve surgery using pre-operative cardiac models. In: Proc. of IEEE Eng. Med. Biol. Soc., pp. 475–478 (2007)
9. Guiraudon, G., Jones, D., Bainbridge, D., Peters, T.: Mitral valve implantation using off-pump closed beating intracardiac surgery: a feasability study. Interact Cardiovasc Thorac. Surg. 6, 603–607 (2007)
10. Zhang, Q., Eagleson, R., Peters, T.M.: Rapid voxel classification methodology for interactive 3d medical image visualization. In: Proc. of Med. Image Comput. Comput. Assist Interv. Lect. Notes Comput. Sci., vol. 4792, pp. 86–93 (2007)
11. Vogt, S., Khamene, A., Niemann, H., Sauer, F.: An AR system with intuitive user interface for manipulation and visualization of 3D medical data. In: Proc. of Medicine Meets Virtual Reality. Stud. Health Technol. Inform., vol. 98, pp. 397–403 (2004)
12. Birkfellner, W., Figl, M., Matula, C., Hummel, J., Hanel, R., Imhof, H., Wanschitz, F., Wagner, A., Watzinger, F., Bergmann, H.: Computer-enhanced stereoscopic vision in a head-mounted operating binocular. Phys. Med. Biol. 48, 49–57 (2003)

Joint Registration and Segmentation of Serial Lung CT Images in Microendoscopy Molecular Image-Guided Therapy

Zhong Xue, Kelvin Wong, and Stephen Wong

Department of Radiology, The Methodist Hospital and The Methodist Hospital
Research Institute, Weill Cornell Medical College, Houston, TX, USA
{zxue, kwong, stwong}@tmhs.org

Abstract. In lung cancer image-guided therapy, a real-time electromagnetic tracked microendoscopic optical imaging probe is guided to the small lung lesion of interest. The alignment of the pre-operative lung CT images as well as the intra-operative serial images is often an important step to accurately guide and monitor the interventional procedure in the diagnosis and treatment of these small lung lesions. Registering the serial images often relies on correct segmentation of the images and on the other hand, the segmentation results can be further improved by temporal alignment of the serial images. This paper presents a joint serial image registration and segmentation algorithm. In this algorithm, serial images are segmented based on the current deformations, and the deformations among the serial images are iteratively refined based on the updated segmentation results. No temporal smoothness about the deformation fields is enforced so that the algorithm can tolerate larger or discontinuous temporal changes that often appear during image-guided therapy. Physical procedure models could also be incorporated to our algorithm to better handle the temporal changes of the serial images during intervention. In experiments, we apply the proposed algorithm to align serial lung CT images. Results using both simulated and clinical images show that the new algorithm is more robust compared to the method that only uses deformable registration.

1   Introduction

Lung cancer is the most common causes of cancer death in the world and peripheral lung cancer constitutes more than half of all lung cancer cases. Decades of research in new detection and treatment methods have failed to impact the long term survival of patients with lung cancer [1]. It is now believed that the key to improving long term survival of patients with lung cancer is better early detection, localization and novel therapies [1,2]. The once-promising approach of Computed Tomography (CT) screening for lung cancer now appears to result in high false positive rates. On initial screening of high risk populations, most studies report false positive rates between 10% and 20% [3]. The Mayo Clinic experience showed that when high risk individuals are screened for lung cancer

T. Dohi, I. Sakuma, and H. Liao (Eds.): MIAR 2008, LNCS 5128, pp. 12–20, 2008.

with CT, the likelihood that they undergo a thoracic resection for lung cancer is increased by 10-fold [4]. These observations suggest that a better theranostic strategy is needed to make CT screening of lung cancer cost-effective [5] and to eliminate unnecessary surgeries.

To tackle the common difficulties in identifying small lung lesions ($< 1.5cm$) at an early stage, an image-guided therapy approach is most promising. This approach relies on pre-operative CT images and real-time electromagnetic (EM) tracking to guide a fiberoptic microendoscope to the small lesion of interest in real-time to provide a molecular imaging diagnosis, and it also offers the possibility to treat the small lung lesion simultaneously, thus eliminating unnecessary surgeries and the procedure related mortality. Molecular imaging is obtained at microscopic resolution using a fiberoptic microendoscope, coupled with optical molecular contrast agents, to highlight cancerous lesions. In order to achieve the high precision real-time guidance for the microendoscope and incorporate the prior knowledge of suspected lung cancer, accurate deformable registration of pre-procedural lung CT images with annotated suspected cancer location and serial images during interventional procedure are critical in order to lower the overall radiation dose and procedure time.

Traditional pairwise [6,7,8] and groupwise [9,10] image registration algorithms have been used in these applications. However the pairwise algorithms warp each image separately and they often cause unstable measures of the serial images because no temporal information of the serial images has been used in the registration procedure. Groupwise image registration methods simultaneously process multiple images, however they often consider the images as a group, not a time series, thus the temporal information has not been used efficiently. For serial image registration, the relationship between temporally neighboring images is much more important than that of the images with larger time intervals, since both anatomical structure and tissue properties of neighboring images tend to be more similar for neighboring images than others; moreover these temporal changes can be characterized using specific physical processes models.

Accurate registration of serial images often relies on correct extraction and matching of robust and distinctive image features. Thus it is a very important step to segment the image into different tissue regions, which act as additional features in the image registration to further improve the temporal alignment of the serial images. Moreover the deformations across serial images also provide more robust image segmentation. This paper presents a joint serial image registration and segmentation, wherein serial images are segmented based on the current temporal deformations so that the temporally corresponding tissues tend to be segmented into the same tissue type, and at the same time, temporal deformations among the serial images are iteratively refined based on the updated segmentation results. The simultaneous registration and segmentation framework had been studied in [11,12,13] for MR images. The previous work, CLASSIC [13], relies on a temporal smoothness constraint and it is particularly suitable for longitudinal analysis of MR brain images of normal healthy subjects, where the changes from one time-point to another is small. Nevertheless, in that algorithm the registration is purely dependent on the segmented images.

In this paper, no temporal smoothness about the deformation fields is enforced so that our algorithm can tolerate larger or discontinuous temporal changes that often appear during image-guided therapy. Moreover, physical procedure models could also be incorporated to our algorithm to better handle the temporal changes of the serial images during intervention. We first demonstrate that, based on the Bayes' rules, the registration of the current time-point image is not only related to the baseline image, but also to its temporally neighboring images. Based on this principle, a new serial image similarity measure is defined, and the deformation is modeled using the traditional Free Form Deformation (FFD) [7]. Based on the current estimate of temporal deformations, a 4-D clustering algorithm is applied for segmenting the serial images. No adaptive centroids are used because of relatively small effect of inhomogeneity in CT. The proposed joint algorithm then iteratively refines the serial deformations and segments the images until convergence. The advantage of the proposed method is that it is particularly suitable for registering serial images in image-guided therapy applications with possible large and discontinuous temporal deformations.

We have applied the proposed algorithm to both simulated and real serial lung CT images and compared it with the FFD. The results show that the proposed algorithm yields more robust registration results and more stable longitudinal measures.

2   Method

2.1   The Serial Image Registration Algorithm

Given a series of images I_t, $t = 0, ..., T$ (I_0 is usually called the baseline, and all the subsequent images have been globally aligned onto the space of the baseline by applying the rigid registration in Insight Toolkit (ITK)), we often need to estimate the deformations from the baseline onto each image, $i.e.$, $\mathbf{f}_{0 \to t}$ or simply denoted as $\mathbf{f}_t$. Since no longitudinal information is used in pairwise registration, the temporal stability of the resultant serial deformations can not be preserved. Groupwise registration jointly registers all the images with the baseline, however no temporal information has been considered effectively.

In this work, we formulate the serial image registration in the Bayes' framework, so that the registration of the current time-point image is related to not only the previous but also the following images (if available). No longitudinal smoothness constraints are applied to the serial deformations so that our algorithm can tolerate temporal anatomical and tissue property changes. For the current image I_t, if the deformation of its previous image I_{t-1}, $\mathbf{f}_{t-1}$, and that of the next image I_{t+1}, $\mathbf{f}_{t+1}$, are known, the posterior probabilities of the current deformation $\mathbf{f}_t$ can be defined as $p(\mathbf{f}_t | I_0, I_{t-1}, I_t, \mathbf{f}_{t-1})$ and $p(\mathbf{f}_{t+1} | I_0, I_t, I_{t+1}, \mathbf{f}_t)$, respectively. By jointly considering both the previous and the next images, we calculate the deformation of the current image, $\mathbf{f}_t$, by maximizing the combined posterior probabilities,

$$\mathbf{f}_t^* = \arg\max\{p(\mathbf{f}_t|I_0, I_{t-1}, I_t, \mathbf{f}_{t-1})p(\mathbf{f}_{t+1}|I_0, I_t, I_{t+1}, \mathbf{f}_t)\}. \tag{1}$$

Using the chain rule of probability equations, and assuming that the temporal deformations are independent, we can easily calculate Eq.(1) as,

$$\mathbf{f}_t^* = \arg\max\{\lambda(t)p(I_{t+1}|I_0, I_t, \mathbf{f}_t, \mathbf{f}_{t+1})p(I_t|I_0, I_{t-1}, \mathbf{f}_{t-1}, \mathbf{f}_t)p(\mathbf{f}_t)\}, \tag{2}$$

where $\lambda(t)$ gives other probability terms (including $p(\mathbf{f}_{t-1}|\mathbf{f}_t)p(\mathbf{f}_{t+1}|\mathbf{f}_t)$), which are not considered in the study). $\mathbf{f}_t^*$ can be calculated by minimizing,

$$\mathbf{f}_t^* = \arg\min\{E_{s,t}(I_0, I_{t-1}, I_t, I_{t+1}, \mathbf{f}_{t-1}, \mathbf{f}_t, \mathbf{f}_{t+1}) + \lambda_r(t)E_r(\mathbf{f}_t)\}, \tag{3}$$

where $E_{s,t}()$ is the new serial image difference/similarity measure, and $E_r()$ is the regularization term of the deformation field. λ_r is the weight of E_r. The serial image difference measure can be defined as,

$$E_{s,t} = \sum_{\mathbf{v}\in\Omega}\{|\mathbf{e}[I_t(\mathbf{f}_t(\mathbf{v}))] - \mathbf{e}[I_0(\mathbf{v})]|^2$$
$$+ \sum_{i=-1,1}|\mathbf{e}[I_t(\mathbf{f}_t(\mathbf{v}))] - \mathbf{e}[I_{t+i}(\mathbf{f}_{t+i}(\mathbf{v}))]|^2\}, \tag{4}$$

where $\mathbf{e}[]$ is the operator for calculating a feature vector, and Ω is the image domain. In this work, the feature vector for each voxel consists of the intensity, gradient magnitude, and the fuzzy membership functions calculated from the segmentation step. When a physical process model is available, it can be incorporated into the second term of Eq.(4) or the conditional probabilities of deformations, so that any feature changes from one image onto another can be considered. Further, the deformations of neighboring images might not be independent by embedding a temporal model of deformations according to the physical model. However that is out of the scope of this study. E_r in Eq.(3) is the regularization energy of deformation field $\mathbf{f}_t$, and it can be derived from the prior distribution of the deformation. If no prior distribution is available, the regularization term can be some continuity and smoothness constraints. In this work, since the cubic B-Spline is used to model the deformation field, the continuity and smoothness is guaranteed, thus the regularization term E_r is omitted.

The serial image registration algorithm then iteratively calculates/refines the deformation field $\mathbf{f}_t$ of each time-point image by minimizing the energy function in Eq.(3) until convergence. Notice that in the first iteration, since the registration results for neighboring images are not available, only the first term of Eq.(4) is used, which is essentially a pairwise FFD.

2.2   The 4-D Clustering Algorithm for Image Segmentation

Given the serial images I_t, $t = 0, 1, ..., T$ and the longitudinal deformations $\mathbf{f}_t$, $t = 1, ..., T$, the purpose of the 4-D segmentation is to calculate the segmented images $I_t^{(\text{seg})}$ by considering not only the spatial but also the temporal neighborhoods.

The clustering algorithm is performed to classify each voxel of the serial image into different tissue types by minimizing the objective function,

$$E(\mu, c) = \sum_{t=0}^{T} \sum_{\mathbf{v} \in \Omega} \sum_{k=1}^{K} \{ \mu_{(t,\mathbf{v}),k}^{q} (I_{(t,\mathbf{v})} - c_{t,k})^2]$$

$$+ \frac{\alpha}{2} \rho_{(t,\mathbf{v})}^{(s)} \sum_{k=1}^{K} [\mu_{(t,\mathbf{v}),k}^{q} \bar{\mu}_{(t,\mathbf{v}),k}^{(s)}] + \frac{\beta}{2} \rho_{(t,\mathbf{v})}^{(t)} \sum_{k=1}^{K} [\mu_{(t,\mathbf{v}),k}^{q} \bar{\mu}_{(t,\mathbf{v}),k}^{(t)}] \}, \quad (5)$$

where voxel $\mathbf{v}$ in image I_0 corresponds to voxel $\mathbf{f}_t(\mathbf{v})$ in image I_t, referred to as voxel $(t, \mathbf{v})$, and μ, c, q, K follow the FCM formulation [15].

$$\bar{\mu}_{(t,\mathbf{v}),k}^{(s)} = \frac{1}{N_1} \sum_{(t,\mathbf{u}) \in N_{(t,\mathbf{v})}^{(s)}} \sum_{m \in M_k} \mu_{(t,\mathbf{u}),m}^{q}, \quad \bar{\mu}_{(t,bfv),k}^{(t)} = \frac{1}{N_2} \sum_{(\tau,\mathbf{v}) \in N_{(t,\mathbf{v})}^{(t)}} \sum_{m \in M_k} \mu_{(\tau,\mathbf{v}),m}^{q}.$$

$N_{(t,\mathbf{v})}^{(s)}$ and $N_{(t,\mathbf{v})}^{(t)}$ are the spatial and temporal neighborhoods of voxel $(t, \mathbf{v})$, and $M_k = \{m = 1, ..., K; m \neq k\}$. The fuzzy membership functions μ are subject to, $\sum_{k=1}^{K} \mu_{(t,\mathbf{v}),k} = 1$, for all t and $\mathbf{v}$.

The second term of Eq.(5) reflects the spatial constraints of the fuzzy membership functions, which is analogous to the FANTASM algorithm [14]. The difference is that an additional weight $\rho_{(t,\mathbf{v})}^{(s)}$ is used as an image-adaptive weighting coefficient, thus stronger smoothness constraints are applied in the image regions that have more uniform intensities, and vice versa. $\rho_{(t,\mathbf{v})}^{(s)}$ is defined as, $\rho_{(t,\mathbf{v})}^{(s)} = \exp\{-\sum_r [(D_r * I_t)_{(t,\mathbf{v})}^2 / 2\sigma_s^2]\}$, where $(D_r * I_t)_{(t,\mathbf{v})}$ refers to first calculating the spatial convolution $(D_r * I_t)$, and then taking its value at location $(t, \mathbf{v})$, where D_r is a spatial differential operator along axis r. Similarly, the third term of Eq.(5) reflects the temporal consistency constraints, and $\rho_{(t,\mathbf{v})}^{(t)}$ is calculated as, $\rho_{(t,\mathbf{v})}^{(t)} = \exp\{-(D_t * I_{(t,\mathbf{v})})_t^2 / 2\sigma_t^2\}$, where D_t is the temporal differential operator, and $(D_t * I_{(t,\mathbf{v})})_t$ refers to first calculating the temporal convolution $(D_t * I_{(t,\mathbf{v})})$ and then taking its value at t. It is worth noting that the temporal smoothness constraint herein does not mean that the serial deformations have to be smooth across different time-points.

Using Lagrange multipliers to enforce the constraint of fuzzy membership function in the objective function Eq.(5), we get the following two equations to iteratively update the fuzzy membership functions and calculate the clustering centroids,

$$\mu_{(t,\mathbf{v}),k} = \frac{[(I_{(t,\mathbf{v})} - c_{t,k})^2 + \alpha \rho_{(t,\mathbf{v})}^{(s)} \bar{\mu}_{(t,\mathbf{v}),k}^{(s)} + \beta \rho_{(t,\mathbf{v})}^{(t)} \bar{\mu}_{(t,\mathbf{v}),k}^{(t)}]^{\frac{-1}{q-1}}}{\sum_{m=1}^{K} [(I_{(t,\mathbf{v})} - c_{t,m})^2 + \alpha \rho_{(t,\mathbf{v})}^{(s)} \bar{\mu}_{(t,\mathbf{v}),m}^{(s)} + \beta \rho_{(t,\mathbf{v})}^{(t)} \bar{\mu}_{(t,\mathbf{v}),m}^{(t)}]^{\frac{-1}{q-1}}}, \quad (6)$$

$$c_{t,k} = \frac{\sum_{\mathbf{v} \in \Omega} \mu_{(t,\mathbf{v}),k}^{q} I_{(t,\mathbf{v})}}{\sum_{\mathbf{v} \in \Omega} \mu_{(t,\mathbf{v}),k}^{q}}. \quad (7)$$

In summary, the proposed joint registration and segmentation algorithm iteratively performs the serial registration and the segmentation algorithms until the difference between two iterations is smaller than a prescribed value.

3   Experimental Results

The dataset used in the experiments consists of anonymized serial lung CT images of lung cancer patients (n=6). The spatial resolutions of the images from the same patient are different due to different settings and imaging protocols. The typical voxel spacing in our data is $0.81mm \times 0.81mm \times 5mm$, $0.98mm \times 0.98mm \times 5mm$, and $0.7mm \times 0.7mm \times 1.25mm$. For the serial images of the same patient, all the subsequent images have been globally aligned and re-sampled onto the space of the first image using the ITK package.

Fig. 1 gives an example of the segmentation results of our dataset. It can be seen that after global registration of the original images in Fig. 1 (a), the lung regions can be roughly aligned in Fig. 1 (b). By performing the joint registration and segmentation for such serial images, the lung region can be precisely aligned as shown in Fig. 1 (c) and (d). The parameters used in the experiments are as follows: $K = 3$, $\alpha = 200$, $\beta = 200$, $\sigma_s = 2$, $\sigma_t = 1$, and the spatial and temporal neighboring voxels are used. All algorithms have been implemented using the

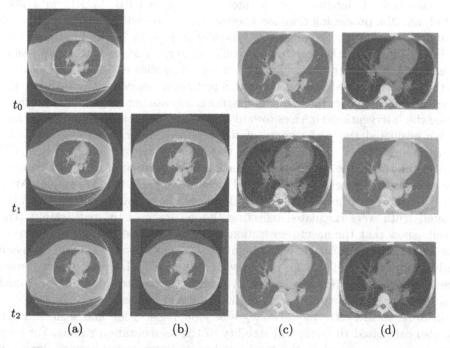

Fig. 1. Illustration of the joint registration and segmentation algorithm. (a) Input serial images, (b) the globally registered images, (c) the results of the proposed algorithm, and (d) the corresponding segmented images.

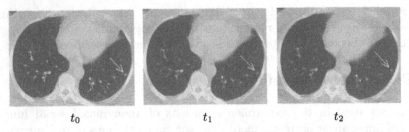

t_0 t_1 t_2

Fig. 2. Registration results of serial images with lesion. The arrows point to the lesion.

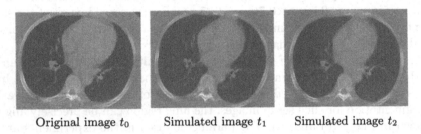

Original image t_0 Simulated image t_1 Simulated image t_2

Fig. 3. Example of the simulated serial images

standard GNU C language on an Intel Core 2 Duo CPU 2.2GHz with 2GB RAM, and the processing time for a series of 3 images with size $512 \times 512 \times 55$ is about 2.5 minutes. The algorithm typically stops with 2 or 3 iterations.

Fig. 2 illustrates the registration results of serial images with small lesion. It can be seen that the lesion appears in the same slice and the same location in the registered serial images. Using this technique, we can easily calculate the longitudinal changes of the lesion for diagnosis and assessment, and also precisely guide the interventional devices toward the lesion during image-guided therapy.

We evaluated the performance of the proposed algorithm using simulated images. First, the demon's algorithm was used to register the real lung CT images, and then the resultant deformation fields were applied to the baseline image in order to generate the simulated images (see Fig. 3 for an example). After applying the algorithm on the simulated images, the registration errors with the ground truth were calculated reflecting the accuracy of the registration. The results show that the mean registration errors are related to the resolutions of the serial images. For images with resolution $0.7mm \times 0.7mm \times 1.5mm$, the mean registration error is $0.9mm$, for images with resolution $0.81mm \times 0.81mm \times 5mm$, the mean registration error is $4.1mm$. In general, the registration errors are found less than the largest voxel spacing of the simulated images.

In order to illustrate the advantages of joint registration and segmentation, we also calculated the temporal stability of the segmentation results. For each image series, we calculate the total number of tissue type changes along the serial deformation fields and normalize this number by the total number of voxels. It turns out that for 6 series of images we tested, the proposed algorithm has about 26% voxels with tissue type changes across the temporal domain, while the FFD yields about 32% tissue type changes across the image series. The results indicate that the joint registration and segmentation generates relatively stable measures for serial images.

4 Conclusion

This paper proposes a joint registration and segmentation algorithm for serial image processing in lung cancer molecular image-guided therapy. The serial image registration and segmentation procedures are performed iteratively to improve the robustness and temporal stability for serial image processing. Experimental results using both simulated and real lung CT images show the accuracy and robustness compared to the free form deformation. Future work include incorporation of physical procedure models into our algorithm to better handle the temporal changes of the serial images during intervention, and the integration to the real-time EM-guided fiberoptic microendoscope system.

Acknowledgement

The research of STCW is partially supported by a grant NIH NLM G08LM008937.

References

1. McWilliams, A., MacAulay, C., Gazdar, A.F., Lam, S.: Innovative molecular and imaging approaches for the detection of lung cancer and its precursor lesions. Oncogene 21(45), 6949–6959 (2002)
2. Hicks, R.J., Lau, E., Alam, N.Z., Chen, R.Y.: Imaging in the diagnosis and treatment of non-small cell lung cancer. Respirology 12(2), 165–172 (2007)
3. Wardwell, N.R., Massion, P.P.: Novel strategies for the early detection and prevention of lung cancer. Semin Oncol 32(3), 259–268 (2005)
4. Bach, P.B., Jett, J.R., Pastorino, U., Tockman, M.S., Swensen, S.J., Begg, C.B.: CT screening and lung cancer outcomes. Jama 297(9), 953–961 (2007)
5. Black, C., de Verteuil, R., Walker, S., Ayres, J., Boland, A., Bagust, A., Waugh, N.: Population screening for lung cancer using CT, is there evidence of clinical effectiveness? A systematic review of the literature. Thorax 62(2), 131–138 (2007)
6. Duncan, J., Ayache, N.: Medical image analysis: Progress over two decades and the challenges ahead. IEEE Trans. Pattern Anal. Mach. Intell. 22(1), 85–106 (2000)
7. Rueckert, D., Sonoda, L., Hayes, C., Hill, D., Leach, M., Hawkes, D.J.: Nonrigid registration using free-form deformations: application to breast MR images. IEEE Trans. Med. Imaging 18(8), 712–721 (1999)
8. Johnson, H., Christensen, G.: Consistent landmark and intensity-based image registration. IEEE Trans. Med. Imaging 21(5), 450–461 (2002)
9. Bhatia, K., Hajnal, J., Puri, B., Edwards, A., Rueckert, D.: Consistent groupwise non-rigid registration for atlas construction. In: ISBI, pp. 908–911 (2004)

10. Marsland, S., Twining, C., Taylor, C.: A minimum description length objective function for groupwise non-rigid image registration. Image Vision Comput. 26(3), 333–346 (2008)
11. Wang, F., Vemuri, B.: Simultaneous registration and segmentation of anatomical structures from brain MRI. In: Duncan, J.S., Gerig, G. (eds.) MICCAI 2005. LNCS, vol. 3749. Springer, Heidelberg (2005)
12. Chen, X., Brady, M., Lo, J., Moore, N.: Simultaneous segmentation and registration of contrast-enhanced breast MRI. In: Christensen, G.E., Sonka, M. (eds.) IPMI 2005. LNCS, vol. 3565, pp. 126–137. Springer, Heidelberg (2005)
13. Xue, Z., Shen, D., Davatzikos, C.: CLASSIC: Consistent longitudinal alignment and segmentation for serial image computing. Med. Image Anal. 30, 388–399 (2006)
14. Pham, D., Prince, J.: FANTASM: Fuzzy and noise tolerant adaptive segmentation method, http://iacl.ece.jhu.edu/projects/fantasm/
15. Bezdek, J., Hall, L., Clarke, L.: Review of MR image segmentation techniques using pattern recognition. Med. Phys. 20(4), 1033–1048 (1993)

Perceptual Docking for Robotic Control

Guang-Zhong Yang, George P. Mylonas, Ka-Wai Kwok, and Adrian Chung

Royal Society/Wolfson Medical Image Computing Laboratory
Institute of Biomedical Engineering
Imperial College London, London, United Kingdom
{g.z.yang, george.mylonas, k.kwok07, a.chung}@imperial.ac.uk

Abstract. In current robotic surgery, dexterity is enhanced by microprocessor controlled mechanical wrists which allow motion scaling for reduced gross hand movements and improved performance of micro-scale tasks. The continuing evolution of the technology, including force feedback and virtual immobilization through real-time motion adaptation, will permit complex procedures such as beating heart surgery to be carried out under a static frame-of-reference. In pursuing more adaptive and intelligent robotic designs, the regulatory, ethical and legal barriers imposed on interventional surgical robots have given rise to the need of a tightly integrated control between the operator and the robot when autonomy is considered. This paper outlines the general concept of *perceptual docking* for robotic control and how it can be used for learning and knowledge acquisition in robotic assisted minimally invasive surgery such that operator specific motor and perceptual/cognitive behaviour is acquired through *in situ* sensing. A gaze contingent framework is presented in this paper as an example to illustrate how saccadic eye movements and ocular vergence can be used for attention selection, recovering 3D tissue deformation and motor channelling during minimally invasive surgical procedures.

Keywords: perceptual docking, minimally invasive surgery, perceptual feedback, eye tracking, machine vision, deformation recovery, 3D tracking, autonomous robot, robotic control, haptics, human-robot interfacing.

1 Introduction

In robotic control, current research is generally carried out under the dichotomy between autonomous and manipulator technologies. Intelligence of the robot is typically pre-acquired through high-level abstraction and environment modelling. With the increasing maturity of master-slave technology in robotic surgery, manual dexterity is enhanced by microprocessor controlled mechanical wrists that allow motion scaling for reduced gross hand movements and improved performance of micro-scale tasks. The continuing evolution of the technology, including force feedback and virtual immobilization through real-time motion adaptation, will permit more complex procedures such as beating heart surgery to be carried out under a static frame-of-reference. The quest for performing ever-complex surgical tasks has given rise to the need of more autonomous control in order to augment the capabilities of the surgeon

T. Dohi, I. Sakuma, and H. Liao (Eds.): MIAR 2008, LNCS 5128, pp. 21–30, 2008.

by taking the best from the robot and human. However, the regulatory, ethical and legal barriers imposed on interventional surgical robots dictate the need of a tightly integrated control between the operator and the robot.

It is well recognised that the success of Minimally Invasive Surgery (MIS) is coupled with an increasing demand on surgeons' manual dexterity and visuomotor control due to the complexity of instrument manipulations. Tissue deformation combined with restricted workspace and visibility of an already cluttered environment imposes significant challenges on surgical ergonomics related to surgical precision and safety. With the availability of robotic assisted MIS, existing research has explored the use of motion stabilisation to simplify the execution of delicate surgical tasks such as small vessel anastomosis. The stereoscopic optics provided by systems such as the daVinci (Intuitive Surgical CA), also offer an ideal platform for incorporating computer vision methods for improving surgical workflow through enhanced visualisation.

Although the fine manipulation capabilities of MIS robots in performing scaled down, steady, tremor-free motion are well appreciated, the future clinical impact of the technology relies heavily on machine intelligence of the system and its ability in bridging the sensory information such as tactile feedback between the tool tip and human hands. Recently, the concept of *perceptual docking* has been developed by researchers at Imperial College London, UK for more effective surgical robotic control. The word docking is different in meaning to the conventional term used in mobile robots - it represents a fundamental paradigm shift of perceptual learning and knowledge acquisition for robotic systems in that operator specific motor and perceptual/cognitive behaviour is acquired *in situ* through human-robot interaction. Humans have unexcelled flexibility and hand-eye coordination, as well as finely developed sense of touch. Our vision system is particularly superior in image understanding, feature tracking, 3D perception, morphological registration, and integrating diverse sources of visual cues. Whilst the use of conventional computer vision techniques for 3D structural recovery and registration for intra-operative guidance has encountered major difficulties in the presence of large tissue deformation, there has been very limited work in making effective use of the human vision system for simplifying, as well as augmenting, some of the complex visual processing tasks.

In this paper, we will provide an overview of the research related to *perceptual docking* and outline some example applications of the system for shifting the computational burden towards perceptually enabled channels.

2 Modes of Human-Robot Interface

Although the introduction of the term *perceptual docking* is relatively recent, the basic idea of bridging the sensory information between human and machine has been around for many years. William Grey Walter, who discovered contingent negative variation (CNV) effect - an increasing negative shift of the cortical electrical potentials associated with an anticipated response to an expected stimulus, and created *Machina Speculatrix* (a light seeking robotic tortoise), already contemplated the use of brain waves for machine control nearly 50 years ago. Whilst creating direct neural interface, either one-way or bi-directional, still remains a major research challenge, researchers are increasingly focussed on natural, non-intrusive methods that are practically useful.

In brain-computer interface, there is a large number of input features that can be measured. These include electrical, magnetic, metabolic, chemical, thermal, mechanical responses to brain activity in both frequency and time-domains. The measurement method is mainly determined by the type of input signals to be measured, their location, spatial resolution, the degree of required signal-to-noise-ratio (SNR), and the potential invasiveness involved. Among these, Electroencephalography (EEG) is one of the most researched modalities. Initially it was used for studying auto-regulation and cognitive feedback. Back in the 70s, Jacques Vidal had already demonstrated the use of computer-generated stimulus to visually evoke potentials to control the movement of a cursor through a two-dimensional maze.

There are other methods based on measuring electrical activity like epidural electrodes and electrocorticography (ECoG), but these are generally invasive, requiring electrodes to be inserted into the brain or spine. Chemical activity in the neurons and glia is also a measurable input by using magnetic resonance spectroscopy and invasive probes. It is worth noting that current techniques are mainly geared towards improving the quality of life of the disabled [1-3]. They are still in their infancy and generally not suited for controlling complex tasks.

With the maturity of non-invasive methods, particularly imaging/spectroscopy based techniques, alternative methods such as magnetoencephalography (MEG) are increasingly being used to measure neural activities. Metabolic features can also be used as input channels and they generally rely on measuring changes in blood flow which can be quantified by fMRI [4], PET and more recently NIRS (Near Infrared Spectroscopy). NIRS can measure changes in cortical oxygenation using refraction of light in living tissues with high circulation density [5]. It is non-invasive and relatively inexpensive. For example, Coyle et al. [6] demonstrated a fNIRS based brain-computer interface that used motor imagery as a "mindswitch". A similar application is proposed by Tsubone et al [7]. Sitaram et al. [8] demonstrated a spelling task via online control of sensorimotor brain areas in a small group of healthy subjects. More recently, Leff et al. demonstrated how NIRS could be effectively used to identify cortical activation patterns between novice and experienced surgeons [9-12]. Dynamic topographs of cortical oxyhaemoglobin intensity changes have been used to study prefrontal response to surgical tasks. The prefrontal cortex is known to be vital for acquisition of visuomotor skills, but its role in the attainment of complex technical skills in terms of both perceptual and motor components, remains poorly understood. It has been shown that its response is highly dependent on technical expertise and manifold embedding has been used to depict practice dependent reorganisation of cortical behaviour in surgical novices [11].

Although these studies have provided insight into certain cortical activation patterns in surgical tasks, their practical use in *perceptual docking* for robotic control still remains farfetched. For practical applications, the input channels need to be non-intrusive and can be naturally (or pervasively) integrated into the working environment. In this regard, the use of remote eye-tracking provides a practical way forward.

3 Gaze-Contingent Perceptual Docking

One of the strongest depth cues available to human is the horizontal disparity that exists between the two retinal images. During surgery, the operating surgeons constantly perform saccadic eye movements and fixations which reflect their attention and cognitive visual search strategies. There is a close relationship between the horizontal disparity and depth perception, which varies with the viewing distance. More specifically, as the fixation point moves away from the observer, the horizontal disparity between the two retinal images decreases. In order to extract quantitative information regarding the depth of the fixation point, ocular vergence needs to be measured, thus providing a veridical interpretation of stereoscopic depth. One technique of achieving this is video-oculography. This is a non-intrusive video based approach used to measure the corneal reflection from a fixed infrared light source in relation to the centre of the pupil, which can be mapped to a unique eye gaze direction. The combined tracking of both eyes provides a binocular vergence measure, which in turn can determine the 3D fixation point.

Eye tracking research has a long history in experimental psychology and it provides objective and quantitative evidence of the user's visual and (mostly overt) attention processes. Visual search is the act of searching for a target within a scene and the myriad of visual search tasks performed in surgery is so large that it has become a reactive rather than deliberative process for most common tasks. During visual searches for a defined target there is evidence for both parallel search, with the target being the first and only fixation point, and for sequential search, in which several fixation points are found leading to the target. The intrinsic dynamics of eye movement are complex, and saccadic eye movement is the most important to consider when studying visual search [13]. The modelling of visual search and information seeking behaviour has attracted significant research interests as it is essential for elucidating the idiosyncrasy behind individual search patterns. Currently, there is a widespread use of eye tracking techniques for art, engineering, psychology, cognitive science, behaviour science, human-machine interfacing, ergonomics, market research, and medical imaging. Related to visual information processing, it has been used for devising gaze contingent systems for medical imaging, image communication, virtual reality displays, image analysis, and robotic vision. The reason for its recent, accelerated use beyond psychological laboratory settings is largely due to advances in CMOS sensors and computing technologies, which make the accuracy, robustness, and calibration processes of the eye-tracking device amenable to practical use.

One of the important uses of the eye tracking information is to reveal the underlying cognitive process involved in surgery. The richness of information provided by eye tracking provides both opportunities and challenges to human robot interaction. Current research in gaze contingent perceptual docking is focussed on the use of eye tracking for commanding instrument control. In MIS, this includes simple instrument manoeuvres such as automatic targeting and panning of the laparoscope, and extracting the intention and visual search strategies of the operator for characterising the visual pathways in deploying hand-eye controls. This allows the design of gaze-adapted user interface for intelligent instrument manipulation. Specific research issues

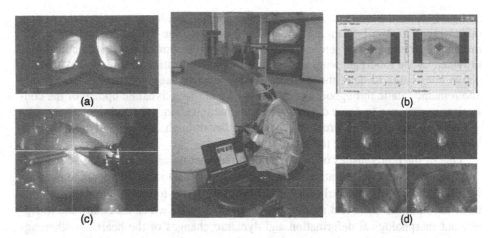

Fig. 1. The experimental setup for the gaze-contingent perceptual docking studies (centre). A binocular eye tracker (a, b, c) is integrated in the daVinci surgical console and a 6-DOF haptic device is used for the experiments. d) Eye tracking is also used for gaze-contingent augmented reality [16].

currently being addressed include how to deal with visual relevance feedback (which in many cases could be implicitly applied), how to deal with overt and covert attention, and how to detect visual saliency and attention. Extensive results have already been generated for using binocular eye tracking for extracting depth from the soft tissue, continuous tracking of tissue deformation [14-15], controlling articulated surgical tools and providing the surgeon with gaze-contingent augmented reality [16]. An example setup of the binocular eye tracking on a daVinci system is shown in Fig. 1.

4   Gaze-Contingent Motor Channelling

Executing dexterous surgical tasks under a static frame of reference for a moving object is one of the ultimate goals of robotic surgery. Current approaches to motion stabilisation are mainly achieved through a mechanical endoscopic stabilizer which provides intracorporeal articulation and facilitates placement of the device to the target vessel. To avoid tools entering unsafe anatomical regions, the concept of active constraints (or virtual fixtures, surgical macros) has been introduced. If the tool approaches a volume of space previously defined to be forbidden, the robot can prevent further motion in that direction. In its early implementation of virtual fixtures, the method only relied on pre-operative registered data and fiducial markers without incorporating force sensors. The surgeon can differentiate between cutting hard or soft tissues via the control instrument. They can also manually define safe regions in order to limit the manipulator movement by directing the tool either perpendicularly or tangentially away from a forbidden boundary. This manipulation constraint was first proposed by Rosenberg [17].

In practice, active constraint is a perceptual overlay of abstract sensory information on a workspace in order to improve the fidelity of the link between the operator and environment. Similar to a ruler guiding a pencil, the idea is to reduce the human sensory workload in performing remote-control tasks. The synergistic use of visual-motor cooperation allows perceptual-motor skills to be combined with the constraints provided by the robot, allowing an accurate and safe operation. In implementations of active constraints to date, the boundaries have always been defined pre-operatively and remained static throughout the operation. To perform dynamic update of the constraints in response to tissue deformation and changing surgical conditions, it requires accurate extraction of 3D structural changes either through intra-operative imaging or biomechanical modelling of the target anatomy.

One of the prerequisites of image guided intervention and introducing active constraints is the correct registration and fusion of the 3D data to the target anatomy. This is difficult in MIS, particularly for cardiac procedures due to the deflation of the lung, insufflation of the chest and application of surgical tools, which all contribute to significant morphological deformation and dynamic changes of the heart. Another significant challenge of beating heart surgery is the destabilization introduced by cardiac and respiratory motion, which severely affects precise tissue-instrument interactions and the execution of complex grafts. Mechanical stabilizers permit off-pump procedures by locally stabilizing the target area while the rest of the heart supports blood circulation. Despite this, residual motion remains, which still complicates delicate tasks such as small vessel anastomosis. These problems are compounded with reduced access to the internal anatomy inherent in MIS, which impose difficulties on target localization.

Based on binocular eye-tracking, we have recently proposed the concept of gaze-contingent motor channelling for augmenting the surgeon's motor abilities in controlling the surgical instruments with the aid of human vision [18]. With this framework, tissue geometry and deformation recovery can be obtained through binocular eye tracking by measuring ocular vergence during robotic assisted MIS. Through the known intrinsic and extrinsic parameters of the calibrated stereo laparoscopic camera, the 3D distance between the surgeon's eye fixation point on the tissue and the laparoscopic instrument can be recovered. By implementing force interactions based on the relative separation between the fixation point and the position of the surgical instrument, there is a strong indication that manipulation of the instrument is enhanced and hand-eye coordination is significantly improved.

Fig. 2a illustrates a haptic-master surgical manipulation station which consists of a stereoscopic console, a binocular eye tracker and two haptic devices used to control the surgical instrument. The exerted attractive forces are based on the separation between the fixation point and the instrument. It has been shown that the amount of improvement achieved in instrument manipulation with and without the use of visual-motor channelling is significant. It is expected that this approach can also benefit many of the existing human-computer interfaces used in tele-presence robot manipulation. As shown in Fig. 2b, a haptic boundary comprising cones and a plate is formed and located on the eye-fixation point on the tissue surface. This is used to confine the instrument working space into a safe region such that the operator is only allowed to approach the deforming tissue (epicardial surface in this example) through the conical pathway defined [18].

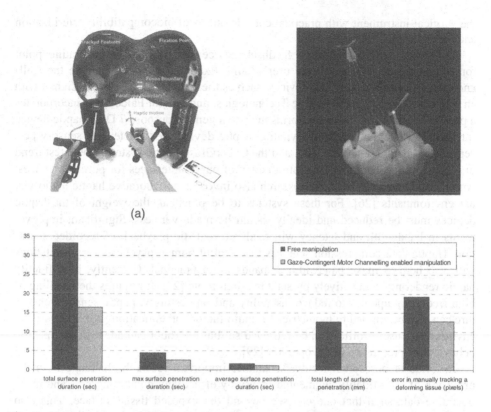

Fig. 2. (a) The conceptual design of a haptic and eye tracking enabled manipulation control station; (b) the conical pathways carved out underneath the safety boundary based on the fixation point of the surgeon; the graph demonstrates the improvement achieved in terms of instrument manipulation during a motor tracking task of a deforming tissue with and without gaze contingent motor channelling

5 Improved Haptics and Perceptual Feedback

In robotic surgery, the use of master-slave technology has created a physical separation between the surgeon and the patient. The use of servo controller also introduces a missing link between the visual and the motor sensory channels. To reconnect the visuomotor sensory feedback, both cutaneous tactile and kinesthetic forces have to be incorporated into the control interfaces. Some early psycho-haptic experiments designed by Okamura *et al.* characterized the problem with the deficiency of haptic feedback in tele-manipulation surgery [19]. Although there is substantial research work on haptic feedback [20-23], this is mainly limited to simulating the force reactions between tissue and surgical instruments. Realistic *in vivo* haptic sensing is difficult to obtain in complicated robot manipulation environments since the instruments are usually interacting with many objects concurrently (*e.g.* trocar, tissue and other tools). Because of this, multiple miniaturised force sensors need to be embedded in the surgical instrument with practical considerations of biocompatibility, sterilization and interactive tactile displays.

Currently, most haptic force feedback devices are limited to generating point forces and torque reaction to the user's hand. Example platforms include the well-known 6 DOF haptic feedback devices, such as the PHANTOM device designed with an articulated joint from SensAble Technologies, and Novint Falcon that incorporates a parallel mechanism. Other platforms include a general purpose 7 DOF haptic device for surgery [24], the magnetic levitation haptic device used for texture sensory perception and haptic rendering [25], and the CyberGrasp haptic system. The latest trend in perceptual feedback is in the introduction of haptic interfaces for portable devices. An emerging concept in haptic research also involves collaborative haptic audio visual environments [26]. For these systems to be practical, the weight of the haptic devices must be reduced and ideally should be made wireless. Significant improvements in bandwidth and latency will facilitate realistic playback of recorded sensation. Haptic data compression schemes that exploit human psychosensory limitations will also help to make bandwidth demands more practical. Currently, high fidelity haptic rendering is an actively pursued research topic [27]. It requires the handling of high frequency updates to reduce instability and interestingly, haptic sensor architecture can also be applied to biometrics for multi factor authentication [28]. In a surgical environment, user profiles can be retrieved so that the robot can adapt to the specific behaviour or preference of the operator [29].

In terms of perceptual feedback, another important research challenge is in the provision of high-fidelity augmented reality by effectively combining pre- and intra-operative data such that one can see beyond the exposed tissue surface. This also entails accurate modelling and simulation of soft tissue combined with direct *in vivo*, *in situ* sensing and imaging. Current research has already made significant in roads into real-time AR systems and the development of *in situ* tissue characterisation techniques based on multi-excitation, multi-spectral imaging to permit simultaneous morphological and functional mapping. It also permits multi-scale image integration such that the visual perceptual capability of the surgeon is significantly enhanced.

6 Conclusions

Empowering robots with human intelligence represents one of the ultimate goals of robotic research. The regulatory, ethical and legal barriers imposed on interventional surgical robots give rise to the need of a tightly integrated control between the operator and robot when autonomy is pursued. The concept of *perceptual docking* represents a new way of knowledge acquisition for robotic systems by using *in situ* learning of operator specific motor and perceptual/cognitive behaviour. In robotic surgery, the technology has developed to a stage that improved motion stabilisation, intra-operative guidance, and active constraints need to be deployed to ensure operating accuracy and consistency. The use of *perceptual docking* naturally avoids some of the major technical hurdles of existing approaches and the technique is also expected to benefit other applications of robotic control beyond surgery.

References

1. Moore, M.M.: Real-World Applications for Brain-Computer Interface Technology. IEEE Trans. on Neural Systems and Rehabilitation Engineering 11(2), 162–165 (2003)
2. Wolpaw, J.R., McFarland, D.J.: Control of a Two-Dimensional Movement Signal by a Noninvasive Brain-Computer Interface in Humans. NeuroScience 101(51), 17849–17854 (2004)
3. Serruya, M.D., Hatsopoulos, N.G., Paninski, L., Fellow, M.R., Donoghue, J.P.: Instant Neural Control of a Movement Signal. Nature 416, 141–142 (2002)
4. Yoo, S.S., Fairneny, T., Chen, N.K., Choo, S.E., Panych, L.P., Park, H., Lee, S.Y., Jolesz, F.A.: Brain-Computer Interface Using fMRI: Spatial Navigation by Thoughts. Neuroreport 15(10), 1591–1595 (2004)
5. Franceschini, M.A., Boas, D.A.: Noninvasive Measurement of Neuronal Activity with Near-Infrared Optical Imaging. NeuroImage 21(1), 372–386 (2004)
6. Coyle, S.M., Ward, T.E., Markham, C.M.: Brain-Computer Interface Using a Simplified Functional Near-Infrared Spectroscopy System. Journal of Neural Eng. 4(3), 219–226 (2007)
7. Tsubone, T., Muroga, T., Wada, Y.: Application to Robot Control Using Brain Function Measurement by Near-Infrared Spectroscopy. In: Proc. of IEEE Eng. Med. Biol. Soc., pp. 5324–5345 (2007)
8. Sitaram, R., Zhang, H., Guan, C., Thulasidas, M., Hoshi, Y., Ishikawa, A., Shimizu, K., Birbaumer, N.: Temporal Classification of Multichannel Near-Infrared Spectroscopy Signals of Motor Imagery for Developing a Brain-Computer Interface. Neuroimage 34(4), 1416–1427 (2007)
9. Leff, D., Koh, P.H., Aggarwal, R., Leong, J., Deligiani, F., Elwell, C., Delpy, D.T., Darzi, A., Yang, G.Z.: Optical Mapping of the Frontal Cortex During a Surgical Knot-Tying Task, a Feasibility Study. In: Medical Imaging Augmented Reality, pp. 140–147 (2006)
10. Leff, D.R., Leong, J.J., Aggarwal, R., Yang, G.Z., Darzi, A.: Could Variations in Technical Skills Acquisition in Surgery be Explained by Differences in Cortical Plasticity? Annals of Surgery 247(3), 540–543 (2008)
11. Leff, D.R., Orihuela-Espina, F., Atallah, L., Darzi, A., Yang, G.Z.: Functional Near Infrared Spectroscopy in Novice and Expert Surgeons - a Manifold Embedding Approach. In: Ayache, N., Ourselin, S., Maeder, A. (eds.) MICCAI 2007, Part II. LNCS, vol. 4792, pp. 270–277. Springer, Heidelberg (2007)
12. Leff, D.R., Elwell, C.E., Orihuela-Espina, F., Atallah, L., Delpy, D.T., Darzi, A.W., Yang, G.Z.: Changes in Prefrontal Cortical Behaviour Depend Upon Familiarity on a Bimanual Co-Ordination Task: an fNIRS Study. Neuroimage 39(2), 805–813 (2008)
13. Yang, G.Z., Dempere-Marco, L., Hu, X.-P., Rowe, A.: Visual Search: Psychophysical Models and Practical Applications. Image and Vision Computing 20, 291–305 (2002)
14. Mylonas, G.P., Darzi, A., Yang, G.Z.: Gaze Contingent Depth Recovery and Motion Stabilisation for Minimally Invasive Robotic Surgery. In: Yang, G.-Z., Jiang, T. (eds.) MIAR 2004. LNCS, vol. 3150, pp. 311–319. Springer, Heidelberg (2004)
15. Mylonas, G.P., Stoyanov, D., Deligianni, F., Darzi, A., Yang, G.-Z.: Gaze-Contingent Soft Tissue Deformation Tracking for Minimally Invasive Robotic Surgery. In: Duncan, J.S., Gerig, G. (eds.) MICCAI 2005. LNCS, vol. 3749, pp. 843–850. Springer, Heidelberg (2005)
16. Lerotic, M., Chung, A.J., Mylonas, G., Yang, G.-Z.: pq-Space Based Non-Photorealistic Rendering for Augmented Reality. In: Ayache, N., Ourselin, S., Maeder, A. (eds.) MICCAI 2007, Part II. LNCS, vol. 4792, pp. 102–109. Springer, Heidelberg (2007)

17. Rosenberg, L.B.: Virtual Fixtures: Perceptual Tools for Telerobotic Manipulation. In: Proc. of the IEEE Annual International Symposium on Virtual Reality, pp. 76–82 (1993)
18. Mylonas, G.P., Kwok, K.-W., Darzi, A., Yang, G.Z.: Gaze-Contingent Motor Channelling and Haptic Constraints for Minimally Invasive Robotic Surgery. In: Proceedings of the 11th International Conference on Medical Image Computing and Computer Assisted Intervention, MICCAI 2008, New York (to appear, 2008)
19. Okamura, A.M.: Methods for Haptic Feedback in Teleoperated Robot-Assisted Surgery. Industrial Robot: An International Journal 31(6), 499–508 (2004)
20. Mendoza, C., Laugier, C.: Tissue Cutting Using Finite Elements and Force Feedback. In: Proc. of International Symposium on Surgery Simulation and Soft Tissue Modeling, pp. 175–182 (2003)
21. Crouch, J.R., Schneider, C.M., Wainer, J., Okamura, A.M.: A Velocity-Dependent Model for Needle Insertion in Soft Tissue. In: Duncan, J.S., Gerig, G. (eds.) MICCAI 2005. LNCS, vol. 3750, pp. 624–632. Springer, Heidelberg (2005)
22. Heverly, M., Dupont, P., Triedman, J.: Trajectory Optimization for Dynamic Needle Insertion. In: Proc. of the 2005 IEEE International Conf. on Robotics and Automation, pp. 1646–1651 (2005)
23. Kennedy, C.W., Hu, T., Desai, J.P., Wechsler, A.S., Kresh, J.Y.: A Novel Approach to Robotic Cardiac Surgery Using Haptics and Vision. Cardiovascular Engineering: An International Journal 2(1), 15–21 (2002)
24. Tholey, G., Desai, J.P.: A General Purpose 7 DOF Haptic Device: Applications Towards Robot-Assisted Surgery. IEEE/ASME Trans. on Mechatronics 12(6), 662–669 (2007)
25. Unger, B., Hollis, R., Klatzky, R.: JND Analysis of Texture Roughness Perception Using a Magnetic Levitation Haptic Device. In: Proc. Of the 2nd Joint Eurohaptics Conference and Symposium on Haptic Interfaces for Virtual Environment and Teleoperator Systems, pp. 9–15 (2007)
26. Saddik, E.: The Potential of Haptics Technologies. IEEE Instrumentation and Measurement Magazine 10(1), 10–17 (2007)
27. Lin, M., Salisbury, K.: Haptic Rendering-Beyond Visual Computing. IEEE Computer Graphics and Applications 24(2), 22–23 (2004)
28. Orozco, M., Asfaw, Y., Shirmohammadi, S.S., Adler, A., Saddik, A.E.: Haptic-Based Biometrics: A Feasibility Study. In: Proc. of the Symposium on Haptic Interfaces for Virtual Environment and Teleoperator Systems, pp. 265–271 (2006)
29. Tsagarakis, N.G., Petrone, M., Testi, D., Mayoral, R., Zannoni, C., Viceconti, M., Clapworthy, G.J., Gray, J.O., Caldwell, D.G.: Pre-Operative Planning for Total Hip Arthroplasty Using a Haptic Enabled Multimodal Interface and Framework. IEEE Trans. of Multimedia and Visualization: Special issue in Haptics 13(3), 40–48 (2006)

An Integration of Statistical Deformable Model and Finite Element Method for Bone-Related Soft Tissue Prediction in Orthognathic Surgery Planning

Qizhen He[1,2], Jun Feng[2], Horace H.S. Ip[2], James Xia[3], and Xianbin Cao[1]

[1] Department of Computer Science and Technology, University of Science & Technology of China, Hefei, China
[2] Image Computing Group, Department of Computer Science, City University of Hong Kong, Hong Kong, China
[3] Surgical Planning Laboratory, Department of Oral and Maxillofacial Surgery, The Methodist Hospital Research Institute, U.S.A
rainy@mail.ustc.edu.cn, feng@cs.cityu.edu.hk,
cship@cityu.edu.hk,
JXia@tmhs.org, xbcao@ustc.edu.cn

Abstract. In this paper, we propose a novel statistical deformable model for bone-related soft-tissue prediction, which we called Br-SDM. In Br-SDM, we have integrated Finite Element Model(FEM) and Statistical Deformable Model(SDM) to achieve both accurate and efficient prediction for orthognathic surgery planning. By combining FEM-based surgery simulation for sample generation and SDM for soft tissue prediction, we are able to capture the prior knowledge of bone-related soft-tissue deformation for different surgical plans. Then the post-operative appearance can be predicted in a more efficient way from a Br-SDM based optimization. Our experiments have shown that Br-SDM is able to give comparable soft-tissue prediction accuracy with respect to conventional FEM-based prediction while only requires 10% of its computational cost.

Keywords: Orthognathic Surgery; Surgery Planning; Operation Prediction; Finite Element Method; Statistical Deformable Model.

1 Introduction

Traditional surgical planning for orthognathic surgery is determined by cephalometric analysis, as well as clinical and aesthetic judgments. Frequently there is a huge demand from surgeons to be able to predict the facial outlook after the surgery preoperatively, and to improve the communication with patients. Although there exists software for surgical planning and post-operation prediction based on 2D images, eg. lateral and frontal skull X-rays [1], accurate and efficient three-dimensional postoperative prediction remains a highly challenging problem. Previous approaches to 3D post-operative prediction are mostly based on the Mass Spring Models (MSM)

T. Dohi, I. Sakuma, and H. Liao (Eds.): MIAR 2008, LNCS 5128, pp. 31–39, 2008.

[2], and Finite Element Models (FEM) [3]. FEM, as a general discretization procedure of continuum problems, has been shown to give an accurate model when simulating deformations of living tissues [4]. However, the approach is not particularly applicable to real-time surgical planning due to its high computational cost and large memory. On the other hand, the low computational time and space complexity of MSM make it very attractive for real-time simulation. However, the parameters in a MSM, such as the spring constant [5], typically do not bear direct relation to the biomechanical properties of human soft tissues. To harness FEM's accuracy and, at the same time, to reduce its computational cost, a Mass Tensor Model (MTM) has been proposed [6]. Quantitative validation results show that MTM can achieve the same accuracy as FEM, while nearly half the computation time [4]. Unfortunately, this comes at the expense of intensive pre-computation.

In order to learn the prior knowledge of tissue deformation from the training samples, Meller, in 2005, has applied Statistical Deformable Model (SDM) for maxillofacial prediction [7]. To capture the basic shape and the major variations of a certain class, point distribution model has been established from the pre- and post- operative facial skins. While SDM seems a promising approach for simulating soft tissue movements and requires much less computations compared with FEM, it suffers from a number of problems when applied to soft tissue prediction in surgical planning. The accuracy of SDM in soft tissue prediction depends to a large extent on the number of pre-operative and post-operative samples available, and the lack of sufficient training samples is a major issue in the application of SDM in the medical domain [8]. In [7], the authors by-passed this problem by using only pre-operational facial data and a joint SDM to predict the post-operational facial changes. More significantly, the work assumed that all patients underwent the same standard surgery. In orthognathic surgery, the facial change is the result of maxillofacial bone movements and the SDM developed in [7] which does not take bone movements into account is not particularly applicable to orthognathic surgical planning where different surgical plans would be investigated.

The primary contribution of this paper is that we propose an integrated approach of *FEM* and *SDM* to construct a SDM of bone-related soft tissue prediction which we called Bone-related SDM or *Br-SDM* to achieve both accurate and efficient prediction for orthognathic surgery planning. In our approach, FEM-based surgery simulation is used to generate a large sample sets of soft-tissue deformations; then the generated set of deformation samples are used to train a Statistical Deformable Model (SDM) for subsequent surgical planning. The advantage of this approach is that the prior knowledge of bone-related planning and the corresponding facial changes have been incorporated into the training samples, the resulting Br-SDM can yield accurate prediction results in a computationally efficient way that facilitates interactive surgical plan generation. The proposed Br-SDM enables surgeons to simulate different operating strategies, and to acquire the bone-related changes of the soft-tissue in real time. The experimental results demonstrate that the Br-SDM has comparable accuracies with FEM while using only 10% of the computational time and memory of conventional FEM.

The rest of this paper is organized as follows. Section 2 and 3 present the construction of the integration model and facial prediction algorithm respectively. The experimental results are shown in section 4. We conclude our paper in the end.

2 An Integrated Approach of FEM and SDM

2.1 Sample Definition

In order to incorporate the prior knowledge of the bone deformation, and to capture the relationship between the bone movement and the soft-tissue variations, we define the sample of the integrated model as: $X = (\delta_1, ..., \delta_m, \delta_{m+1}, ..., \delta_{m+n})^T$, where δ_i is the displacement of vertex i of two 3D (polygonal) meshes, with the first m vertices on the jaw mesh, and the remaining n vertices on the soft-tissue mesh.

We define those soft-tissue vertices that overlap with the jaw surface as boundary points. These boundary points are assumed to have the same displacements with their counterparts on the jaw during surgical planning. Therefore, X can be reduced from $(m+n)$ dimensions to n by re-arranging the surface vertices of the soft-tissue models: $X = (\delta_{boundary}, \delta_{non-boundary})^T = (\delta_1, ..., \delta_m, \delta_{m+1}, ..., \delta_n)^T$, where the first m vertices are the boundary points and the remaining $n-m$ points are the non-boundary points. We show the meshes of deforming area of the soft-tissue in Fig. 1, in which the boundary points are highlighted in yellow.

2.2 FEM Based Sample Generation

In order to capture the relationship between the jawbone operation and the corresponding facial deformation, here we propose to perform Finite Element Method (FEM) based surgical prediction to generate training samples for further statistical analysis. Different cutting planes are simulated randomly, and for each cutting strategy, cut pieces of the jawbone are moved virtually to their target positions. Accordingly, the corresponding facial variations are computed from the FEM, which give rise to a sample defined in section 2.1.

To construct the FEM for soft-tissue movement prediction, soft-tissue is modeled as homogeneous, linear and elastic material [8]. Through Hooke's law, we obtain:

$$\begin{pmatrix} \sigma_x \\ \sigma_y \\ \sigma_z \\ \tau_{xy} \\ \tau_{yz} \\ \tau_{xz} \end{pmatrix} = \frac{E}{(1+v)(1-2v)} \begin{pmatrix} 1-v & v & v & 0 & 0 & 0 \\ v & 1-v & v & 0 & 0 & 0 \\ v & v & 1-v & 0 & 0 & 0 \\ 0 & 0 & 0 & \frac{1-2v}{2} & 0 & 0 \\ 0 & 0 & 0 & 0 & \frac{1-2v}{2} & 0 \\ 0 & 0 & 0 & 0 & 0 & \frac{1-2v}{2} \end{pmatrix} \begin{pmatrix} \varepsilon_x \\ \varepsilon_y \\ \varepsilon_z \\ \gamma_{xy} \\ \gamma_{yz} \\ \gamma_{zx} \end{pmatrix} \quad (1)$$

$$\Leftrightarrow \{\sigma\} = [D]\{\varepsilon\}$$

with stress components $\sigma_x, \sigma_y, \sigma_z, \tau_{xy}, \tau_{yz}, \tau_{xz}$, strain components $\varepsilon_x, \varepsilon_y, \varepsilon_z, \gamma_{xy}, \gamma_{yz}, \gamma_{zx}$, Young's modulus E and Poisson coefficient v.

Under linear assumption, the displacement $\vec{u}$ of the points within the element can be approximated by a linear interpolation of the nodal displacements, i.e. $\vec{u} = \sum N_i \delta_i$, with the nodal displacement δ_i and the interpolating weight N_i for each node. Then from the Green-Lagrange strain tensor we can relate the strain ε with the nodal displacement $\{\delta\}$, such that:

$$\{\varepsilon\} = \begin{pmatrix} \varepsilon_x & \varepsilon_y & \varepsilon_z & \gamma_{xy} & \gamma_{yz} & \gamma_{xz} \end{pmatrix}^T$$
$$= \left(\frac{\partial u}{\partial x} \quad \frac{\partial v}{\partial y} \quad \frac{\partial w}{\partial z} \quad \frac{\partial u}{\partial y} + \frac{\partial v}{\partial x} \quad \frac{\partial v}{\partial z} + \frac{\partial w}{\partial y} \quad \frac{\partial u}{\partial z} + \frac{\partial w}{\partial x} \right)^T = [B]\{\delta\} \tag{2}$$

with the three components (u, v, w) of $\vec{u}$ and the nodal displacement vector $\{\delta\}$.

According to the virtual energy's principle, we have $\delta U = \iint \{\varepsilon\}^T \{\sigma\} dx dy = \{\delta\}^T \{F\} = \delta V$, which leads to $\{F\} = [k]\{\delta\}$ with the virtual strain energy δU, the virtual work of the nodal force δV, the external force $\{F\}$ and the stiffness matrix $[k] = \iiint [B]^T [D][B] dV$.

Recalled that we choose those soft-tissue points that overlap with the jaw surface as the boundary conditions and they are therefore fixed with respect to the jaw surface, the rest of the points of the soft-tissue are free to deform. Accordingly, $\{F\} = [k]\{\delta\}$ can be written as

$$\begin{pmatrix} f \\ 0 \end{pmatrix} = \begin{pmatrix} k_{aa} & k_{ab} \\ k_{ba} & k_{bb} \end{pmatrix} \begin{pmatrix} \delta_{boundary} \\ \delta_{non-boundary} \end{pmatrix} \tag{3}$$

Then we can have

$$\delta_{non-boundary} = -k_{bb}^{-1} k_{ba} \delta_{boundary} \tag{4}$$

with $m*m$ matrix k_{aa}, $m*n$ matrix k_{ab}, $n*m$ matrix k_{ba}, $n*n$ matrix k_{bb}.

From equation (4), given the jaw movement, which can be considered as the displacements of the boundary points of the soft-tissue ($\delta_{boundary}$), we can easily compute the displacements for the rest of the points of the soft-tissue ($\delta_{non-boundary}$).

2.3 Integrating FEM and SDM for a Br-SDM

To build our Br-SDM for soft tissue prediction, correspondence of the points on the soft tissue should be established and all the samples should be aligned. Traditional Iterative Closest Point (ICP) can be applied here [10]. Having achieved approximate

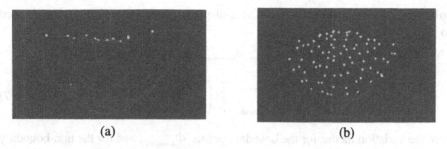

(a)   (b)

Fig. 1. Part of the volume mesh of the facial soft tissue, with "bone-soft tissue" boundary points shown in yellow, (a) anterior (front) view and (b) posterior (back) view of the soft tissue mesh

alignment for all the samples, the mean shape $\overline{X}$ and covariance matrix S can be calculated as :

$$\overline{X} = \frac{1}{N}\sum_{i=1}^{N} X_i \ , \ S = \frac{1}{N}\sum_{i=1}^{N} dX_i dX_i^{\ T} \tag{5}$$

where N is the size of the sample set, and dX_i is the deviation from the mean, i.e. $dX_i = X_i - \overline{X}$ .The modes of variation of the points can then be described by p_i, the unit eigenvectors of S . Following the Principal Component Analysis (PCA), we choose the eigenvectors $(p_1,...,p_t)$ corresponding to the largest t eigenvalues of S to capture the major variation modes among the samples. Then a new sample can be represented as

$$X = \overline{X} + \Phi b \tag{6}$$

with the mean of the sample $\overline{X}$, the variation matrix $\Phi = (p_1,...,p_t)$ and the variation parameter b .

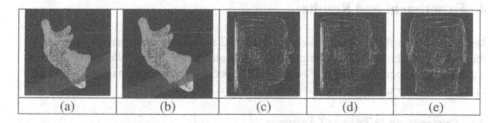

(a)   (b)   (c)   (d)   (e)

Fig. 2. The process of the surgical simulation. (a) the cutting plane, (b) the movement of the jaw piece, (c) the pre-operative model of the face (d) the side view of the post-operative model of the face calculated by FEM (e) the front view of the post-operative model.

3   Bone-Related Soft-Tissue Prediction Based on Br-SDM

Given a statistical deformable model for bone-related soft tissue prediction, a surgery plan can be expressed in terms of the cutting plane of the jaw model and the displacement of the jawbone pieces. These displacements can be further transformed into $\delta_{boundary}$ to predict $\delta_{non-boundary}$.

As defined in section 2, $X = (\delta_{boundary}, \delta_{non-boudary})$, we can rewrite (6) as

$$\begin{pmatrix} \delta_{boundary} \\ \delta_{non-boundary} \end{pmatrix} = \begin{pmatrix} \overline{\delta}_{boundary} \\ \overline{\delta}_{non-boundary} \end{pmatrix} + \begin{pmatrix} \Phi_{boundary} \\ \Phi_{non-boundary} \end{pmatrix} b \qquad (7)$$

where the variation modes for the boundary points $\Phi_{boundary}$, and for the non-boundary modes $\Phi_{non-boundary}$. To fit $\delta_{boundary}$ into Br-SDM, we minimize

$$D(b) = \left\| \delta_{boundary} - (\overline{\delta}_{boundary} + \Phi_{boundary} b) \right\|^2 \qquad (8)$$

This optimization result can be found by a Singular Value Decomposition $\Phi_{boundary} = UWV^T$, with a diagonal matrix $W = diag(w_i)$, and $U^T U = V^T V = I$. The pseudo-inverse of $\Phi_{boundary}$ is $\Phi_{boundary}^+ = VW^+ U^T$

$$W^+ = diag \begin{pmatrix} w_i^{-1} & if & w_i \neq 0 \\ 0 & otherwise \end{pmatrix} \qquad (9)$$

The minimum of $D(b)$ can be computed with the pseudo-inverse:

$$b = \Phi_{boundary}^+ (\delta_{boundary} - \overline{X}_{boundary}) \qquad (10)$$

Then the computation of $\delta_{non-boundary}$ becomes:

$$\delta_{non-boundary} = \overline{\delta}_{non-boundary} + \Phi_{non-boundary} b \qquad (11)$$

4   Experiment and Results

Using the above method, we have generated 300 soft tissue deformation samples for the training of the Br-SDM. The number of the surface points is 596. In this section, we present the performance of Br-SDM based prediction and compared it with FEM in terms of accuracy and computational efficiency.

4.1   Comparison in Terms of Accuracy

We use the prism as the volumetric element and the soft-tissue volume model is composed of 627 prisms [9]. The predicting difference of FEM and our Br-SDM for vertex i is given by $e(i) = \left\| d_{FEM}(i) - d_{Br-SDM}(i) \right\|$ with the displacement of vertex i calculated from FEM $d_{FEM}(i)$, and from Br-SDM $d_{Br-SDM}(i)$. In the experiment, we have designed 9 surgical plans, with bone advancement range from 2.2mm to 8.1mm, and left movement range from 0.9mm to 5.4mm. The prediction difference between FEM and Br-SDM based surgery simulation are compared in Table 1. The result shows that for the mean soft-tissue deformation of around 5mm, the prediction difference of Br-SDM and FEM is less than 1mm for 90% of the vertices. For 70% of the points, the difference is below 0.5mm. The mean difference is about 0.4mm. Additionally we can see the predicting differences remain relatively low (less than 10%) comparing with the average deformation.

4.2 Comparison of Computational Efficiency

Since, in our integrated approach, FEM is applied to generate samples to train our Br-SDM, the dominant computation time is consumed in FEM calculation, specifically in the computation of stiffness matrix. However, in our approach, such calculations are done off-line instead of on-line as in the case of conventional FEM-based prediction, the actual soft-tissue deformation and prediction process can be done very efficiently using the resulting Br-SDM.

Using a PC with Intel Pentium M processor and 2Gbyte RAM, Br-SDM requires only on average 2 seconds to compute correspondence matching, comparing with several hours required for the stiffness matrix computing in FEM for each patient. And when predicting soft-tissue deformation for a given surgical plan, Br-SDM only takes on average 15 milli-second while FEM takes 130 milli-seconds. Even when much more details have to be taken into the model (typically around 100,000 elements) Br-SDM based surgery simulation required only a very low time cost of within 1 second, while FEM spent more than 20 seconds according to [4]. Our experiments confirm that Br-SDM is well-suited to real-time surgical planning. Table 2 compares the pre-computation and real-time prediction of Br-SDM with FEM methods respectively.

Table 1. Predicting Difference between FEM and Br-SDM based Surgery Simulation

Surgery plan(mm)	Mean deformation	Mean difference (E)
F+2.2	1.5	0.16
F+3.1	2.2	0.23
F+4.9	3.4	0.37
F-5.8,L+1.3	4.2	0.48
F-5.8,L+2.2	4.4	0.52
F-5.8,L+5.4	5.8	0.66
F+8.1,L+0.9	5.7	0.62
F+8.1,L-1.3	5.8	0.64
F+8.1,L+2.2	5.9	0.68

* F+ is for Mandible Advancement, F- is for Mandible Setback, L+ is Mandible Right and L- is for Mandible Left. The mean difference is defined as $E = \dfrac{1}{n}\sum_{i=1}^{n} e(i)$

Table 2. The comparison of computational time between two models

Method	Pre-computation Time	Computation time
Br-SDM	2s	15ms
FEM (627 prisms)	>20 hours	130ms

5 Conclusion

In this paper, we have proposed an integrated approach of FEM and SDM to develop a novel statistical deformation model for bone-related soft tissue prediction called *Br-SDM*. Specifically, through this integrated approach. The prior knowledge of maxillo-facial bone surgery and the resulting soft-tissue deformation have been incorporated into the training samples for the Br-SDM.

Our experiments have shown that, for surgical plans that involve bone movement of 2 to 10 mm which are typical for orthognathic surgery, Br-SDM can achieve accurate soft-tissue prediction compared with conventional FEM-based prediction but at a significantly much reduced computation costs for the prediction process. This makes Br-SDM suitable for interactive surgical planning. For surgical plans that involve large bone movements, we found that the prediction differences between FEM and Br-SDM increase. This can be explained that for large bone displacement, the relationship between the bone and the soft tissue become non-linear and cannot be sufficiently captured by Br-SDM which is essentially a linear model. Nevertheless, for typical orthognathic surgery, during which the displacements of the jaw are usually around 10mm or less, Br-SDM can achieve an accuracy of less than 1mm comparing with Finite Element Method.

Acknowledgement

The work described in this paper was supported by a grant from the Research Grants Council of Hong Kong SAR, China. [Project No: CityU113706].

References

1. Zhu, M.: Simulation and Prediction of Orthognathic Surgery on Skeletal Class III Deformation. In: 3rd Chinese International Congress on Oral and Maxillofacial Surgery, in conjunction with 6th National Congress on Oral and Maxillofacial Surgery, Kunming, Yunan, PRC, p. 338 (2002)
2. Keeve, E., Girod, S., et al.: Deformable Modeling of Facial Tissue for Craniofacial Surgery Simulation. Computer Aided Surgery 3, 228–238 (1998)
3. Bro-Nielsen, M., HTM Inc., Rockville, M.D.: Finite Element Modeling in Surgery Simulation. Proceedings of the IEEE 86(33), 490–503 (1998)
4. Mollemans, W., Schutyser, F., et al.: Predicting soft-tissue deformations for a maxillofacial surgery planning system: From computational strategies to a complete clinical validation. Medical Image Analysis 11(3), 282–301 (2007)

5. Roose, L., De Maerteleire, W., Mollemans, W., Suetens, P.: Validation of different soft tissue simulation methods for breast augmentation. In: Proceedings of CARS, pp. 485–490 (2005)
6. Cotin, S., et al.: A hybrid elastic model allowing real-time cutting, deformations and force feedback for surgery training and simulation. The Visual Computer 16(88), 437–452 (2000)
7. Meller, S., Nkenke, E., Kalender, W.: Statistical Face Models for the Prediction of Soft-tissue Deformations after Orthognathic Osteotomies. In: Duncan, J.S., Gerig, G. (eds.) MICCAI 2005. LNCS, vol. 3750, pp. 443–450. Springer, Heidelberg (2005)
8. Fung, Y.C.: Biomechanics: Mechanical Properties of Living Tissues, pp. 242–320. Springer, Heidelberg (1993)
9. Keeve, E., Girod, S., Pfeifle, P., Girod, B.: Anatomy-Based Facial Tissue Modeling Using the Finite Element Method. In: Proceedings of IEEE visualization 1996, p. 21 (1996)
10. Besl, P.J., Mckay, N.D.: A Method for Registration of 3D Shapes. IEEE Trans. on Pattern Anal. & Mach. Intell. 14(2), 239–256 (1992)

Automated Preoperative Planning of Femoral Component for Total Hip Arthroplasty (THA) from 3D CT Images

Itaru Otomaru[1], Masahiko Nakamoto[2], Masaki Takao[2], Nobuhiko Sugano[2],
Yoshiyuki Kagiyama[1], Hideki Yoshikawa[2], Yukio Tada[1], and Yoshinobu Sato[2]

[1] Graduate School of Engineering, Kobe University, Kobe, Japan
[2] Graduate School of Medicine, Osaka University, Suita, Japan

Abstract. This paper describes a method for 3D automated preoperative planning of the femoral stem in total hip arthroplasty (THA). The stem planning is formulated as a problem to determine the optimal position, rotation, and size, on the 3D surface model of femur reconstructed from CT images. We obtain the parameters that maximize the fitness between the femoral canal and stem surfaces subject to the positional and rotational constraints. The maximization is performed by local optimization from multiple initial positions. The proposed method was experimentally evaluated by the difference from planning results of an experienced surgeon in 7 cases. The average positional and rotational differences were 1.9 mm and 2.5 deg., respectively, and there was size difference only in 1 case for the proposed method while these differences were 2.8 mm, 5.0 deg., and 5 cases for an existing method. The proposed method showed better performance than the existing method.

Keywords: computer assisted surgery, stem fitness, anteversion angle, orthopaedic implant.

1 Introduction

Recently, surgical navigation and robotic systems have been developed for total hip arthroplasty (THA) for the purpose of accurate placement of the orthopaedic implants in preoperatively determined 3D position and orientation [1-3]. This fact means that preoperative planning is becoming important because the preoperative plan can be accurately executed using these systems. In preoperative planning of THA, anatomical compatibility of each implant component with host bone is essential for stable fixation and good clinical results. Especially, the fit and fill of the cementless femoral component (stem) in the femoral canal are important factors for component stability [4-6]. Recently, CT-based interactive systems for preoperative 3D planning have been developed in order to quantitatively visualize the fit and fill [7]. However the interactive 3D planning is subjective as well as involves time-consuming, which limit its clinical use.

T. Dohi, I. Sakuma, and H. Liao (Eds.): MIAR 2008, LNCS 5128, pp. 40–49, 2008.

In order to solve these problems, we have been developing the automated preoperative planning system for THA, which automatically select optimal size, position, and orientation of the stem.

In our previous work, we have defined the objective function which describes the "fitness" value of the stem from surgeon's expertise and his planning results. And we have determined the solution by one-by-one search at the interval of 1.0 mm and 1.0 deg. in each axis [8-9]. However, this procedure of search is not appropriate because there is a possibility that the system overlook the solution which maximizes the fitness. On the other hand, related to our efforts, Viceconti et al. proposed the use of volume registration between the femoral canal and stem [10] for automated placement of the stem. However, image matching criteria used in volume registration were not derived from stem fitness criteria used by the experienced surgeon.

In this study, we propose an automated preoperative planning system of the femoral stem using 3D CT data. We use the definition of the "fitness" which we have used in previous work. In addition, we propose the constraints which describes the surgeon's expertise of the positional relation of the stem and the femur, and the optimization procedure to maximize the fitness. To evaluate the performance of the proposed system, we apply our method and the existing method [10] to 7 cases, and measure the difference between automated planning results and those of the experienced surgeon.

2 Methods

2.1 Preconditions

Block diagram of proposed system is shown in Fig. 1. As the patient information, we assume that 3D CT image of hip joint of the patient is given. The 3D model of the femoral canal is reconstructed from CT images, and the femoral coordinate system and the anatomical feature points are determined on its 3D models. As the implant information, we assume that the 3D shape models of all the variations in the femoral stems are given. Outputs of this system is the set of parameters ($\mathbf{z} = [\mathbf{t}, \mathbf{r}, s]$), of the position $\mathbf{t}$, orientation $\mathbf{r}$, and size s of stem.

The femur coordinate system is defined as Fig. 2. In specification of the femur coordinate system, we use the table top plane of the femur and the peak of the lesser trochanter. The z-axis of femur coordinate system is defined as the canal long axis estimated from the 3D model of femoral canal. The x-axis is orthogonal to the z-axis, and parallel to the table top plane. The y-axis is defined as the axis orthogonal to both x and z-axes. The origin is defined as the intersection point between the z-axis and the line which is perpendicular to the z-axis and passes through the peak of the lesser trochanter (Fig. 2, sagittal view).

2.2 Definition of Objective Function of Stem Fitness

We formulate the preoperative planning of the stem as the optimization problem that obtain the parameter $\mathbf{z}$ that maximizes the stem fitness evaluate function. The criteria in stem planning are defined as follows:

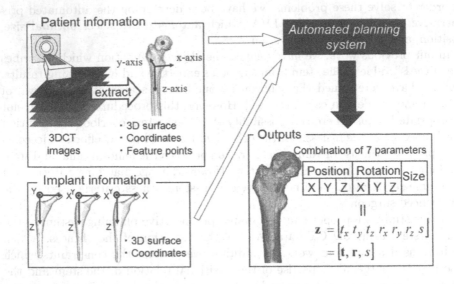

Fig. 1. Block diagram of proposed system

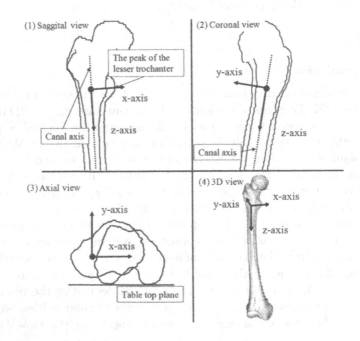

Fig. 2. Definition of the femur coordinate system ((1) Sagittal view, (2) Coronal view, (3) Axial view, (4) 3D view))

1. Overlap of the femoral canal and the stem surface is prohibited for the whole stem area.
2. Strong contact with the host bone in specific area of the stem is desirable.
3. Keep the positional and rotational relation with the femur.
4. Select the largest stem size unless the stem is not overlapped with the canal.

In proposed method, we use the distance from the femoral canal and the stem surface to describe these criteria. When the distance value is negative, the femoral canal and the stem surface is overlapped, and when the distance value is positive, there is a gap between the canal and the stem surface. Especially, when the gap is small, we consider that there is a strong fixation. At the same time, we define the positional and rotational constraints derived from anatomical compatibility between the host bone and the stem other than the stem fitness. In determination of the automated plan, first we obtain the candidates of parameters in each stem size, and then select the maximum size.

In our formulation, first we describe the $\mathbf{t}$ and $\mathbf{r}$ of the $\mathbf{z}$ as the transformation matrix of position and rotation $\mathbf{T}$. In addition, $\mathbf{t}$ and $\mathbf{r}$ are collectively described as the 6 parameters vector $\mathbf{q} = [t_x, t_y, t_z, r_x, r_y, r_z]$. We determine the parameters $\mathbf{T}$ in stem size s, which maximizes the objective function of stem fitness $F(\mathbf{T})$, and then select the maximum stem size. The derivation of the optimal $\mathbf{T}$ is defined as the following optimization problem

$$\text{maximize} : F(\mathbf{T}) = \iint_S f(\pm|C - \mathbf{Tx}|)dS, \quad (\mathbf{x} = [x, y, z])$$
$$\text{subject to} : \pm|C - \mathbf{Tx}| \geq 0, \forall \mathbf{x}$$
$$\mathbf{q}_0 - \mathbf{q}_r \leq \mathbf{q} \leq \mathbf{q}_0 + \mathbf{q}_r$$

where S describes the stem surface, and C describes the femoral canal. $\mathbf{x}$ is the coordinates of the stem surface point, and $\mathbf{Tx}$ is the coordinates of $\mathbf{x}$ when the position and orientation of the stem is $\mathbf{T}$. $\pm|C - \mathbf{Tx}|$ describes the shortest distance between the C and the $\mathbf{Tx}$, where negative values apply when the $\mathbf{Tx}$ is internal to the host bone. The first expression of the constraints describes the constraint of the prohibiting of the overlap for the whole stem area. $\mathbf{q}_0$ is the central position and rotation of the range of limitation, and the range of limitation is described as $\mathbf{q}_r$.

To define the function f, we divide the stem surface into three regions. The proximal region of surface is named as zone 1, and the distal region is named as zone 2 (Fig. 3)D Zone 1 is the specific area that the strong contact with the host bone is demanded. Both zone 1 and zone 2 are demanded not to be overlapped with the femoral canal. On the other hand, Other parts of stem surface are not evaluated. In objective function, the fitness value is maximized when the gap is smaller than the constant value, and if the gap is larger than the constant, the fitness value decreases according to the distance. The objective function is defined as (Fig. 4)

$$f(d) = \begin{cases} 1 & (0 \leq d < c_{th}) \\ -\exp\{-\frac{(d-c_{th})^2}{2\sigma^2}\} & (c_{th} \leq d) \end{cases}, \quad (d = \pm|C - \mathbf{Tx}|)$$

where c_{th} is the threshold of distance whose fitness value is maximized, and σ is the parameter of the Gaussian function which describes the decreasing of fitness if the distance is larger than c_{th}.

2.3 Definition of the Constraints

The positional and rotational constraints used in stem planning are the height of the stem position and the anteversion angle. The height of the stem position affects the difference of leg length between before and after the surgery. This change of the height should be small. The change of the height is defined as the difference between the height of the femoral head center and the height of the tip of the stem neck. Anteversion angle is the angle of the femoral neck against the body of femur. This angle affects the range of motion (ROM) of the hip joint After the surgery, femoral neck is removed, and replaced by the stem neck. Therefore, the anteversion angle after the surgery is redefined using the stem neck. This change of the angle should be minimum.

To define the constraints parameters q_0 and q_r, we refer the conventional study of the prediction of the height of the femoral head center and anteversion angle. In the prediction of the femoral head center, it is not appropriate to apply the sphere fitting to the deformed femoral head such as intended in our study. Therefore, we use the height of femoral neck saddle instead, and limit the range as 8.3 mm of the height difference from femoral neck saddle by referring the conventional study (Fig. 6)[11]. Anteversion angle is defined as the angle of of the femoral neck axis against the table top plane when the femur is put on ground (Fig. 5)[12], and we fix this angle during the automated planning.

In proposed method, the initial position q_0 is defined as whose height accords with that of stem neck, and whose anteversion angle accords with that before the surgery. In our definition of the coordinate axes, the height corresponds to the translation along the z axis, and anteversion angle corresponds to the rotation around the z axis. Using criteria of the range of limitation in each axis around q_0, q_r is defined as

$$q_r = [\infty,\ \infty,\ 8.3[mm],\ \infty,\ \infty,\ 0]^T$$

2.4 Optimization Procedure

The derivation of the candidate in each stem size is performed by the Powell method using initial values equally sampled within the possible solution space. We define the range of initial positions using q_0 as

$$q_0 - q_s \le q_I \le q_0 + q_s,\quad q_s = [P_t\ P_t\ P_t\ P_r\ P_r\ 0]^T$$

where q_I is the set of the initial positions, and P_t and P_r are the constant which describe the range of initial position. In proposed method, the $P_t = 8.0$ mm and $P_t = 4.0$ deg.. This range is inside the constraints, and we have already confirmed experimentally that this range includes the appropriate position and

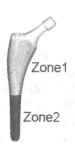

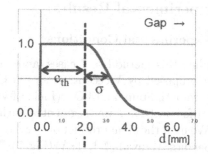

Fig. 3. Evaluation areas   **Fig. 4.** Definition of $f(d)$ of stem fitness

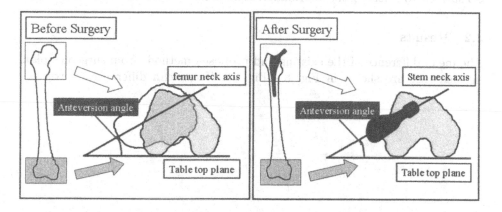

Fig. 5. ConstraintsFAgreement of "anteversion angle"

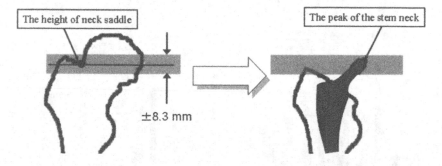

Fig. 6. ConstraintsFLimitation of height of femoral neck saddle and tip of stem neck

rotation enough. We define the sample rate of initial position as 4.0 mm and 4.0 deg. We have also experimented the sample rate of 1.0 mm and 1.0 deg., and 2.0 mm and 2.0 deg., and we have confirmed that there is few risk to failed to find the optimal solution in the sample rate of initial position of 4.0 mm and 4.0 deg.

3 Experimental Results

3.1 Experimental Conditions

We applied this method to 7 cases, and compared the results with the existing method proposed by Viceconti et al. [9]. CT slice thickness and reconstruction pitch were both 3mm, and FOV (Field of view) was 421 mm × 421 mm. The 3D model of femoral canal was segmented with a threshold of 800 Hounsfields Units (HU). We used the stem product of size 3 to 8 of Centpillar GB HA Stem (Stryker Orthopaedics, Mahwah, NJ, USA) (Fig. 7). The parameter tuning of evaluate function was $c_{th} = 2.0$ [mm]C $\sigma = 1.0$. The difference of the planning result was calculated from the experienced surgeon's plan, in position, rotation, and size selection. Surgeon's plan was planned using the complex system of the MPR images and the 3D surface, by referring the information of distance between the canal and stem.

3.2 Results

The mean difference of the existing and proposed methods from surgeon's plan in each case are shown in Fig. 8 - Fig. 10. The mean difference of existing

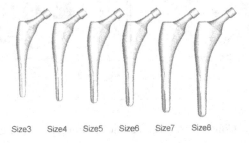

Size3   Size4   Size5   Size6   Size7   Size8

Fig. 7. Centpillar GB HA Stem (Size 3 ∼ 8)

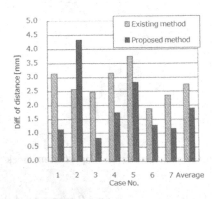

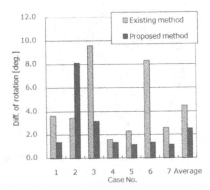

Fig. 8. Mean difference between existing methods and proposed method in each case (distance)

Fig. 9. Mean difference between existing methods and proposed method in each case (rotation)

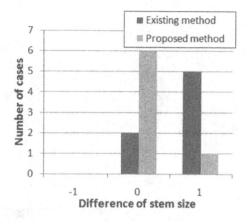

Fig. 10. Mean difference between existing methods and proposed method in each case (size selection)

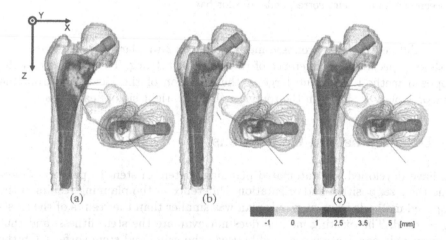

Fig. 11. Visualization of each planning results of case 3 ((a) existing method, (b) proposed method (c) surgeon planning). The color map on stem surface indicates distance between canal and stem, corresponds to color bar.

method in 7 cases of distance was 2.8 mm, rotation was 5.0 deg., and 2 cases are matched with surgeon's plan. On the other hand, the mean difference of proposed method of distance was 1.9 mm, rotation was 2.5 deg., and 5 cases are matched with surgeon's plan. The planning results of case 3 is shown in Fig. 11. The color map on the stem surface indicates the distance between the canal and stem, corresponds to the color bar in the bottom of the figure. In the result of existing method (a), there was some undesirable regions of the stem surface which distance is negative.

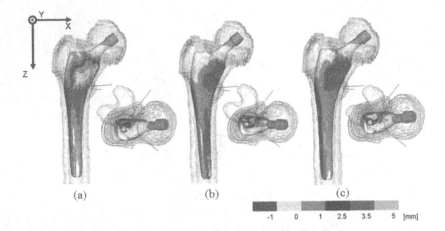

Fig. 12. Visualization of each planning results of case 2 ((a) existing method, (b) proposed method (c) surgeon planning). The color map on stem surface indicates distance between canal and stem, corresponds to color bar.

The difference of the proposed method in case 2 was larger than the existing method, especially the difference of rotation was 8.1 deg. The difference of the proposed method was quite large in the direction of the stem neck from the surgeon's plan as shown in the top view (Fig. 12, right side of each figure).

4   Discussions and Conclusions

We have developed the automated planning system of stem to properly determine the size, position and orientation. Difference of the planning results of the proposed methods from surgeon's plan was smaller than the results of the existing method. The existing method does not evaluate the stem fitness, and thus unacceptable penetration occurred between the canal and stem surface. On the other hand, the proposed method measures and optimizes the fitness and thus the system is able to determine the plan which is near to the experienced surgeon's one. And, in the size selection, difference of proposed method was smaller than the existing method. Because, the scaling factors of the femur shape which is used as criteria in size selection in existing method, does not completely correspond to the suitable size selection. On the other hand, the proposed method shows the higher performance in size selection.

However, the difference in rotation of the proposed method from surgeon's plan was quite large in case 2. From the visualization of the planning result, we found out that the difference of the anteversion angle was larger than the other axes. We consider that this result was caused by the failure of estimation of the anteversion angle which was not optimized by Powell method in the proposed method. This is the limitation of the current method.

As future work, we will add the learning function to this system, to learn the aspects of planning due to surgeon's trend or to automate the parameter tuning when the unknown stem model is given.

References

1. Sugano, N.: Computer-assisted orthopedic surgery. Journal of Orthopaedic Science 8(3), 442–448 (2003)
2. Bargar, W.L., Bauer, A., Borner, M.: Primary and revision total hip replacement using the Robodoc system. Clinical Orthopaedics & Related Research 354, 82–91 (1998)
3. Nishihara, S., Sugano, N., Nishii, T., Miki, H., Nakamura, N., Yoshikawa, H.: Comparison Between Hand Rasping and Robotic Milling for Stem Implantation in Cementless Total Hip Arthroplasty. The Journal of Arthroplasty 21(7), 957–966 (2006)
4. Laine, H.J., Puolakka, T.J.S., Moilanen, T., Pajamaki, K.J., Wirta, J., Lehto, M.U.K.: The effects of cementless femoral stem shape and proximal surface texture on fit-and-fill characteristics and on bone remodeling. International Orthopaedics 24(4), 184–190 (2000)
5. Nishihara, S., Sugano, N., Nishii, T., Tanaka, H., Yoshikawa, H., Ochi, A.: Comparison of the fit and fill between the Anatomic Hip femoral component and the VerSys Taper femoral component using virtual implantation on the ORTHODOC workstation. Journal of Orthopaedic Science 8(3), 352–360 (2003)
6. Howard, J.L., Hui, A.J., Bourne, R.B., McCalden, R.W., MacDonald, S.J., Rorabeck, C.H.: A quantitative analysis of bone support comparing cementless tapered and distal fixation total hip replacements. The Journal of Arthroplasty 19(3), 266–273 (2004)
7. Lattanzi, R., Viceconti, M., Zannoni, C., Quadrani, P., Toni, A.: Hip-Op: an innovative software to plan total hip replacement surgery. Medical Informatics and the Internet in Medicine 27(2), 71–83 (2002)
8. Nakamoto, M., Sato, Y., Sugano, N., Sasama, T., Nishii, T., Pak, P.S., Akazawa, K., Tada, Y., Yoshikawa, H., Tamura, S.: Automated CT-based 3D surgical planning for total hip replacement: a pilot study. International Congress Series, vol. 1256, pp. 389–394 (2003)
9. Otomaru, I., Takao, M., Nakamoto, M., Sugano, N., Kagiyama, Y., Sato, Y.: Automated Preoperative Planning System of Total Hip Arthroplasty Using Anatomical Femoral Components. In: 6th Annual Meeting of CAOS-International Proceedings, pp. 419–423 (2006)
10. Viceconti, M., Testi, D., Simeoni, M., Zannoni, C.: An automated method to position prosthetic components within multiple anatomical spaces. Computer Methods and Programs in Biomedicine 70(2), 121–127 (2003)
11. Sugano, N., Noble, P.C., Kamaric, E.: Predicting the Position of the Femoral Head Center. The Journal of Arthroplasty 14(1), 102–107 (1999)
12. Sugano, N., Noble, P.C., Kamaric, E.: A comparison of alternative methods of measuring femoral anteversion. Journal of Computer Assisted Tomography 22(4), 610–614 (1998)

Validation of Viscoelastic and Nonlinear Liver Model for Needle Insertion from in Vivo Experiments

Yo Kobayashi[1], Akinori Onishi[2], Takeharu Hoshi[2], Kazuya Kawamura[2], Makoto Hashizume[3], and Masakatsu G. Fujie[4]

[1] Consolidated Research Institute for Advanced Science and Medical Care, Waseda University, Japan, Tokyo, Shinjuku-ku, Ohkubo, 3-4-1
[2] Graduate School of Science and Engineering, Waseda University, Japan
[3] Center for the Integration of Advanced Medicine and Innovative Technology, Kyushu University Hospital
[4] Graduate School of Science and Engineering, Waseda University, and Faculty of Science and Engineering, Waseda University, Japan

Abstract. This paper shows the viscoelastic and nonlinear liver model for organ model based needle insertion, in which the deformation of an organ is estimated and predicted, and the needle trajectory is decided with organ deformation taken into consideration. An organ model including detailed material characteristics is important in order to achieve the proposed method. Firstly, the material properties of the liver are modeled from the measured data and its viscoelastic characteristics are represented by differential equations, including the term of the fractional derivative. Nonlinearity in terms of the stiffness was measured, and modeled using the quadratic function of strain. Next, a solution of an FE(Finite element) model using such material properties is shown. We use the sampling time scaling property as the solution for the viscoelastic system, while the solution for a nonlinear system using the Euler method and the Modified Newton-Raphson method is also shown. Finally, the deformation of liver model is calculated and pig liver of in vivo situation is obtained from medical ultrasound equipment. Comparing the relationship between needle displacement and force on real liver and liver model, we validate the proposed model.

Keywords: Needle insertion, Physical modeling, Liver, Robot surgery.

1 Introduction

As a cancer treatment method, percutaneous therapy is now a focus of attention. For instance, PEIT (Percutaneous Ethanol Injection Therapy) and RFA (Radio Frequency Ablation) are performed for liver cancer. Such treatment is a method to necrotize cancer cells existing inside the organ by delivering the needle tip to the cancer cells to either inject ethanol (PEIT) or ablate (RFA). Percutaneous therapy has become a major trend in liver cancer treatment with a feature of significantly minimally invasive but sufficient results.

Recently, robot assisted surgery systems have been developed under cooperation between domestic and international medicine and engineering as a measure to realize

T. Dohi, I. Sakuma, and H. Liao (Eds.): MIAR 2008, LNCS 5128, pp. 50–59, 2008.
© Springer-Verlag Berlin Heidelberg 2008

minimally invasive surgeries. Research on robotic systems to assist needle insertion also has been conducted with the purpose of improving of needle placement accuracy and expansion of approach path. The author and his team are carrying out research to develop robot assisted surgery systems based on the physical organ model as shown in Fig.1 [1]-[2].

Medical procedures such as PEIT and RFA require the insertion of a needle into a specific part of the diseased area. In all cases, the needle tip should be as close as possible to the center of target cancer. However, it is difficult to maneuver the needle toward the target cancer due to organ deformation. The needle insertion site, for example, in the case of the liver, is very soft, and it is easy for the force of the needle to deform the tissues, whereupon the position of the target cancer will be displaced due to organ deformation. Therefore, needle is required to be inserted, corresponding to the risk of cancer displacement. With this in mind, precise needle insertion is very difficult. Therefore, it is necessary to make a plan for insertion position and angle taking into account of organ deformation. For the above planning method, a simulation method in virtual surgery environment reproduced with physical models of organs may be used to predict and visualize the organ deformation.

1.1 Organ Modeling

Physical organ modeling has aroused considerable recent attention, with various pieces of research on this topic having been conducted by numerous researchers. Conventional research into the modeling of living bodies mainly concerns deformation analysis using a finite element method (FEM). These researches mainly target surgical simulation and training. For example, Alterovitz et al. have researched the simulation of needle insertion for prostate brach therapy [3].

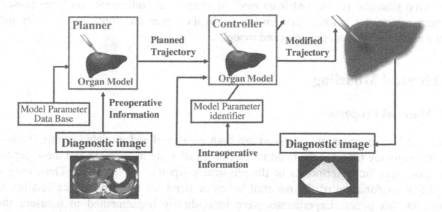

Fig. 1. Organ model based needle insertion system

Meanwhile, DiMaio et al. illustrate a system for measuring the extent of planar tissue phantom deformation during needle insertion, using a linear elastic material model [4].

The accurate organ model to estimate and visualize organ state occupies the key role of the proposed system. However, creating an accurate organ model remains a challenging problem due to the complexity of organ properties and is still the subject of much research. In general, tissue is inhomogeneous and exhibits nonlinear, anisotropic elastic and viscous behavior, meaning models are relatively complex. An accurate model of the target object, including its essential properties and proper features, is important because the model accuracy of the target object determines the performance of the planning system. In particular, the viscoelastic and nonlinear properties are important for precise needle insertion for the liver. The nonlinear properties affect the response of liver deformation when there is large deformation, while the viscoelastic properties affect the insertion velocity dependence of liver deformation. Thus, the liver model, including viscoelastic and nonlinear properties, is required for precise needle insertion.

1.2 Objectives

Detailed data on viscoelasticity and the nonlinearity of the organ have been presented in a few reports, while several reports also show the organ model based on detailed material properties such as viscoelasticity or nonlinearity. In previous work[1]-[2], we have been developed an physical liver model based on the detailed material properties of tissues, namely in terms of viscoelasticity and nonlinearity. The originality of this paper lies in the validation experiment of proposed model to compare the deformation of a pig liver of in vivo situation and the proposed liver model. The flow of this paper is listed as follows:

Chapter 2) Physical Modeling: the material properties of the liver considering the viscoelasticity and nonlinearity are modeled based on the measured data. The liver deformation model is developed based on the material properties.

Chapter 3) Simulation: the deformation of liver model is calculated and pig liver of in vivo situation is obtained from medical ultrasound equipment and force sensor. Comparing the relationship between needle displacement and force on real liver and liver model, we validate the proposed model.

2 Physical Modeling

2.1 Material Properties

The material properties of a pig liver are both measured and modeled in this section. We have already reported the material properties of a pig liver in [1] and these papers also gave specific descriptions of the physical properties of the liver. Thus, only a simplified explanation of the material behavior used for deformation calculation is shown in this paper. Experiments were individually implemented to measure the physical properties of the pig's interior liver using a rheometer (TA-Instrument: AR550). The shear modulus, shear stress and shear strain are then calculated based on these results.

1)Viscoelastic properties: A dynamic viscoelastic test was carried out to measure the frequency response of the liver. Sine-wave stress from 0.1 to 250 rad/s, providing 3 % strain amplitude, was loaded on the liver, while the mechanical impedance of the pig liver obtained from the result of a dynamic viscoelastic test is shown in Fig. 2. G^*

is a complex shear modulus, G' the storage elastic modulus, and G'' the loss elastic modulus. The needle is generally inserted into the organ at low velocity; hence the response is mainly affected by the low frequency characteristics. Thus, we use the viscoelastic model using the fractional derivative described in (1) which takes only low frequency characteristics into consideration.

$$ G\frac{d^k\gamma}{dt^k} = \tau \tag{1} $$

where t is time, τ is the shear stress, γ is the shear strain and G is the viscoelasticity, k is the order of derivative.

The derivative order k is approximately equal to 0.1 based on the slope of G' and G'' in Fig. 2.

2) Nonlinear properties (Strain dependence of elastic modulus): Nonlinear characteristics of liver as material are investigated based on the creep test, where the step response is measured. The steady state of the step response following sufficient elapsed time exhibits the low-frequency characteristics described in (1) and equation (1) becomes (2) if (1) is solved by the condition of the creep test.

$$ \gamma = \frac{\tau_c}{G\ \Gamma(1+k)} t^k = \gamma_c t^k \tag{2} $$

where τ_c is constant shear stress, γ_c is the coefficient deciding the strain value and $\Gamma()$ is the gamma function.

The creep test for each stress was carried out repeatedly while the viscoelasticity G and strain ε_c for each stress are calculated using (2). Fig. 3 shows the viscoelasticity G - strain γ_c diagram from these results. A liver with a low strain of less than about 0.35 displays linear characteristics, and a viscoelasticity G at a constant 400 Pa. A liver with a high strain of more than about 0.35 displays nonlinear characteristics and an increased degree of viscoelasticity. Then, strain dependence is modeled using the quadratic function of strain shown by (3):

$$ G(\gamma) = \begin{cases} G_o & (\gamma < \gamma_0) \\ G_0(1 + a_\gamma(\gamma - \gamma_0)^2) & (\gamma > \gamma_0) \end{cases} \tag{3} $$

where G_o is the viscoelastic modulus of linear part, γ_0 is the strain in which the characteristics of liver change to show nonlinearity and a_γ is the coefficient deciding the change of stiffness.

3) Shear stress-strain relationship: The material properties of the liver are modeled using (4) from the discussion in 1) and 2).

$$ G(\gamma)\frac{d^k\gamma}{dt^k} = \tau \tag{4} $$

4) Stress-strain relationship: In general, elastic modulus E is used to construct the deformation model. The relation between elastic modulus E and the shear modulus G is calculated using Poisson's ratio v as in the following equation:

$$ E = 2(1+v)G \tag{5} $$

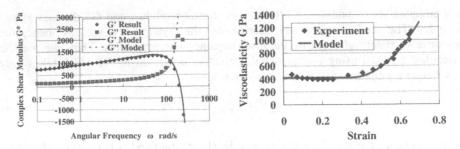

Fig. 2. Mechanical impedance of the liver [1]   **Fig. 3.** Strain dependence of G [1]

In the experiment of rheometer, only shear modulus is loaded on the test material. However, the stress state is more complex in the situation of deformation simulation. We assume that the nonlinearity of elastic modulus is decided by the relative strain calculated in (6).

$$\varepsilon_r = \sqrt{\frac{1}{2}\left\{(\varepsilon_1 - \varepsilon_2)^2 + (\varepsilon_2 - \varepsilon_3)^2 + (\varepsilon_3 - \varepsilon_1)^2\right\}} \tag{6}$$

where ε_1, ε_2, ε_3 is the principal strain.

Thus, the material properties using organ model is described in (7) - (8) from these consideration.

$$E(\varepsilon_r)\frac{d^k \varepsilon}{dt^k} = \sigma \tag{7}$$

$$E(\varepsilon) = \begin{cases} E_o & (\varepsilon < \varepsilon_0) \\ E_0(1 + a_\varepsilon(\varepsilon_r - \varepsilon_0)^2) & (\varepsilon > \varepsilon_0) \end{cases} \tag{8}$$

where σ is the stress vector, ε is the strain vector.

2.2 FEM Based Modeling

This section shows the solution to the FEM model using the material properties described in section 2.1. We have already reported the solution to the FEM model in [2] and these papers also gave specific descriptions. Thus, only a simplified explanation for the solution is shown in this paper.

The expression between the displacements at all the nodal points and all the applied loads is written in (9)-(11) from the result of (8).

$$K(U)D^{(k)}U = F \tag{9}$$

where

$$K(U) = \sum_{all\ element} k(\varepsilon_r) \tag{10}$$

$$k(\varepsilon_r) = \begin{cases} k_0 & (\varepsilon_r < \varepsilon_0) \\ k_0(1 + a_\varepsilon(\varepsilon_r - \varepsilon_0)^2)(\varepsilon_r > \varepsilon_0) \end{cases} \qquad (11)$$

where k is the nonlinear element stiffness matrix, k_0 is the element stiffness matrix when the liver tissue shows linear characteristics, a_ε is the coefficient deciding the change of stiffness and ε_r is the relative strain.

In the following sentence, firstly, the solution for viscoelastic system is shown in 1), followed by the solution for the nonlinear system, which is described in 2). Finally, the solution for (9) is shown from both discussions 1) and 2).

1) Solution for the viscoelasticitc system: The analysis can be considerably simplified when the following conditions are fulfilled [5]:
- The derivative operator of (9) is a common factor in all element stiffness.
- Only the external loads influence the stresses.
Then, equation (12) is derived from (9).

$$K(U)U = F' \quad (F' = D^{(-k)}F) \qquad (12)$$

where $D^{(-k)}$ means the kth-order integration.

Equation (12) is identical to the elastic problem when the virtual external force vector F' is used. The fractional calculation (12) for each component of the external force vector F is implemented in order to obtain the virtual external force vector F'. We use the sampling time scaling property introduced in [6] to realize a discrete fractional calculation.

2) Nonlinear system: Incremental approaches are important to obtain the significant answer because the answer is not unique for many nonlinear situations. The incremental form of discretized nonlinear model is generally is written by (13).

$$K_r(U_n)\Delta U_n = \Delta F_n \qquad (13)$$

where K_t is the tangential stiffness matrix, ΔU_n is an increment of the overall displacement vector and ΔF_n is an increment of the overall external force.

The tangential matrix K_t is described by (14) from equation (11) .

$$K_t(U) = \sum_{all\ element} k_t(\varepsilon_r) \qquad (14)$$

$$k_t(\varepsilon_r) = \begin{cases} k_0 & (\varepsilon_r < \varepsilon_0) \\ [1 + a_\varepsilon(\varepsilon_r - \varepsilon_0)^2 + 2a_\varepsilon(\varepsilon_r - \varepsilon_0)\varepsilon_r]k_0 & (\varepsilon_r > \varepsilon_0) \end{cases} \qquad (15)$$

where k_t is the tangential element stiffness matrix, k_0 is the element stiffness matrix when the liver tissue shows linear characteristics.

We use both Euler method and Modified Newton-Raphson method to solve the nonlinear system.

3) Calculation process: Based on these discussions, the solution for the system (9) is described as follows: Firstly, the virtual external force F' is calculated, then the incremental of F' ($\Delta F'$) is computed. The solution to the nonlinear system described in 2) is then carried out using $\Delta F'$.

$$K(U_n)\Delta U_n = \Delta F_n' \qquad (16)$$

3 Simulation

3.1 Methods

The deformation of liver model is calculated and pig liver of in vivo situation is obtained from medical ultrasound equipment and force sensor. Comparing the relationship between needle displacement and force on real liver and liver model, we validate the proposed model.

1) In vivo experiment: The needle was inserted into a pig liver at a constant speed of 5 [mm/s] using needle insertion manipulator with a medical ultrasound equipment (Fig.4). Inferior vena cava in the liver is set to be the virtual target of this experiment. Then, the needle displacement and force during needle insertion was collected and ultrasound image was captured.

2) Analysis using liver model: Fig.5 shows the shape of the liver model and the mesh used for this simulation. In order to create the shape of the liver model, the images of liver sections of human (horizontal plane) taken with X-ray CT, those several outlines were manually extracted. Using Delaunay method with extracted outline data, mesh was created. In Fig.5, green colored nodes are set as fixed ends taking into consideration of restriction from ribs and spine existing at dorsal aspect of the abdomen. A red node in Fig.5 is defined as the target position. The actual liver is non-uniform tissue including cirrhosis and cancer cells. However, as the first step in this study, the liver shall be assessed as though it is uniform. The stiffness parameters such as E_o, ε_0 and a_ε of normal tissue part is set manually to fit the measured data.

The needle is assumed to be inserted at a constant speed of 5 [mm/s]. The time-series data of needle displacement and displace of virtual target was collected during numerical experiment.

3.2 Results and Discussions

Figure 6 shows the relationship between needle displacement and force of real liver and liver model. Figure 6 show the data on in vivo liver also displays the nonlinear relationship of needle displacement and force. As shown in previous work[7], the main puncture event is designated by a peak in force after a steady rise, followed by a sharp decrease. This data explains that when the needle puncture the liver it does not cut the tissue with a certain force, instead 1) it pushes the tissue and then 2) the tissue is punctured instantaneously.

The liver model proposed in this paper reproduces the relationship between needle displacement and force of in vivo liver with high accuracy. The liver model proposed in this paper is suggested to reproduce *in vivo* situation from these discussion.

Figure 7 shows the ultrasound image captured during in vivo experiment and the deformation of liver model. In Fig.7, the color of each element implies the stress. The liver model estimate and visualize the deformation and stress state of in vivo liver.

This validation using this liver model is not rigorous because the real shape of pig liver is not same as the human one to create the liver model and boundary condition is

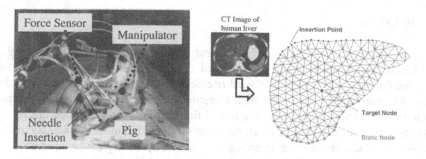

Fig. 4. Experimental setup of in vivo experiment   **Fig. 5.** Physical model of the liver

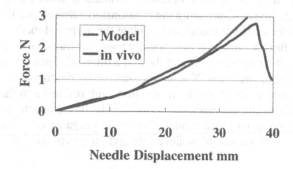

Fig. 6. Relationship between needle displacement and force: in vivo experiment

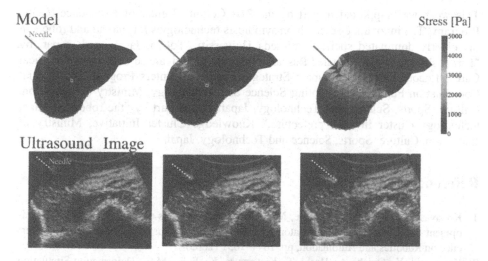

Fig. 7. Comparison of model deformation with the ultrasound image

more complex as a matter of course. Then, the deformation analysis of liver model with real shape of pig liver and complex boundary condition should be carried out in future work for the more detailed evaluation.

4 Conclusion

This paper shows a viscoelastic and nonlinear liver deformation model for organ model based needle insertion and validation of the proposed model was carried out. Firstly, the concept of organ model based needle insertion for needle insertion is described, whereupon the importance of the organ model, including detailed material characteristics, is shown. Secondly, we model the detailed material properties of the liver based on the measured data. Next, the solution of the FE model using such material properties is shown. We use sampling time scaling property as the solution for a viscoelastic system and the Euler method and Modified Newton-Raphson method is used as a solution to the nonlinear system. Finally, the deformation of liver model is calculated and pig liver of in vivo situation is obtained from medical ultrasound equipment and force sensor. Comparing the relationship between needle displacement and force on real liver and liver model, we validate the proposed model.

In future work, further precise organ modeling will be carried out. For example, a 3D organ model will be constructed, and the acquisition of organ geometries will be researched for actual applications. The model parameter identification method using intra-operative information will also be researched, with reference to the ambiguity of the model parameter, while the method of organ model based needle insertion will be realized using a constructed organ model. Finally, the organ model based needle insertion system will be developed to achieve safe and precise treatment.

Acknowledgement

This work was supported in part by the 21st Century Center of Excellence (COE) Program "The innovative research on symbiosis technologies for human and robots in the elderly dominated society", Waseda University, Tokyo, Japan ,and in part by "Establishment of Consolidated Research Institute for Advanced Science and Medical Care", Encouraging Development Strategic Research Centers Program, the Special Coordination Funds for Promoting Science and Technology, Ministry of Education, Culture, Sports, Science and Technology, Japan and in part by "the robotic medical technology cluster in Gifu prefecture," Knowledge Cluster Initiative, Ministry of Education, Culture, Sports, Science and Technology, Japan.

References

1. Kobayashi, Y., Okamoto, J., Fujie, M.G.: Physical Properties of the Liver and the Development of an Intelligent Manipulator for Needle Insertion. In: IEEE International Conference on Robotics and Automation, pp. 1644–1651 (2005)
2. Kobayashi, Y., Onishi, A., Hoshi, T., Kawamura, K., Fujie, M.G.: Deformation Simulation using a Viscoelastic and Nonlinear Organ Model for Control of a Needle Insertion Manipulator. In: 2007 IEEE International Conference on Intelligent Robotics and Systems, pp. 1801–1808 (2007)
3. Alterovitz, R., Lim, A., Goldberg, K., Chirikjian, G.S., Okamura, A.M.: Steering Flexible Needles under Markov Motion Uncertainty. In: International Conference on Intelligent Robots and Systems, pp. 120–125 (2005)

4. DiMaio, S.P., Salcudean, S.E.: Interactive Simulation of Needle Insertion Model. IEEE Transaction on Biomedical Engineering 52(7), 1167–1179 (2005)
5. Zienkiewicz, O.C., Cheung, Y.K.: The Finite Element Method in Structural and Continuum Mechanics (1967)
6. Ma, C., Hori, Y.: The Application of Fractional Order Control to Backlash Vibration Suppression. In: Proceedings of American Control Conference, pp. 2901–2906 (2004)
7. Okamura, A.M., Simone, C., O'Leary, M.D.: Force modeling for needle insertion into soft tissue. IEEE Transaction on Biomedical Engineering 51(10), 1707–1716 (2004)

Simulation of Active
Cardiac Electromechanical Dynamics

Ken C.L. Wong[1], Linwei Wang[1], Heye Zhang[2], Huafeng Liu[3],
and Pengcheng Shi[1]

[1] B. Thomas Golisano College of Computing and Information Sciences,
Rochester Institute of Technology, Rochester, New York, USA
{kenclwong, maomaowlw}@mail.rit.edu, pengcheng.shi@rit.edu
[2] Bioengineering Institute, University of Auckland, New Zealand
heye.zhang@auckland.ac.nz
[3] State Key Laboratory of Modern Optical Instrumentation,
Zhejiang University, Hanzhou, China
liuhf@zju.edu.cn

Abstract. While finite element methods have been extensively used
for computational cardiology, the complicated and computationally expensive meshing procedures largely increase the difficulties of improving
numerical accuracy. Furthermore, as the complexity of the element structure increases with the order of polynomial can be handled, the finite element procedures are either simple but numerically inaccurate or accurate
but labor intensive. In view of these problems, we adopt the meshfree
methods for computational cardiology. Using the meshfree methods, the
heart is represented by a set of nodes distributed in the myocardium
without any mesh, thus spatial refinements only involve distribution of
extra nodes to the area of interest. Furthermore, as the order of polynomial is not limited by elements, it can be increased with relatively ease.
These are desirable features as they provide the flexibility for improving
numerical accuracies. In this paper, the simulation of the cardiac electromechanical dynamics using the meshfree methods will be introduced.
Experiments have been done on a cubical object to provide an insight
into the electromechanical dynamics, and also on a canine heart model
to show the physiological plausibility of the simulation.

1 Introduction

Study on cardiac physiology shows that at the beginning of each cardiac cycle,
pacemaker cells in the heart generate action potentials which are conducted to
the whole heart through the conduction fibers spreading throughout the myocardium [1]. The myocardial contractile cells are then excited by the action
potentials and contract according to the sequence of excitations, and the heart
beats in a rhythmic motion. Thus, in order to properly model the cyclic dynamics of the heart, the cardiac electric wave propagation model (E model) that
describes the spatiotemporal propagation pattern of the action potentials [2],

T. Dohi, I. Sakuma, and H. Liao (Eds.): MIAR 2008, LNCS 5128, pp. 60–69, 2008.
© Springer-Verlag Berlin Heidelberg 2008

the electromechanical coupling model (EM model) which transforms the excitation into myocardium contractile stresses [3], and the biomechanical model (BM model) which captures the deformation caused by the contractile stresses through the system dynamics [4] are all required. Since the integration of these three models gives a more complete macroscopic description of the physiological behavior of the heart, it is called the *cardiac physiome model* [5]. Several experiments have been done on the simulations of the heart cycle using the cardiac physiome model and validated through different criteria [3,6], this shows that the cardiac physiome model provides a very useful tool for analyzing cardiac physiology and pathology.

In order to solve the formulations of the cardiac physiome model which do not have closed form solutions, the continuous space of the heart has to be discretized so that numerical methods can be applied. In computational cardiology, the finite element methods (FEM) have been extensively used. In [6], tetrahedral elements are used, for which the meshing algorithm is relatively simple, and the procedures of assembling the system matrices are also computationally efficient. Nevertheless, as tetrahedral elements are usually associated with linear interpolation, strains approximated are constant within an element and thus a relatively large number of elements are required to achieve numerically accurate results. In [3], high order elements are used with spherical polar coordinate system which provides good accuracy for approximating different cardiac quantities. Nevertheless, the complicated meshing procedures cannot be done automatically, thus mesh refinements for improving numerical accuracy can be very labor-intensive. In consequence, it is hard to make a balance between numerical accuracy and algorithmic complexity with the finite element methods.

In view of these problem, we adopt the meshfree methods for computational cardiology [7]. Using the meshfree methods, the heart is represented by a set of nodes bounded by surfaces representing the heart boundaries. As no meshing is involved, the distribution of the nodes is more flexible, and thus facilitates adaptive refinements to improve regional numerical accuracy. Furthermore, its intrinsic *hp*-adaptivity makes it relatively easy to incorporate high order polynomials. In this paper, a meshfree method based on moving least squares (MLS) will be described, followed by the cardiac physiome model and its matrix representation. Experiments have been done on a cubical object and a canine heart model to show the physiological plausibility of the simulation.

2 Methodology

In this section, the meshfree method based on moving least squares will be introduced, followed by the cardiac physiome model and its matrix representation based on the meshfree method.

2.1 Meshfree Methods

In the computational environment, the heart is represented by a set of nodes distributed in the myocardium bounded by surfaces representing the epicardium

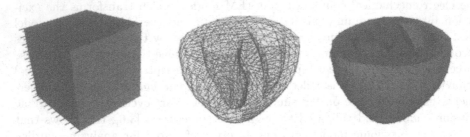

Fig. 1. Meshfree representations. Left: a cubical object with nodes (red) and fibers (blue) pointing along the z-axis. Middle: a set of nodes distributed in the myocardium bounded by surfaces of the heart boundaries. Right: fiber orientations of the canine heart model.

and the endocardia (Fig. 1). Thus simulating the deformation of the heart is equivalent to solving the governing cardiac system dynamics for the nodal displacements. In order to approximate the continuous cardiac system dynamics from the node set, the spatial relations between these nodes must be defined. For FEM, such relations are provided by the elements, and all nodes of an element are responsible for the approximation of the value of any point within that element. As there is no element for the meshfree methods, the nodal relations are provided through a different way.

For the meshfree methods, every node has an influence domain specifying the spatial region that it can influence [7]. The values of any point in the myocardium are approximated by the nodes which influence domains covering this point. Thus, the influence domains of all nodes together have to cover the whole myocardium, so that the values of any point can be approximated. The shapes of the influence domains can be spherical, rectangular, or any arbitrary shape. FEM is actually a special case of the meshfree methods which has the influence domains defined by the elements. For simplicity, we use the spherical shape influence domain. In this case, the radius of the influence domain of every node is determined by searching for enough other nodes to be covered, which is equivalent to ensuring every point in the myocardium can be approximated.

In order to approximate the values of any point from the nodes, the moving least squares method is being used because of its compatibility and consistency. Compatibility means the approximated field is smooth and continuous, and consistency means the approximated field can exactly represent the polynomial with desired order.

Let $u(\mathbf{x})$ be the value of a point we want to approximate at coordinate $\mathbf{x}$, and u_I be the value of node I located at $\mathbf{x}_I$. $u(\mathbf{x})$ can be approximated as:

$$u(\mathbf{x}) = \sum_{j=1}^{m} p_j(\mathbf{x}) a_j(\mathbf{x}) \equiv \mathbf{p}^T(\mathbf{x}) \mathbf{a}(\mathbf{x}) \tag{1}$$

where $p_j(\mathbf{x})$ are the monomial basis functions, m is the number of bases, and $a_j(\mathbf{x})$ are the unknown coefficients. $p_j(\mathbf{x})$ are the bases of the polynomial we want to exactly represent. In our case, we use the simple linear bases:

$$\mathbf{p}^T(\mathbf{x}) = [1 \; x \; y \; z] \tag{2}$$

where x, y and z are the cartesian coordinates. By minimizing the weighted, discrete L_2 norm:

$$J = \sum_{I=1}^{n} w(\mathbf{x} - \mathbf{x}_I)[\mathbf{p}^T(\mathbf{x}_I)\mathbf{a}(\mathbf{x}) - u_I]^2 \tag{3}$$

where n is the number of nodes, and $w(\mathbf{x} - \mathbf{x}_I)$ is the weight function, we have $\mathbf{a}(\mathbf{x}) = \mathbf{A}^{-1}(\mathbf{x})\sum_{I=1}^{n}\mathbf{B}_I(\mathbf{x})u_I$, and thus:

$$u(\mathbf{x}) = \sum_{I=1}^{n}(\mathbf{p}^T(\mathbf{x})\mathbf{A}^{-1}(\mathbf{x})\mathbf{B}_I(\mathbf{x}))u_I \equiv \sum_{I=1}^{n}\phi_I(\mathbf{x})u_I \tag{4}$$

where

$$\mathbf{A}(\mathbf{x}) = \sum_{I=1}^{n}w_I(\mathbf{x})\mathbf{p}(\mathbf{x}_I)\mathbf{p}^T(\mathbf{x}_I); \quad \mathbf{B}_I(\mathbf{x}) = w_I(\mathbf{x})\mathbf{p}(\mathbf{x}_I); \quad w_I(\mathbf{x}) \equiv w(\mathbf{x} - \mathbf{x}_I)$$

and ϕ_I is called the shape function of node I. The weight function $w_I(\mathbf{x})$ can be given as:

$$w(r) = \begin{cases} \frac{2}{3} - 4r^2 + 4r^3, & \text{for } r \leq \frac{1}{2} \\ \frac{4}{3} - 4r + 4r^2 - \frac{4}{3}r^3, & \text{for } \frac{1}{2} < r \leq 1 \\ 0, & \text{for } r > 1 \end{cases} \tag{5}$$

with $r = \|\mathbf{x} - \mathbf{x_I}\|/d_I$, the distance between $\mathbf{x}$ and $\mathbf{x_I}$ normalized by the size of the influence domain d_I.

From the above equations, we can see that MLS possesses good hp-adaptivity. h stands for the size of the influence domain and p stands for the order of polynomial. If we want to increase the numerical accuracy of a particular region, we simply distribute extra nodes to it with respective size reductions of the related influence domains, which only involves a simple node searching procedure. If we want to increase the order of the polynomial, which means to increase the number of bases of $\mathbf{p}(\mathbf{x})$, what we have to do is to increase the sizes of the influence domains so that $\mathbf{A}(\mathbf{x})$ is invertible. In contrast, for the case of FEM, the change of numerical accuracy requires re-meshing, and the change of the order of polynomial even leads to the change of the element type, both involve complicated algorithms which usually cannot be done automatically.

2.2   Cardiac Physiome Model

The cardiac physiome model comprises the electric wave propagation model, the electromechanical coupling model, and also the biomechanical model. These three models are connected together through the cardiac system dynamics.

Electric Wave Propagation Model. After leaving the Purkinje fibers, the action potentials propagate throughout the myocardium through the myocytes. To model the electric wave propagation in the myocardium, a simplified reaction system based on FitzHugh-Nagumo model has been chosen [8]. It is able to reproduce the basic excitation propagation pattern through:

$$\frac{\partial u}{\partial t} = \nabla \cdot (D \nabla u) + c_1 u(u-a)(1-u) - c_2 uv;$$
$$\frac{\partial v}{\partial t} = b(u-dv) \tag{6}$$

where u is the transmembrane potential, v is the recovery variable, D is the diffusion tensor, and a, b, c_1, c_2 and d are parameters that define the shape of the action potential. These parameters are constant in time but not necessary in space. Using the meshfree method, (6) can be converted into a matrix equation as described in detail in [9], which can then be solved for the nodal values of the action potentials u.

Electromechanical Coupling Model. When a myocyte is excited by the action potential, it generates the active force for the contraction of the heart through *electromechanical coupling*. Although realistic complex models are available [4,3], because of the computational efficiency, a simple ordinary differential equation (ODE) proposed in [6] is used as our electromechanical coupling model:

$$\frac{\partial \sigma_c}{\partial t} + \sigma_c = u\sigma_0 \tag{7}$$

where σ_c is a scalar related to the stress tensor, and σ_0 is a constant for scaling the stress. With (7), the action potential can be converted to σ_c. And then the contraction Cauchy stress tensor can be obtained by:

$$\sigma = -\sigma_c f \otimes f \tag{8}$$

with f the fiber orientation vector under the current configuration of the heart geometry, and $\otimes$ the tensor product. The minus sign is necessary as σ_c is always positive while a *contraction* stress tensor is required. In the implementation, as (7) is not related to spatial derivative, σ_c of a node can be calculated using only the action potential on the same node. As the nodal fiber orientations are provided, σ on every node can be calculated, and thus the Cauchy stress tensor at very point can be approximated using the meshfree shape functions. With the stress tensor available, the active body and surface forces can be calculated as:

$$R_{body} = J\text{div}(\sigma_c f \otimes f); \quad R_{surface} = J\sigma(\mathbf{F}^{-1})^T \mathbf{N} \tag{9}$$

with $\mathbf{F}$ the deformation gradient matrix, $J = \det(\mathbf{F})$, and $\mathbf{N}$ the outward normal of the heart surface.

Biomechanical Model. The biomechanical model characterizes the material properties of the myocardium, which relates the active forces generated by the EM model with the resulted deformation of the myocardium through the cardiac system dynamics. Assuming the myocardium is elastic, the stress-strain relation obeys the Hooke's Law [10]:

$$\mathbf{S} = C\epsilon, \tag{10}$$

where $\mathbf{S}$ the second Piola-Kirchhoff stress tensor and ϵ the Green-Lagrangian strain tensor. C is the stiffness matrix containing the material properties. Let C_o be the 3D stiffness matrix of a point in the myocardium under the local fiber coordinate system, it is defined as:

$$C_o = \begin{bmatrix} \frac{1}{E_f} & -\frac{\nu_f}{E_{cf}} & -\frac{\nu_f}{E_{cf}} & 0 & 0 & 0 \\ -\frac{\nu_f}{E_{cf}} & \frac{1}{E_{cf}} & -\frac{\nu_{cf}}{E_{cf}} & 0 & 0 & 0 \\ -\frac{\nu_f}{E_{cf}} & -\frac{\nu_{cf}}{E_{cf}} & \frac{1}{E_{cf}} & 0 & 0 & 0 \\ 0 & 0 & 0 & \frac{1}{G} & 0 & 0 \\ 0 & 0 & 0 & 0 & \frac{1}{G} & 0 \\ 0 & 0 & 0 & 0 & 0 & \frac{2(1+\nu_{cf})}{E_{cf}} \end{bmatrix}^{-1}$$

where E_f, E_{cf}, ν_f, ν_{cf} are the Young's moduli and Poisson's ratios along and cross the fiber respectively, $G \approx E_f/(2(1+\nu_f))$ describes the shearing property.

With C_o defined, the stiffness matrix at any point with known fiber orientation can be obtained using the tensor transformation:

$$C = T^{-1}C_oRTR^{-1} \tag{11}$$

where T is a tensor transformation matrix related to the fiber orientation, and R is a diagonal matrix responsible for the transformation between the strain tensor components and the engineering strain tensor components [11]. During implementation, the fiber orientation at a point is approximated by the nodal fiber orientations using the shape functions.

Cardiac System Dynamics. The cardiac system dynamics acts as a central link between the E, EM and BM models. The active forces provided by the E and EM models can be related to the strains through the BM model, which can then be further related to the cardiac kinematics. The total-Lagrangian formulation is chosen to be the cardiac system dynamics, which matrix representation is [10]:

$$\mathbf{M\ddot{U}} + \mathbf{C\dot{U}} + (\mathbf{K}_L + \mathbf{K}_{NL})\Delta\mathbf{U} = \mathbf{R}_c - \mathbf{R}_i \tag{12}$$

with $\Delta\mathbf{U}$, $\dot{\mathbf{U}}$, and $\ddot{\mathbf{U}}$ the nodal incremental displacement, velocity and acceleration vectors. The matrices $\mathbf{M}$, $\mathbf{C}$, $\mathbf{K}_L$ and $\mathbf{K}_{NL}$ are derived using the nodal approximations with the meshfree method. $\mathbf{M}$ is the mass matrix:

$$\mathbf{M} = \int_V \rho\Phi^T\Phi \, dV \tag{13}$$

where

$$\Phi = \begin{bmatrix} \phi_1 & 0 & 0 & \dots & \phi_n & 0 & 0 \\ 0 & \phi_1 & 0 & \dots & 0 & \phi_n & 0 \\ 0 & 0 & \phi_1 & \dots & 0 & 0 & \phi_n \end{bmatrix} \tag{14}$$

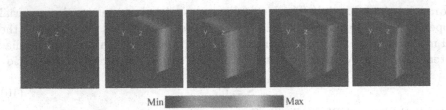

Min [gradient bar] Max

Fig. 2. Cubical object. Normalized active contraction stress propagation computed from simulated action potentials, shown together with the deformations. The action potentials were initiated from the fixed face normal to the z-axis, and propagate along the fibers. Left to right: 0 ms, 100 ms, 200 ms, 300 ms, and 400 ms.

and ρ is the density of the myocardium. $\mathbf{K}_L$ and $\mathbf{K}_{NL}$ are the stiffness matrices comprising the BM model:

$$\mathbf{K}_L = \int_V \mathbf{B}_L^T\, C\, \mathbf{B}_L\; \mathrm{d}V; \quad \mathbf{K}_{NL} = \int_V \mathbf{B}_{NL}^T\, \mathbf{S}\, \mathbf{B}_{NL}\; \mathrm{d}V \tag{15}$$

C is the matrix of Rayleigh damping:

$$C = \alpha \mathbf{M} + \beta(\mathbf{K}_L + \mathbf{K}_{NL}) \tag{16}$$

with α and β controlling the low and high frequency damping respectively. $\mathbf{R}_c$ contains the active contraction force while $\mathbf{R}_i$ contains the current internal stress:

$$\mathbf{R}_c = \int_V \boldsymbol{\Phi}^T R_{body}\; \mathrm{d}V + \int_S \boldsymbol{\Phi}^T R_{surface}\; \mathrm{d}S; \tag{17}$$

$$\mathbf{R}_i = \int_V \mathbf{B}_L^T\, \hat{\mathbf{S}}\; \mathrm{d}V \tag{18}$$

with V and S the volume and surface of the heart, and

$$\mathbf{B}_L = \mathbf{B}_{L0} + \mathbf{B}_{L1} = [\mathbf{B}_{L01} \ldots \mathbf{B}_{L0n}] + [\mathbf{B}_{L11} \ldots \mathbf{B}_{L1n}];$$

$$\mathbf{B}_{L0I} = \begin{bmatrix} \phi_{I,x} & 0 & 0 \\ 0 & \phi_{I,y} & 0 \\ 0 & 0 & \phi_{I,z} \\ \phi_{I,y} & \phi_{I,x} & 0 \\ \phi_{I,z} & 0 & \phi_{I,x} \\ 0 & \phi_{I,z} & \phi_{I,y} \end{bmatrix};$$

$$\mathbf{B}_{L1I} = \begin{bmatrix} l_{xx}\,\phi_{I,x} & l_{yx}\,\phi_{I,x} & l_{zx}\,\phi_{I,x} \\ l_{xy}\,\phi_{I,y} & l_{yy}\,\phi_{I,y} & l_{zy}\,\phi_{I,y} \\ l_{xz}\,\phi_{I,z} & l_{yz}\,\phi_{I,z} & l_{zz}\,\phi_{I,z} \\ (l_{xx}\,\phi_{I,y} + l_{xy}\,\phi_{I,x}) & (l_{yx}\,\phi_{I,y} + l_{yy}\,\phi_{I,x}) & (l_{zx}\,\phi_{I,y} + l_{zy}\,\phi_{I,x}) \\ (l_{xx}\,\phi_{I,z} + l_{xz}\,\phi_{I,x}) & (l_{yx}\,\phi_{I,z} + l_{yz}\,\phi_{I,x}) & (l_{zx}\,\phi_{I,z} + l_{zz}\,\phi_{I,x}) \\ (l_{xy}\,\phi_{I,z} + l_{xz}\,\phi_{I,y}) & (l_{yy}\,\phi_{I,z} + l_{yz}\,\phi_{I,y}) & (l_{zy}\,\phi_{I,z} + l_{zz}\,\phi_{I,y}) \end{bmatrix};$$

$$\mathbf{B}_{NL} = \begin{bmatrix} \tilde{\mathbf{B}}_{NL} & \tilde{\mathbf{0}} & \tilde{\mathbf{0}} \\ \tilde{\mathbf{0}} & \tilde{\mathbf{B}}_{NL} & \tilde{\mathbf{0}} \\ \tilde{\mathbf{0}} & \tilde{\mathbf{0}} & \tilde{\mathbf{B}}_{NL} \end{bmatrix}; \quad \tilde{\mathbf{B}}_{NL} = \begin{bmatrix} \phi_{1,x} & 0 & 0 & \phi_{2,x} & \cdots & \phi_{n,x} \\ \phi_{1,y} & 0 & 0 & \phi_{2,y} & \cdots & \phi_{n,y} \\ \phi_{1,z} & 0 & 0 & \phi_{2,z} & \cdots & \phi_{n,z} \end{bmatrix}; \quad \tilde{\mathbf{0}} = \begin{bmatrix} 0 \\ 0 \\ 0 \end{bmatrix};$$

$$\mathbf{S} = \begin{bmatrix} \tilde{\mathbf{S}} & \bar{\mathbf{0}} & \bar{\mathbf{0}} \\ \bar{\mathbf{0}} & \tilde{\mathbf{S}} & \bar{\mathbf{0}} \\ \bar{\mathbf{0}} & \bar{\mathbf{0}} & \tilde{\mathbf{S}} \end{bmatrix}; \quad \tilde{\mathbf{S}} = \begin{bmatrix} S_{xx} & S_{xy} & S_{xz} \\ S_{yx} & S_{yy} & S_{yz} \\ S_{zx} & S_{zy} & S_{zz} \end{bmatrix}; \quad \bar{\mathbf{0}} = \begin{bmatrix} 0 & 0 & 0 \\ 0 & 0 & 0 \\ 0 & 0 & 0 \end{bmatrix};$$

$$\hat{\mathbf{S}}^T = \begin{bmatrix} S_{xx} & S_{yy} & S_{zz} & S_{xy} & S_{xz} & S_{yz} \end{bmatrix}$$

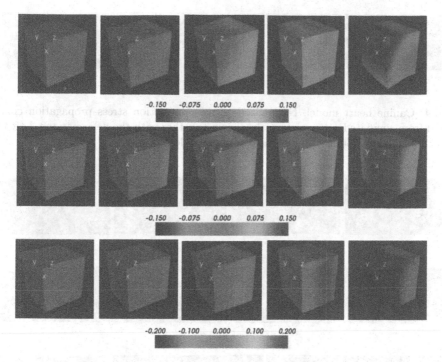

Fig. 3. Cubical object. Strain maps of the simulated deformations, with positive and negative values indicating extensions and contractions respectively. Top to bottom: normal strains along the x, y and z axes. Left to right: 0 ms, 100 ms, 200 ms, 300 ms, and 400 ms.

where $\phi_{I,j} = \partial\phi_I/\partial j$ and $l_{ij} = \sum_{I=1}^{n} \phi_{I,j} \, u_{iI}$, with u_{iI} the i-component of the nodal displacement of node I. In consequence, with the nodes representing the heart geometry, the nodal fiber orientations mapped from anatomical heart model or diffusion tensor magnetic resonance images, and also the material properties obtained through cardiac physiology, the cardiac system dynamics (12) can be well defined. By using the Newmark method and Newton-Raphson iteration, (12) can be solved and the active cardiac deformation can be simulated.

3   Results

3.1   Regular Cubical Object

In order to understand the local cardiac physiome behaviors, a regular cubical object with 1331 nodes has been used to emulate a piece of heart muscle. The geometry and fiber orientations are shown in Fig. 1. The action potentials were initiated from a fixed face normal to the fibers, and propagated throughout the whole object. One cycle of 700 ms was simulated. It can be seen that stresses were induced by the electric wave propagation, and the object deformed accordingly (Fig. 2). Because the Poisson's ratios were set to simulate incompressibility,

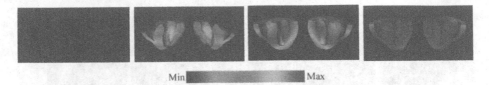

Fig. 4. Canine heart model. Normalized active contraction stress propagation computed from simulated action potentials, shown together with the deformations. Left to right: 0 ms, 30 ms, 60 ms, and 90 ms (during systole).

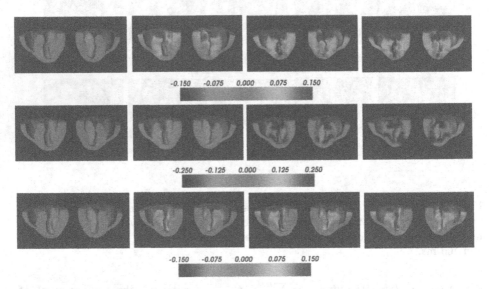

Fig. 5. Canine heart model. Strain maps of the simulated deformations, defined on a cylindrical coordinate system (r, θ, z), with the long axis of the left ventricle as the z-axis. Top to bottom: radial, circumferential, and radial-circumferential strain maps. Left to right: 50 ms, 100 ms, 150 ms, and 200 ms (during systole).

during the contraction, the object shortened along the fiber direction while extended cross the fiber direction (Fig. 3). This actually manifests the heart muscle contraction along the circumferential direction and thickening along the radial direction.

3.2   Canine Heart Model

The canine heart model from the University of Auckland was used [3]. The model was obtained through anatomical experiments on a number of canines, which provides both the *in-vitro* geometry and fiber architecture. A down-sampled version with 2081 nodes was built for the simulation (Fig. 1). The simulation of the electrical propagation using the meshfree method of the canine heart model has been described in detail in [9]. With the action potentials available, the corresponding active contraction stresses were obtained through the EM model

(Fig. 4), and a simulated cardiac cycle in 500 ms was obtained through the cardiac system dynamics with the deformations shown in Fig 5.

From biomechanical literatures, the myocytes are mainly lying on the plane perpendicular to the radial direction. Thus when they contract, the myocardium contracts along the circumferential direction while extends along the radial direction, and the left and right ventricles shrink and pump out the blood. From Fig. 5, we can observe such patterns through the circumferential strain maps and the radial strain maps. The radial-circumferential strain maps also tell that the simulated heart twisted.

References

1. Germann, W.J., Stanfield, C.L.: Principles of Human Physiology. Pearson Benjamin Cummings, London (2005)
2. Knudsen, Z., Holden, A., Brindley, J.: Qualitative modelling of mechano-electrical feedback in a ventricular cell. Bulletin of Mathematical Biology 6(59), 115–181 (1997)
3. Nash, M.: Mechanics and Material Properties of the Heart using an Anatomically Accurate Mathematical Model. PhD thesis, University of Auckland (1998)
4. Glass, L., Hunter, P., McCulloch, A. (eds.): Theory of Heart: Biomechanics, Biophysics, and Nonlinear Dynamics of Cardiac Function. Springer, Heidelberg (1991)
5. McCulloch, A., Bassingthwaighte, J., Hunter, P., Noble, D.: Computational biology of the heart: From structure to function. Progress in Biophysics and Molecular Biology 69, 153–155 (1998)
6. Sermesant, M., Delingette, H., Ayache, N.: An electromechanical model of the heart for image analysis and simulation. IEEE Transactions on Medical Imaging 25(5), 612–625 (2006)
7. Liu, G.R.: Mesh free methods: moving beyond the finite element method. CRC Press, Boca Raton (2003)
8. Rogers, J., McCulloch, A.: A collocation-Galerkin finite element model of cardiac action potential propagation. IEEE Transactions on Biomedical Engineering 41, 743–757 (1994)
9. Zhang, H., Shi, P.: A meshfree method for solving cardiac electrical propagation. In: 27th Annual International Conference of the IEEE-EMBS, pp. 349–352 (2005)
10. Bathe, K.J.: Finite Element Procedures. Prentice Hall, Englewood Cliffs (1996)
11. Matthews, F., Rawlings, R.: Composite Materials: Engineering and Science. Chapman & Hall, Boca Raton (1994)

Wheelchair Propulsion Analysis System That Incorporates Human Skeletal Muscular Model Analyses on the Flat Floor and Slope

Akihiko Hanafusa[1], Motoki Sugawara[1], Teruhiko Fuwa[1],
Tomozumi Ikeda[1], Naoki Suzuki[2], and Asaki Hattori[2]

[1] Polytecnic University,
4-1-1 Hashimotodai, Sagamihara, Kanagawa 229-1196, Japan
[2] Jikei University School of Medicine,
4-11-1 Izumihoncho, Komae, Tokyo 201-8601, Japan

Abstract. A wheelchair propulsion analysis system that can be used to generate the motion of propulsion and calculate the driving force and the muscular force using a human model having a skeleton and muscles was developed. To evaluate the driving force and muscular forces calculated by the analysis system, typical forward movement of two cycles of propulsion from the start-up on a flat floor and on a slope were measured and the movement including the trunk was input to the system. In addition, the muscular forces of biceps, triceps, clavicular and acromion deltoids, pectoralis major and extensor carpi radialis were evaluated by electromyogram. The calculated driving force was in good agreement with the measured driving force even on the slope and the trend of calculated muscular force corresponded with measured electromyogram data. The system is effective for analyzing the driving force and load on muscles during the wheelchair propulsion.

Keywords: Wheelchair, Propulsion, Human model, Muscular force.

1 Introduction

Wheelchairs should be fitted to the individual user's body, physical strength, and propulsion ability. To design a custom wheelchair, a wheelchair propulsion analysis system that uses a three-dimensional wheelchair model and a human model with a skeleton and muscles has been developed. To date, research on motion and kinematic analysis of wheelchair propulsion have been conducted in order to fit the wheelchair size to the human body[1]. In addition, measurement analyses of muscular force by electromyogram (EMG) during propulsion have been performed and the results for normal and spinal cord injury subjects have been compared[2]. However, we consider that development of the wheelchair propulsion analysis system in which the wheelchair and human model with a musculoskeletal model are generated and used concurrently for calculation is a novel concept. The feature of the system[3] is that the system can be used to

T. Dohi, I. Sakuma, and H. Liao (Eds.): MIAR 2008, LNCS 5128, pp. 70–80, 2008.

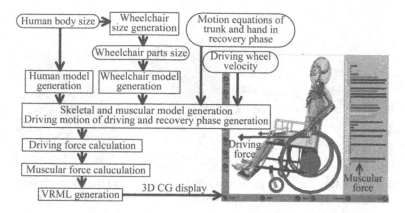

Fig. 1. System flow of the wheelchair propulsion analysis system

generate propulsion motion and calculate the driving force and muscular force according to the input movement of the wheelchair.

The present paper describes an overview of the system and the result of driving force and muscular force evaluation of the entire propulsion period. To evaluate the driving force and muscular forces calculated by the analysis system, typical forward movement of two cycles of propulsion from start-up on a flat floor and on a slope, respectively, were measured, and the movement including the trunk was input to the system. The driving force was calculated considering the human body movement. In addition, the calculated muscular forces were evaluated by measured EMG.

2   Wheelchair Propulsion Analysis System

2.1   System Configuration

Figure 1 shows the system flow of the wheelchair propulsion analysis system. A human model is generated from 25 human body size parameters, and a wheelchair model is generated from 25 wheelchair size parameters. These wheelchair size parameters can be specified manually or generated automatically by the wheelchair parameter generation system based on input body size parameters. The human model is incorporated with skeletal and muscular models for a sitting position on the wheelchair model. According to the input transition of the driving wheel velocity, the propulsion motion of the entire phase is generated based on geometric considerations and approximate polynomials of the trunk and hands in the recovery phase. Equations are derived from experimental three-dimensional measurement of wheelchair propulsion. In addition, the driving force necessary to execute the movement is calculated. Based on the resulting driving force, the muscular forces required to generate the driving force are calculated. Generated models are output in Virtual Reality Modeling Language (VRML) format as an animation of a human model propelling a wheelchair.

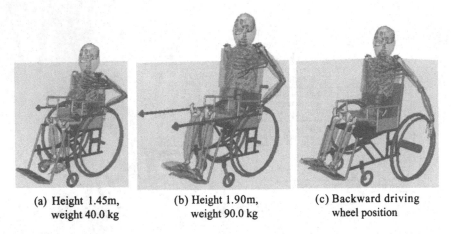

(a) Height 1.45m,   (b) Height 1.90m,   (c) Backward driving
   weight 40.0 kg   weight 90.0 kg   wheel position

Fig. 2. VRML models to analyze human models and wheelchairs of varied sizes

The calculated results are output as arrows or graphs and can be observed from any viewpoint using a World Wide Web browser, as shown in the figure.

By the system, human models or wheelchairs of varied sizes can be analyzed as shown in Figure 2. Figures 2(a) and 2(b) show models for individuals whose height and weight are 1.45 [m], 40.0 [kg] and 1.90 [m], 90.0 [kg] respectively, driving a wheelchair that is fitted to a individual whose height and weight are 1.70 [m] and 60 [kg]. Based on the generated models, the wheelchair is confirmed to be too large for individuals whose height is 1.45 [m], because the user's feet do not reach the footrests and the elbow angles for driving at the top of handrim become very small. In contrast, the wheelchair is too small for individuals whose height is 1.90 [m], because there is a space between the seat and the user's femurs. Figure 2(c) shows the situation in which the driving wheels are positioned to the rear, such that the arms must be extended backward in order to grasp the handrim.

2.2 Human Model

The human model consists of 15 rigid bodies, a head, an upper trunk, a lower trunk, left and right brachia, forearms, hands, femurs, lower legs, and feet. The forearm part is divided into radius and ulna sub-parts to accurately model rotation of the forearm. Dimensions such as the length and width of each body, distances between left and right shoulders, and legs are defined by 25 parameters. The mass, moment of inertia and center of gravity of each part are calculated by the equations in Reference [4].

The skeletal model consists of a triangular surface model of 93 bones prepared from MRI slice data. The bones are divided into separate body parts of the human model, and their position and size are normalized by the size of each part. The muscular model consists of 37 muscles that belong to the arm and are relevant to wheelchair propulsion motion, as shown in Figure 3(a). Their origin, insertion and midpoints connected to body parts are defined. The coordinates of

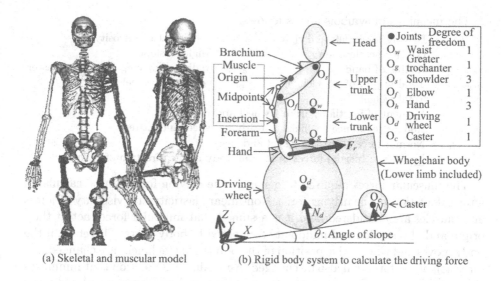

● Joints	Degree of freedom
O_w Waist	1
O_g Greater trochanter	1
O_s Showlder	3
O_f Elbow	1
O_h Hand	3
O_d Driving wheel	1
O_c Caster	1

(a) Skeletal and muscular model   (b) Rigid body system to calculate the driving force

Fig. 3. Defined skeletal muscular human model and rigid body system

the skeletal and muscular model are defined based on the origin and coordinates normalized by the length of each body part. Thus, skeletal and muscular models of different body size parameters can be generated and moved in cooperation with the movement of each body part.

2.3 Driving Force and Muscular Force Calculation

Driving force calculation is based on the rigid body system shown in Figure 3(b). The wheelchair body includes the lower limbs of the human body. The shoulder, elbow and wrist joints of left and right upper limbs have three, one and three degrees of freedom, respectively. The waist and greater trochanter of the trunk each have one degree of freedom. The human body and the wheelchair body are connected at the greater trochanter. The axles of the left and right driving wheels and the casters of the wheelchair each have one degree of freedom. The system has a total of 20 degrees of freedom.

Calculation is based on the equations of translatory motion in the direction of the movement (1)[1] and vertical to the road (2). In the equations below, the term $\sum_i m_i \dot{v}_i$ represents the movement of the human body. Coeffcients K and μ were obtained experimentally.

$$\left(m_{wc} + \frac{2I_d}{r_d^2} + \frac{2I_c}{r_c^2}\right)\dot{v}_{wc} + \sum_i m_i \dot{v}_{xi} - m_{all}g\sin\theta + Kv_{wc}$$

$$= \frac{r_h}{r_d}(F_r + F_l) - \mu_d N_d - \mu_c N_c \qquad (1)$$

$$\sum_i m_i \dot{v}_{zi} - m_{all}g\cos\theta = N_d + N_c \qquad (2)$$

The meanings of symbols are as follows:

F_l, F_r :	Driving force (left and right)	K :	Coefficient of viscosity
g :	Gravity acceleration	θ :	Angle of slope
r_h :	Radius of handrim	r_d, r_c :	Radius of driving wheel and caster
m_{wc} :	Total weight of wheelchair	v_{wc} :	Velocity of wheelchair
m_{all} :	Total weight		

I_d, I_c :   Moment of inertia of driving wheel and caster
μ_d, μ_c :   Rolling resistance coefficient of driving wheel and caster
N_d, N_c :   Normal force of driving wheel and caster
$\sum_i m_i \dot{v}_{xi}, \sum_i m_i \dot{v}_{zi}$: Inertial forces of human body in the direction of x and z

The muscular forces required to generate the driving force can be calculated after calculation of the driving force. Non-linear elasticity and viscosity of joints and muscles are considered, and it is assumed that muscular forces act at their origin and at insertion and midpoints connected to body parts. Therefore, if the body moves and the relative position of the points of attachment are changed, the direction of the force will also be changed. An evaluation function that minimizes the sum of squares of the muscular force is used, and forces are calculated using Lagrange's method of undetermined multipliers under the condition that the equations of translatory motion (3) and rotating motion (4) hold:

$$m\dot{\mathbf{v}} = \mathbf{T}\left[\mathbf{F}_M, \mathbf{F}_J, \mathbf{F}_E, \mathbf{F}_G\right]^T \tag{3}$$

$$\mathbf{I}\dot{\boldsymbol{\omega}} = \mathbf{r} \times \mathbf{T}\left[\mathbf{F}_M, \mathbf{F}_J, \mathbf{F}_E, \mathbf{F}_G\right]^T - \mathbf{M}_M + \mathbf{M}_J \tag{4}$$

where, m is mass of a body part and $\mathbf{v}$ is the corresponding velocity vector, $\mathbf{F}_M$ is the sum of muscular force and the forces caused by the elasticity and viscosity of muscles, $\mathbf{F}_J$ is the force of constraint at the joints, $\mathbf{F}_E$ is the external force, $\mathbf{F}_G$ is the force of gravity, $\mathbf{T}$ is a coefficient matrix that shows the x, y and z components of the forces, $\mathbf{I}$ is the moment of inertia of a body part, $\boldsymbol{\omega}$ is the angular velocity around the coordinate axes, $\mathbf{r}$ is the distance vector between the center of gravity and the points of application of the forces, $\mathbf{M}_M$ is the sum of moments caused by the elasticity and viscosity of joints, and $\mathbf{M}_J$ is the moment of constraint at the joints.

3   Simulated and Experimental Results

3.1   Methods

To evaluate the driving force and muscular forces calculated by the analysis system, typical forward movement of two cycles of propulsion from the start-up on a flat floor and on a slope were measured and the movements were input to the system.

A wheelchair designed specifically for propulsion ability evaluation[6] was used to measure the velocity and force of the driving wheel. A rotary encoder, a torque sensor, a microcomputer and a memory card writer, the total weight of which is 7.75 [kg], are incorporated into the left and right driving wheels. The motion of the human operator was measured by a three-dimensional motion capture

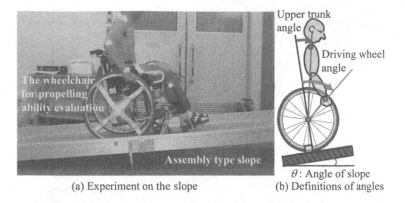

(a) Experiment on the slope   (b) Definitions of angles

Fig. 4. Experiment on the slope and definitions of angles

system (MA2000 Anima Corp.) using infrared markers. Hand and trunk motion equations that approximate the measured movement and measured variation of the driving wheel velocity were input to the analysis system to calculate the driving force and muscular forces. In addition, the electromyogram (EMG) was measured with surface electrodes by the bipolar lead method using a wireless biological signal measuring system (MT11 NEC Medical Corp) and was captured to a MA2000 with a sampling frequency of 240 Hz. The average rectified value of EMG (ARV EMG) is calculated by the processing of full-wave rectification and averaging 31 adjacent data for 0.13 seconds. The result was compared with the muscular forces calculated by the system. The target muscles were the clavicular and acromion deltoids, pectoralis major, biceps, triceps, and extensor carpi radialis. A subject driving the wheelchair for propulsion ability evaluation with attached markers is shown in Figure 4(a). Electrodes for measuring EMG were mounted on the left-hand side of the body. In addition, as shown in Figure 4(a), an assembly type slope of 3.6 [m] in length having an angle 4.5 [°] that can be installed indoors was used.

3.2   Results and Discussion of SC Propulsion on a Flat Floor

For the recovery phase on the flat floor, semicircular (SC)[5] movement by which the elbow is extended and the hand is returned near the center of the driving wheel was used. Figure 5 is a result of SC propulsion on the flat floor. DRV1, DRV2 and RCV in the figure denote the first and second driving phases and the recovery phase, respectively. Figure 5(a) shows the input velocity variation and the calculated and measured driving force. Figure 5(b) shows the variation of the driving wheel angle and upper trunk angle, which is a center angle of the driving wheel between the plumb line and the position of wrist and shoulder, as shown in Figure 4(b). The front side is positive, and the rear side is negative. Figures 5(c)-(d) show ARV EMG data and the calculated muscular force of the biceps and triceps. Figures 5(e)-(f) are the results for the pectoralis major and

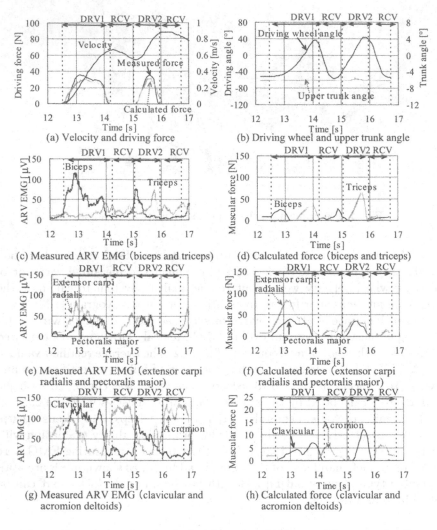

Fig. 5. Experimental and calculated results of SC propulsion on a flat floor

extensor carpi radialis. Figures 5(g)-(h) show the results for the clavicular and acromion deltoids.

As shown in Figure 5(a), the velocity of wheelchair and driving wheel angle increase during the driving phase and decrease during the recovery phase. The calculated driving force was in good agreement with the measured driving force. The range of the driving wheel angle was from −50 to 40 [°]. In this case, the upper trunk angle was fixed to approximately −6 [°]. As for the clavicular deltoid, the pectoralis major and extensor carpi radialis, which function during the driving phase, and the acromion deltoid, which functions during the recovery phase, the trend reported in the literature[2][7] corresponded with both the calculated muscular force and the measured EMG data. However, the calculated muscular

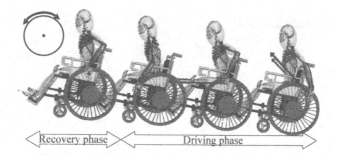

Fig. 6. Propulsion movement on a slope by the generated model

forces of the deltoids are small compared to other muscles. According to the literature[2], the biceps functions from the latter period of the recovery phase until the middle period of the driving phase, and the triceps functions gradually from the earlier to the latter period of the driving phase. The transition of the calculated muscular force of the triceps was coincident with this description. However, the calculated muscular force of the biceps functioned from the earlier period of the recovery phase until the triceps started to function, and the two muscles function alternately. Conversely, the ARV EMG showed that, during a certain period, the two muscles function simultaneously. The difference occurs because the current evaluation formula of muscular force that minimizes the sum of squares tends to avoid simultaneous action of antagonist muscles.

3.3   Results and Discussion of ARC Propulsion on a Slope

The propulsion movement on the slope by the generated model is shown in Figure 6. Arching (ARC)[5] movement was used for the recovery phase. In this movement, the hand returns approximately through the trajectory of the driving phase. Figure 7 shows the results of propulsion on the slope. Figure 7(a) shows the input velocity variation and the calculated and measured driving forces. Compared with the results on the flat floor, the variation of amplitude of the velocity was larger on the slope, ranging from 0.2 to 0.8 [m/s] and the maximum driving force was almost twice that on the flat floor. The calculated driving force was in good agreement with the measured driving force. However, there was a difference of 10 [N] between the calculated and measured driving forces at the start time on the slope. The measured driving force denotes the force to avoid slipping down the slope, while the calculated driving force denotes the force necessary for climbing the slope. Therefore, the directions of friction are opposite to each other. Figure 7(b) shows the variation of the driving wheel and upper trunk angle. The period of the recovery phase was smaller, and the ARC movement by the subject requires the hand to return more quickly on the slope than on the flat floor. The results of the upper trunk angle show that the trunk was bent forward and the angle increases to 14 [°] during the drive phase. Consequently, the range of driving angle shifted forward. These movements, including the upper trunk, are considered in calculating the driving force.

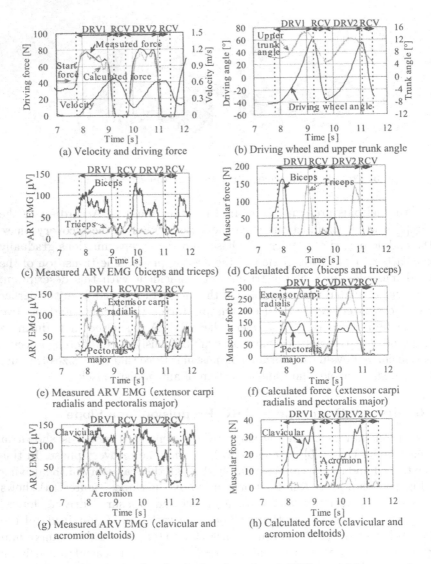

Fig. 7. Experimental and calculated results of ARC propulsion on a slope

Figures 7(c)-(d) show the ARV EMG data and the calculated muscular force of the biceps and triceps. Figures 7(e)-(f) show the results for the pectoralis major and extensor carpi radialis, while Figures 7(g)-(h) show the results for the clavicular and acromion deltoids. In most cases, with the exception of the triceps and acromion deltoid, the ARV EMG increased compared with that on the flat floor, especially during the second driving phase. All of the calculated muscular forces for the case of the slope, except for that of the acromion deltoid, which is effective during the recovery phase, are greater than twice the values of the calculated forces on the flat floor. However the increase of ARV

EMG was smaller than that of simulation. One reason for this is that the muscles of the trunk, such as the abdominal and back muscles, used for propulsion, including the movement of the upper trunk, are not defined in the current human muscular model, and the force cannot be distributed to these muscles. The biceps are dominant during the early period of the driving phase. As for the triceps, both the calculated and measured results show peaks at the end of the driving and recovery phases when the elbow is extended. However, the peak value during the recovery phase is small compared to that during the driving phase. By the calculated and measured result, pectoralis major, extensor carpi radialis and clavicular deltoid functioned during the driving phase. However, the calculated force of the extensor carpi radialis is large, and those of the deltoids are small compared to other muscles. These results indicate the necessity for adopting adequate methods for distributing the calculated force to each muscle.

4 Conclusions

A wheelchair propulsion analysis system that can be used to generate the motion of propulsion and calculate the driving force and the muscular force using a human skeletal muscular model was developed. To evaluate the driving force and muscular forces calculated by the system, typical forward movement of two cycles of propulsion from start-up on a flat floor and a slope were measured, and the movement including the trunk was input to the system. In addition, muscular forces were evaluated by ARV EMG. The calculated driving force was in good agreement with the measured driving force, even on the slope and under the movement of trunk. For the clavicular deltoid, the pectoralis major and extensor carpi radialis, which function during the driving phase, and the acromion deltoid, which functions during the recovery phase, the trend of the calculated muscular force corresponded with measured EMG data. In addition, the trend whereby the biceps function primarily during the earlier period of the driving phase and the triceps function during the latter period of the driving phase was observed for both the calculated and measured EMG data. Both the results of a simulation and an experiment on a slope showed that the load on the clavicular deltoids, biceps, pectoralis major and extensor carpi radialis, which function during the driving phase, increased compared to the results on the flat floor.

It is verified that the system is effective for analyzing the driving force and the load on muscles during wheelchair propulsion. In a future study, the trunk muscles will be defined, and a detailed verification of the calculated values of muscular forces and a method for distributing the force to each muscle must be performed. In addition, the proposed system should be extended to generate efficient propulsion movement considering muscular load and in cases in which there is damage to the muscles.

References

1. Cooper, R.A.: A Systems Approach to the Modeling of Racing Wheelchair Propulsion. J. Rehab. R&D. 27(2), 151–162 (1990)
2. Ookawa, T., Itoh, T., Tanaka, O., Iijima, H.: Wheelchair, Igaku-Syoin, pp. 105–110 (1987) (in Japanese)
3. Hanafusa, A., Sugawara, M., Fuwa, T., Suzuki, N., Otake, Y.: Wheelchair Propulsion Analysis Using a Human Model that Incorporates Muscles Evaluation for Cases When the Seat Positions are Changed. J. Soc. of Comput. Aided Surg. 9(1), 23–35 (2007) (in Japanese)
4. Ae, M., Tan, H., Yokoi, T.: Estimation of Inertia Properties of the Body Segments in Japanese Athletes. Biomechanisms 11, 23–31 (1992) (in Japanese)
5. Shimada, S.D., Robertson, R.N., Bonninger, M.L., Cooper, R.A.: Kinematic Characterization of Wheelchair Propulsion. J. Rehab. R&D 35(2), 210–218 (1998)
6. Kakimoto, A., Suzuki, S., Sekiguchi, Y.: Development of Wheelchair for Propelling Ability Evaluation. J. Soc. of Life Support Tech. 11(4), 14–19 (1999) (in Japanese)
7. Spaepen, A.J., Vanlandewijck, Y.C., Lysens, R.J.: Relationship Between Energy Expenditure and Muscular Activity Patterns in Handrim Wheelchair Propulsion. Int. J. Ind. Ergon. 17(2), 163–173 (1996)

Automatic Detection of Fiducial Marker Center Based on Shape Index and Curvedness

Manning Wang and Zhijian Song*

Digital Medical Research Center, Fudan Uniuversity,
138 Yixueyuan Road, 200032 Shanghai, China
zjsong@fudan.edu.cn

Abstract. Fiducial marker is widely used for registration in image guided neurosurgery. In this paper we propose a novel automatic approach of localizing the center of these markers in CT volume. We first segment the volume into three parts according to shape index and curvedness of each voxel. Part1 includes some voxels on top of the markers, part2 includes some voxels at the bottom of the markers, and part3 is the background. Then we cluster voxels in part1 and part2 separately. The result groups in part1 are candidates for the top of markers, and the groups in part2 are candidates for bottom. For each group in part2, if there is a group in part1 that is close to it, this pair is regarded as a marker and the centroid of the group from part2 is the marker center. Experiments show that the marker center can be localized with sub millimeter accuracy.

Keywords: Shape Index, Curvedness, Image Guided Neurosurgery, Fiducial Marker Detection.

1 Introduction

Image Guided Neurosurgery System (IGNS) makes use of medical images to help surgeon in planning before the surgery, and provide guidance during the surgery. As the development of medical imaging technology and the maturation of IGNS, it integrates more and more information including both the anatomical and the functional, while needs less and less human intervention in clinical application. IGNS has become a routine instrument in the neurosurgical room [1].

For utilizing the images obtained before the surgery in guiding the surgeon during surgery, IGNS has to register the image space to the patient space accurately. In the early days of IGNS, this is accomplished by attaching a stereotaxic frame to the patient during scanning and surgery. But the implanting of the frame is invasive, and the existence of the frame brings a lot of inconvenience to the surgical operation. So, after the emergence of the so-called frameless stereotaxis depending on computer and tracking system, the frameless system becomes the mainstream of the IGNS [2].

In frameless stereotaxic system, the user usually extracts some common features from both the image and the patient, and registers the image space to the patient

---

* Corresponding author.

T. Dohi, I. Sakuma, and H. Liao (Eds.): MIAR 2008, LNCS 5128, pp. 81–88, 2008.

space by matching these features [3]. The features commonly used in IGNS can be classified into 3 categories: fiducial markers, anatomical landmarks, and head surface. [4] pointed out that the registration based on fiducial markers is the most accurate one. In addition, because the operation of registration using fiducial markers is simpler than that using head surface, and the marker is more easily to be identified than anatomical landmarks, fiducial marker based registration is used most widely in clinical application.

In IGNS using fiducial markers for registration, the accuracy of the registration and the guidance depends on the accuracy of the selection of the markers on the images and the patient. This relies to a large degree on the experience of the operator. So if the markers can be automatically and precisely localized on the images, the accuracy of the guidance can be enhanced and the man-made error can be reduced. In addition, the major extra cost of time by introducing IGNS to conventional surgery is the optimization of the marker selection both on the patient and on the images, and this is also a major task in training of the IGNS. An automatic method can also help to cut down the preparation and training time of IGNS.

There have been some researches done for automatic localization of the center of fiducial markers. For example, Chen et al. [5] has proposed a marker localization method for automatic registration of two series, and this method is based on edge detection and curved-based object identification. Tan et al. [6] also proposed a method based on template for series registration. Wang et al. [7] describe a method for identifying implanted markers. But all these methods are based on the processing of section images. The 3D geometric properties of the markers are not fully utilized, and the detection may be influenced by the orientation of the markers in the volume. Gu and Peters [8] has proposed a method based on 3D morphological operation. But they didn't validate their method on real clinical data in their paper.

In this paper, we propose an automatic approach to localize the center of fiducial markers in CT images. This method explores the 3D geometric features of the markers, and didn't rely on the section images. We will describe the method in detail in section 2, and give the experiment results on clinical data in section 3. Finally we'll conclude this paper by discussion and outlook.

2   Method

Several kinds of fiducial markers are used clinically for image guided neurosurgery. At the early days of IGNS, some kinds of markers are implanted to the patient skull, but the implanting process is not only time-consuming but also invasive to the patient. Now almost all fiducial markers are adhered to the patient's skin before scanning and can be easily removed after registration. MM3302 Multi-Modality IGS/CAS Fiducial Marker produced by IZI Medical Products is the most popular one of this kind of fiducial marker. The appearance of the marker is illustrated in Fig.1. The thickness of the ring is 3.5mm. The outer diameter of the ring is 15mm, and the inner diameter is 5mm.The bottom of the marker is adhered to the skin of patient's head before CT scanning, and the center of the bottom serves as the feature for registration. The objective of our approach is to localize the center of the bottom of the marker automatically.

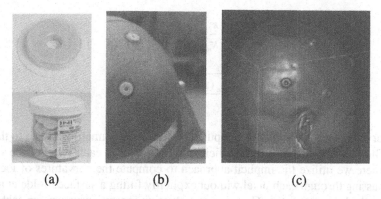

(a)   (b)   (c)

Fig. 1. MM3302 Multi-Modality IGS/CAS Fiducial Marker. (a) Photograph of the markers. (b) Photograph of the markers adhered to the skin of patient's head. (c) Visualization of the markers in CT volume.

Our method includes two major steps. The first step is the calculation of shape index and curvedness for each voxel of the volume. In the second step we segment out two parts from the volume according to the parameters calculated in the first step, and cluster the results of the segmentation. Then we identify the markers by finding cluster pairs from different parts, and locate the center of the marker at the centroid of one cluster of the pair. We will describe in detail of the method in the following two subsections.

2.1   Calculate the Shape Index and the Curvedness in the CT Volume

Shape index and curvedness are used to describe the differential geometric property of a local surface patch at a point. They are both invariant to translation and rotation because the geometric property is intrinsic to the patch. The fiducial markers in the volume data have different orientation, but the shape index and curvedness around each marker possess similar characteristic, and this characteristic is the basis for identifying the marker center in this paper. Napii et al. [9] describe the calculation of shape index and curvedness from Gaussian curvature and mean curvature as follows.

Denote Gaussian curvature as K and mean curvature as H. They can also be defined by

$$K = \kappa_1\kappa_2, \ H = \frac{\kappa_1 + \kappa_2}{2}. \tag{1}$$

Where κ_1 and κ_2 are principal curvatures. From equation (1), it can be derived that at any voxel p, the principal curvatures can be expressed as

$$\kappa_i(p) = H(p) \pm \sqrt{H^2(p) - K(p)}, \quad i = 1,2. \tag{2}$$

If we denote $\kappa_{min} = \min\{\kappa_1, \kappa_2\}$ and $\kappa_{max} = \max\{\kappa_1, \kappa_2\}$, the shape index $S(p)$ and the curvedness $C(p)$ at this voxel are defined as

$$S(p) = -\frac{2}{\pi}\arctan\frac{\kappa_{max}(p) + \kappa_{min}(p)}{\kappa_{max}(p) - \kappa_{min}(p)}. \tag{3}$$

$$C(p) = \frac{2}{\pi}\ln\sqrt{\frac{\kappa_{min}(p)^2 + \kappa_{max}(p)^2}{2}}. \tag{4}$$

The curvatures are traditionally computed by fitting a parametric surface to the data locally. But it is very difficult and inefficient to fit surface at each voxel of the volume data. So here we utilize the implicit approach to compute the curvatures of local iso-surface passing through each pixel without explicitly fitting a surface. Solde et al. [10] gives a method for computing Gaussian curvature and mean curvature for each voxel in volumetric images from 1st and 2nd order difference of a scalar field. This approach is adopted in this paper, and the shape index and curvedness can be calculated by put the Gaussian curvature and mean curvature back into equation (1) to (4). Napii et al. [9] also gives an illustration of how the surface patch looks like with different shape index and curvedness, as illustrated in Fig.2 (a).

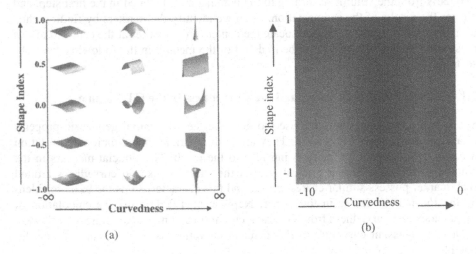

Fig. 2. (a) The outlook of surface patch with different shape index and curvedness. (b) Map from shape index and curvedness to color. The curvature is bounded within -10 to 0.

We construct a map from the 2d space formed by shape index and curvedness to color, as illustrated in Fig.2 (b). To demonstrate the characteristic of differential geometric properties around the marker, we use this map to color the surface of the patient visualized from CT volume. The results are illustrated in Fig.3. In this image, all curvatures above 0 are set to 0, and all curvatures below -10 are set to -10.

From Fig.3 (b), it is clear that the shape index and curvedness around the marker is quite different with other position on the head, and this make it possible to identify the markers based on these two properties.

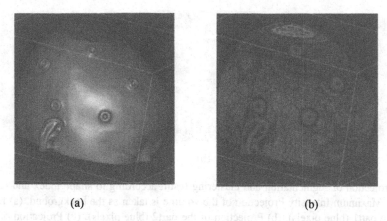

(a)   (b)

Fig. 3. (a) Visualization of patient's head with 5 markers using pseudo color (b) Visualization of the same patient's head using color map in Fig.2 (b)

2.2 Segment the Volume and Identify Markers by Clustering

In Fig.3 (b) we can see that on the top of the markers, there are some voxels with big curvature and small shape index (bright red), and at the bottom of the marker there are some voxels with big curvature and big shape index (dark red). We segment the volume into 3 parts according to the shape index and curvedness of each voxel. Part1 (shape index range:-1~-0.5, curvedness range:-2.5~0) includes the voxels on top of the marker as illustrated in the Fig.4 (a). Part2 (shape index range:0.5~1, curvedness range:-2.5~0) includes the voxels at the bottom of the markers as illustrated in Fig.4 (b). All other voxels form part3.

For localize the center of the markers, we first cluster all voxels in part1. Then pick out the clusters that may correspond to markers based on the distribution of voxels within the group. The clustering is done as follows:

1) Initial partitioning. In the first step, we scan all voxels in part1. For each point, calculate its distance to every existing group (the distance from a point to a group is defined as the minimal distance from the point to each point in the group). If there is a group which is close to the point (close means that the distance from the point to the group is less than a threshold, such as 3mm), add the point to this group. Else, if there isn't any group close to the point, create a new group and make the point as the first element of this group.

2) Delete small group. After step 1, all voxels in part1 are partitioned into different groups. Delete groups with less than 50 voxels.

3) Group Merging. Iteratively scan the remaining groups, and merge two groups if the distance between them is less than a threshold (such as 3mm, the distance between two groups is defined as the minimal distance between two points from different group). When there is no pair of groups to merge, the clustering stop.

In step 2, we delete the small groups which have less than 50 markers. This is done to speed up the merging process and avoid the possibility of small groups around markers to be merged with the marker group. Fig.4 (c) illustrates the result of clustering.

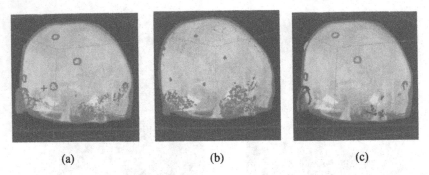

(a)   (b)   (c)

Fig. 4. Projection of segmentation and clustering result according to shape index and curvedness. The Maximum Intensity Projection of the volume is taken as the background. (a) Projection of the part1 (blue pixels). (b) Projection of the part2 (blue pixels). (c) Projection of part1 after clustering. Different groups are marked with different color.

Fig.4 (c) shows that the remaining groups after clustering includes not only the top of markers, but also other groups around ears, eyes, nasal cavity etc. By examining the distribution of voxels in each group, we can find that the points in the marker groups rest on a thin round belt, while the distribution in other groups are fairly random. Here we adopt a simple method to delete group that is impossible to be the top of markers. We first calculate the centroid of each group, and then move a pair of concentric spheres within a small neighborhood of the centroid. The radius of the inner sphere is 3.5mm, and the radius of the outer sphere is 7mm. If there is a position where more than 95% of the voxels of the group rests between the two spheres, this group may be the top of a marker. And if there is not such a position, the group is discarded.

After the processing of groups in part1, we cluster voxels in part2. To speed up the clustering process, only voxels those are close to remaining groups in part1 are included. The clustering procedure is similar with that of part1, except that in step 2 groups with less than 20 voxels are deleted instead of 50. As we can see from Fig.4 (b), the groups in part2 are smaller than those in part1. After clustering of part2, we examine every group in part2. For each group, if we can find another group in part1 that is close to it, this group is regarded as the bottom of a marker and the centroid of the group in part2 is the localized center.

3 Results

We test our method on 21 patients' CT scanning used for image guided neurosurgery from 3 different hospitals. All data are scanned under the imaging protocol for image guided neurosurgery. The volume data contains continuous, non-overlapping slices. The thickness of each slice is constant and no greater than 2.5mm. Scan is performed with standard soft tissue algorithm. Circular or square FOV is adopted, and use the smallest FOV to encompass the whole head. The resolution of the original image is 512*512. After loading original data, the volume is formatted to be isotropic with voxel size about 0.6mm. Before calculating the shape index and curvedness, the volume is filtered by 5*5*5 mean filter.

The center of each marker is first identified by two different experts who are very familiar with Image Guided Neurosurgery. The midpoint of the two centers identified by different expert is regarded as the real center of each marker. Then the automatic approach proposed in this paper is used to identify the centers automatically. If the distance from the automatic identified center to the real center is smaller than 0.6mm, the marker center is regarded as correctly identified. In our experiment, all 113 markers in these 21 volumes are correctly identified, and the mean localization error of the automatic approach is 0.43mm compared with the real center.

Experiments show that the accuracy of our approach is similar with the method described in [5] and [6]. But our method is based on 3D geometric features instead of the characteristics in 2D section image. And our approach should be more robust when the patient's head and the markers possess different orientation in the volume data.

4 Conclusion

We have presented a novel approach to automatically localize the center of fiducial markers used in image guided neurosurgery. The method is based on shape index and curvedness which are invariant to translation and rotation, so this approach is robust and reliable. Experiments on clinical CT data showed that the center of the fiducial markers can be automatically localized with high precision. The automatic approach will help to improve the accuracy in image to patient registration by reducing the man-made error and cut down the preparation time.

We have also tested our method on clinical MRI data, but the results are not as good as that with CT data. This may be due to the fact that most MRI images used in IGNS are very noisy. Major focus of our future work is to find better clustering and localization strategy for MRI data. The idea of target detection by combination of different 3D geometric features may also be extended to detect objects which possess specific 3D characteristics.

Acknowledgements

The authors thank for the grants of Science and Technology Commission of Shanghai Municipality of China (project NO.06dz22103) and NSFC (project 30570506).

References

1. Yaniv, Z., Cleary, K.: Image-Guided Procedures: A Review. Technical report, CAIMR of Georgetown University (2006)
2. Peters, T.M.: Image-Guidance for Surgical Procedures. Phys. Med. Biol. 51, 505–540 (2006)
3. Zitova, B., Flusser, J.: Image registration methods: A survey. Image and Vision Computing 21, 977–1000 (2003)

4. Woerdeman, P.A., Willems, P.W.A., Noordmans, H.J., Tulleken, C.A.F., Sprenkel, J.W.B.: Application accuracy in frameless image-guided neurosurgery: a comparison study of three patient-to-image registration methods. J. Neurosurg. 106, 1012–1016 (2007)
5. Chen, D., Tan, J., Chaudhary, V., Sethi, I.K.: Automatic Fiducial Localization in Brain Images. International Journal of Computer Assisted Radiology and Surgery 1, 45–46 (2006)
6. Tan, J., Chen, D., Chaudhary, V., Sethi, I.K.: A Template Based Technique for Automatic Detection of Fiducial Markers in 3D Brain Images. International Journal of Computer Assisted Radiology and Surgery 1, 47–48 (2006)
7. Wang, M.Y., Maurer, C.R., Fitzpatrick, J.M., Maciunas, R.J.: An Automatic Technique for Finding and Localizing Externally Attached Markers in CT and MR Volume Images of the Head. IEEE Transactions on Biomedical Engineering 43(6), 627–637 (1996)
8. Gu, L., Peters, T.M.: 3D Automatic Fiducial Marker Localization Approach for Frameless Stereotactic Neuro-surgery Navigation. In: Yang, G.-Z., Jiang, T. (eds.) MIAR 2004. LNCS, vol. 3150, pp. 329–336. Springer, Heidelberg (2004)
9. Nappi, J., Frimmel, H., Yoshida, H.: Virtual Endoscopic Visualization of the Colon by Shape-Scale Signatures. IEEE Transactions on Information Technology in Biomedicine 9(1), 120–131 (2005)
10. Soldea, O., Elber, G., Rivlin, E.: Global Segmentation and Curvature Analysis of Volumetric Data Sets Using Trivariate B-spline Functions. IEEE Transaction on Pattern Analysis and Machine Intelligence 28(2), 265–278 (2006)

Modality-Independent Determination of Vertebral Position and Rotation in 3D

Tomaž Vrtovec

University of Ljubljana, Faculty of Electrical Engineering, Slovenia
tomaz.vrtovec@fe.uni-lj.si

Abstract. The determination of the position and rotation of vertebrae is important for the understanding of normal and pathological spine anatomy. Existing techniques, however, estimate the position and rotation parameters from two-dimensional (2D) planar cross-sections, are relatively complex and require a relatively large amount of manual interaction. We have developed an automated and modality-independent method for the determination of the position and rotation of vertebrae in three dimensions (3D) that is based on registration of image intensity gradients, extracted in 3D from symmetrical vertebral parts. The method was evaluated on 52 vertebrae; 26 were acquired by computed tomography (CT) and 26 by magnetic resonance (MR). The results show that by the proposed gradient-based registration of symmetrical vertebral parts, the position and rotation of vertebrae in 3D can be successfully determined in both CT and MR spine images. As the position and rotation of vertebrae in 3D are among the most important spine parameters, the proposed method may provide valuable support in the evaluation of deformities and disease processes that affect the spine.

1 Introduction

The determination of the position and rotation of individual vertebrae is important for the understanding of the nature of normal and pathological spine anatomy. The Cobb technique [1] is the most established method for measuring vertebral rotation from two-dimensional (2D) radiographic images of the spine in cases of scoliotic [2,3,4] and kyphotic/lordotic deformities [5,6,7,8]. Techniques that exploit the information from three-dimensional (3D) images, such as computed tomography (CT) and magnetic resonance (MR) images, were also proposed [9,10,11,12,13,14] and further combined with low level [2,3,8,15] and also more sophisticated image analysis methods [16,17,18]. Rogers et al. [16] measured axial vertebral rotation by registering circular areas in two MR axial cross-sections. The vertebral pose was determined by registering statistical shape models of vertebrae to presegmented vertebral bodies in stereoradiographic images in the study of Benameur et al. [17]. Adam and Askin [18] defined axial vertebral rotation as the axis of maximum symmetry in axial CT cross-sections. The vertebral center of rotation, located in the mid-sagittal plane at the anterior wall of the vertebral canal [19] and at the superior vertebral endplate [20], was

T. Dohi, I. Sakuma, and H. Liao (Eds.): MIAR 2008, LNCS 5128, pp. 89–97, 2008.

inherently included in the estimation of vertebral rotation. Although the afore-mentioned methods aimed to exploit the information in 3D, the measurements were still performed in 2D cross-sections, required a relatively high number of parameters and a relatively large amount of manual interaction. Besides manual determination of the center of rotation, the cross-sections were manually selected either from the original images or, to reduce the effect of virtual rotation [11,14] and vertebral torsion [12,15], from manually reformatted images, yielding cross-sections that were perpendicular or tangent to the spine. Moreover, the measurements were based on manually identified reference points (e.g. the center of the vertebral body and vertebral canal, extreme points of pedicles and processes), which reflect only local characteristics of vertebral anatomy as they are limited to a specific vertebral region. An automated approach to the determination of the location and rotation of vertebrae in 3D was presented by Vrtovec et al. [21], who registered symmetrical parts of vertebrae using an intensity-based similarity measure. However, although the authors reported a relatively high precision of the method, it was applicable only to CT spine images.

The purpose of this study is to develop a method for the determination of the position and rotation of vertebrae in 3D images that does not require man-ual interaction and takes into account the global characteristics of vertebral anatomy, i.e. is not limited to a specific vertebral region. We propose and test the performance of an automated, modality-independent method that is based on registration of image intensity gradients, extracted from symmetrical verte-bral parts in 3D. Automated determination of vertebral parameters in 3D may improve clinical diagnosis of spinal deformities and support high-level image analysis techniques, e.g. the segmentation of vertebrae.

2   Method

2.1   Vertebral Parameters and Vertebral Symmetry

The position and rotation of a vertebra in the coordinate system of a 3D image, denoted by (e_x, e_y, e_z) (sagittal, coronal and axial directions, respectively), can be represented by the vertebral parameters p (Fig. 1):

$$p = (t, \varphi) = (x, y, z, \alpha, \beta, \gamma) \,, \tag{1}$$

where the translation parameters $t = (x, y, z)$ and rotation parameters $\varphi = (\alpha, \beta, \gamma)$ represent the center and the angles of rotation of the vertebra, respec-tively. Symmetrical volume pairs can be obtained by dividing the vertebral body with the following planes (Fig. 1):

- The mid-sagittal plane of the vertebral body splits the whole vertebra into symmetrical left and right parts, i.e. into the volume pair $I_x \leftrightarrow I'_x$.
- The mid-coronal plane of the vertebral body splits the vertebral body into symmetrical anterior and posterior parts, i.e. into the volume pair $I_y \leftrightarrow I'_y$.
- The mid-axial plane of the vertebral body splits the vertebral body into symmetrical cranial and caudal parts, i.e. into the volume pair $I_z \leftrightarrow I'_z$.

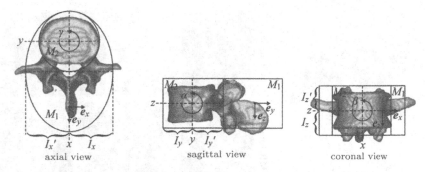

Fig. 1. By dividing the vertebral body with the mid-sagittal, mid-coronal and mid-axial planes, symmetrical volume pairs $I_x \leftrightarrow I_x'$, $I_y \leftrightarrow I_y'$ and $I_z \leftrightarrow I_z'$ are obtained, respectively. The symmetry captured within the vertebral masks M_1 and M_2 is used to determine the vertebral parameters $\boldsymbol{p} = (\boldsymbol{t}, \boldsymbol{\varphi}) = (x, y, z, \alpha, \beta, \gamma)$.

The proposed method is based on the assumption that, if the translation parameters $\boldsymbol{t}$ are defined by the center of the vertebral body and the rotation parameters $\boldsymbol{\varphi}$ are defined by the rotation of the vertebra, the vertebral parameters $\boldsymbol{p}$ can be obtained by evaluating the natural symmetry of vertebral anatomy.

2.2 Registration of Symmetrical Vertebral Parts

The volume of interest of each vertebra is masked by two elliptical cylinders, i.e. by two 3D vertebral masks M_1 and M_2, so that M_1 roughly encompasses the whole vertebra and M_2 roughly encompasses the vertebral body (Fig. 1). By dividing the masks with the mid-sagittal, mid-coronal and mid-axial planes, mirror volume pairs can be extracted from the 3D image. The extracted volume pairs contain symmetrical parts of vertebral anatomy $I_x \leftrightarrow I_x'$, $I_y \leftrightarrow I_y'$ and $I_z \leftrightarrow I_z'$ when the 3D vertebral masks are perfectly aligned with the vertebra, i.e. when the position and rotation of the 3D vertebral masks correspond to the vertebral parameters $\boldsymbol{p}$ (Eq. 1). The maximal symmetry of the volume pairs therefore yields the most correct estimation of the vertebral parameters $\boldsymbol{p}$.

The sagittal $(d = x)$, coronal $(d = y)$ and axial $(d = z)$ symmetry S of the volume pair $I_d \leftrightarrow I_d'$ is estimated by comparing the corresponding image intensity gradients in I_d and I_d' within the 3D vertebral mask M_i (Fig. 2a):

$$S\left(I_d, I_d'\right)\big|_{M_i} = -\frac{1}{K} \sum_{k=1}^{K} (\boldsymbol{v}_k \cdot \boldsymbol{m}_d)(\hat{\boldsymbol{v}}_k' \cdot \boldsymbol{m}_d) = \frac{1}{K} \sum_{k=1}^{K} |\boldsymbol{v}_k| |\boldsymbol{v}_k'| \cos\theta_k \cos\theta_k'. \quad (2)$$

In the equation above, K is the number of voxels in each volume, $\boldsymbol{v}_k$ is the gradient vector at the kth voxel in I_d, and $\boldsymbol{v}_k'$ is its corresponding gradient vector in I_d' ($\hat{\boldsymbol{v}}_k'$ is the vector $\boldsymbol{v}_k'$, mirrored from I_d' to I_d). θ_k and θ_k' are the angles of the gradient vectors $\boldsymbol{v}_k$ and $\boldsymbol{v}_k'$, respectively, against the unit vector $\boldsymbol{m}_d$, which denotes the direction of the estimated symmetry in the coordinate system of the 3D vertebral mask M_i. The symmetry S is therefore a measure of similarity between all corresponding intensity gradient vectors in I_d and I_d', projected in

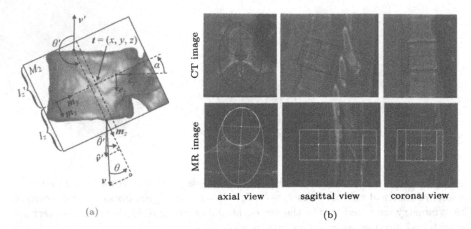

Fig. 2. (a) An illustrative example of the estimation of axial symmetry $S(I_z, I_z')$ for a single voxel within the vertebral mask M_2. (b) Examples of aligned 3D vertebral masks for a T7 vertebra from a CT (top) and an MR (bottom) spine image, shown in their mid-plane cross-sections.

the direction m_d of the estimated symmetry. The larger are the vectors and the more similar are their directions, the higher is the estimated symmetry.

The sum of symmetries over the mid-sagittal plane in M_1, the mid-coronal plane in M_2 and the mid-axial plane in M_2 represents the joint symmetry within the two 3D vertebral masks. To maximize the symmetry of the mirror volume pairs and yield the most correct estimation of the vertebral parameters p, the joint symmetry is used as the criterion function $CF = CF(p)$ for the rigid registration of the corresponding mirror volume pairs:

$$CF = S(I_x, I_x')\big|_{M_1} + S(I_y, I_y')\big|_{M_2} + S(I_z, I_z')\big|_{M_2}. \tag{3}$$

The maximum of the criterion function is reached at vertebral parameters p^{opt}, i.e. when the joint symmetry of the mirror volume pairs, obtained from the 3D vertebral masks, is maximal (Fig. 3).

3   Experiments and Results

3.1   Data and Experiments

The proposed method was evaluated on 26 vertebrae from two CT (voxel size $0.7 \times 0.7 \times 1.0$ mm) and on 26 vertebrae from two T_2-weighted MR (voxel size $0.4 \times 0.4 \times 3.0$ mm) spine images (Table 1). The images were filtered with a Gaussian kernel ($\sigma = 2$ mm) and the intensity gradients were computed for each voxel. For the purpose of quantitative evaluation of the method, the position and rotation of each vertebra were determined manually, yielding the manually determined vertebral parameters p_{man}. The vertebral parameters were normalized to the translation of $t = (1,1,1)$ mm and rotation of $\varphi = (2,2,2)$ degrees, which represented a translation of $p_N = (1,1,1,1,1,1)$ mm in the normalized

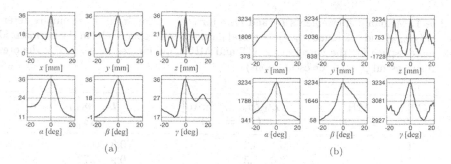

(a)   (b)

Fig. 3. The criterion function $CF = CF(p)$ (i.e. the joint symmetry within the two 3D vertebral masks), evaluated by displacing each of the reference vertebral parameters independently, shown for a T7 vertebra from (a) a CT and (b) an MR spine image. The criterion function has rather large capture ranges and distinctive maxima.

six-dimensional parameter space (displacement $D = \sqrt{6}$ mm). The direction set (Powell's) method in multidimensions ($N_{iter} = 4$, $f_{tol} = 10^{-5}$) was used as the optimization technique for the registration procedure. The 3D vertebral masks of the shape of elliptical cylinders $M_i = (a_i, b_i, c_i)$, where a_i and b_i are the corresponding ellipse half-axes and c_i is the corresponding cylinder half-height, were defined as $M_1 = (30, 50, 25)$ mm and $M_2 = (25, 25, 25)$ mm (Fig. 2b). Basing on vertebral morphometric data [5,22], such dimensions of 3D vertebral masks ensured that vertebrae of above average size would also be encompassed by the 3D vertebral masks.

Manual determination of vertebral parameters is a difficult and error-prone task, affected by the subjective interpretation of the observer, low image resolution, vertebral torsion, imperfect symmetry of vertebral structures and interdependence of parameters (i.e. the center of rotation affects the rotation angles). An initial experiment of $N_1 = 50$ registrations was therefore performed for each vertebra to obtain the reference vertebral parameters. The registrations were initialized in the manually determined vertebral parameters p_{man}, and the starting positions were defined as random displacements, uniformly distributed in the normalized parameter space (maximal displacement $D_{1,max} = 5$ mm). The median of the obtained results represented the reference vertebral parameters p_{ref}, which were used as initialization values in the main experiment of $N_2 = 500$ registrations for each vertebra (maximal displacement $D_{2,max} = 10$ mm). The results represented the basis for the quantitative evaluation of the proposed method.

3.2   Results

The results, presented for all vertebrae in Table 1 as displacements in the normalized parameter space, show that the method was successful on 23 out of 26 vertebrae from CT and on 20 out of 26 vertebrae from MR spine images. The cases of failure were detected by the large median displacement after the initial or main experiment ($\tilde{D} > 10$ mm). Visual verification indicated that the failures probably occurred due to anatomical structures such as ribs and arteries, which

Table 1. Median displacements $\tilde{D}_1$ and $\tilde{D}_2$ after registration from the manually determined (p_{man}) and reference (p_{ref}) vertebral parameters, respectively, in the normalized parameter space for the vertebrae in CT and MR spine images (the mark × denotes the unsuccessful parameter estimations)

CT 1	CT 2	MR 1	MR 2	$\tilde{D}_1 (p_{man})$ [mm] ($N_1 = 50$)				$\tilde{D}_2 (p_{ref})$ [mm] ($N_2 = 500$)			
T1	T1			3.1	3.3			0.8	0.9		
T2	T3			3.6	2.3			0.9	0.7		
T3	T3			2.5	5.0			1.0	1.6		
T4	T4			×	1.5			×	1.5		
T5	T5	T5	T5	3.5	2.5	3.2	3.0	0.7	×	×	1.3
T6	T6	T6	T6	4.6	2.0	4.4	×	0.7	1.1	×	×
T7	T7	T7	T7	2.0	3.0	3.0	1.9	0.9	1.0	1.2	0.9
T8	T8	T8	T8	2.2	3.7	1.9	1.9	1.0	2.5	1.1	0.7
T9	T9	T9	T9	2.2	1.9	3.0	2.7	1.2	1.6	2.3	1.4
T10	T10	T10	T10	1.7	2.6	2.7	4.2	1.0	2.4	1.7	×
T11	T11	T11	T11	2.3	3.9	2.4	3.3	0.7	×	1.2	×
T12	T12	T12	T12	1.1	1.1	1.4	3.9	0.7	0.8	0.8	×
	L1	L1	L1		2.4	4.9	3.3		0.4	0.7	2.5
	L2	L2	L2		1.6	1.9	2.4		0.7	2.3	2.4
		L3	L3			2.6	2.1			1.6	2.4
		L4	L4			3.8	2.8			0.9	1.9
		L5	L5			3.0	5.7			1.7	1.3
mean				2.6		3.0		1.1		1.5	

are less symmetrical than the vertebrae and therefore hamper the evaluation of the natural symmetry of vertebral anatomy. Besides, the symmetry over the axial plane $S(I_z, I_z')$ may reach a high value not only when the axial plane passes through the center of the vertebral body, but also when it passes through the adjacent intervertebral discs, thus affecting the computation of the joint symmetry (Eq. 3). Nevertheless, the method was successful for most vertebrae (43 out of 52; 83%), for which the mean of the median displacements after registration from the manually determined vertebral parameters p_{man} (initial experiment $N_1 = 50$) and from the reference vertebral parameters p_{ref} (main experiment $N_2 = 500$) was 2.8 mm and 1.3 mm, respectively. The results also show that the method is more accurate on CT spine images, which may be due to more distinctive intensity edges and higher image resolution in CT than in MR images used in the experiments.

Success rates, defined as the cumulative ratios of successful registrations against the overall number of registrations, were obtained from the scatter plots of the main registration experiment results (Fig. 4). A registration was considered successful when the displacement after registration was less than the threshold displacement $D_{thresh} = \sqrt{6} \approx 2.45$ mm in the normalized parameter

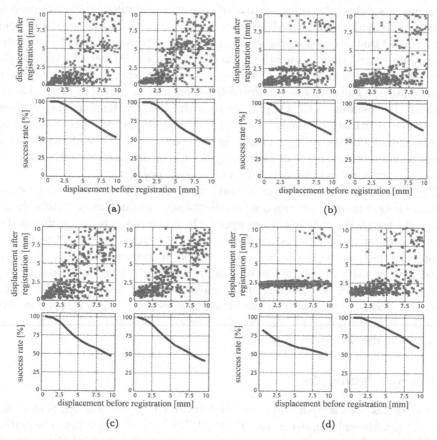

Fig. 4. Scatter plots of the displacements from the reference vertebral parameters p_{ref} in the normalized parameter space after the initial registration experiment ($N_1 = 50$, before the main registration experiment, left column) and after the main registration experiment ($N_2 = 500$, right column), and the corresponding success rates ($D_{thresh} = \sqrt{6} \approx 2.45$ mm). The results are shown for a T7 vertebra from (a) a CT and (b) an MR spine image, and for a T9 vertebra from (c) a CT and (d) an MR spine image.

space, which corresponds to the translation of $t = (1, 1, 1)$ mm and rotation of $\varphi = (2, 2, 2)$ degrees. The obtained success rates indicate that an arbitrary registration converged if the displacement was lower than $D_{conv} \approx 2.5$ mm, which corresponds to a translation of 2.5 mm in a single direction or a rotation of 5.0 degrees around a single axis from the reference vertebral parameters.

4 Discussion

The position and rotation of vertebrae are among the most important parameters in the quantitative evaluation of the deformities and disease processes that affect the spine, and are therefore valuable for the understanding of the nature of normal and pathological spine anatomy, monitoring of the progression of spinal deformities, surgical planning, and analysis of surgical results [20,23]. We propose and test a method for automated determination of the position and rotation of vertebrae in 3D that is based on registration of image intensity gradients, extracted from volume parts that capture the natural symmetry of vertebral anatomy. The proposed method is therefore not limited to a specific vertebral region, but takes into account the global characteristics of 3D vertebral anatomy. The method is also modality-independent, as it is applicable to both CT and MR spine images. Moreover, image reformation, manual selection of cross-sections and a priori knowledge in the form of statistical shape models is not required. The size of the vertebral masks was determined manually, however, it could be obtained by statistical analysis of the vertebral morphometric data of a larger population.

The results show that the position and rotation of vertebrae in 3D can be successfully determined by the proposed gradient-based evaluation of vertebral symmetry. Although the gradient-based approach, if compared to an approach that estimates the vertebral symmetry from image intensities, improves the distinctiveness of the maxima of the criterion function, a combination of the gradient-based and intensity-based approaches may result in a method of relatively high success rate and precision. Our future research will be focused on combining the proposed gradient-based with an intensity-based method and testing the method on normal and pathological (e.g. scoliotic) vertebrae in order to evaluate its performance in disease circumstances.

Acknowledgements

This work has been supported by the Ministry of Higher Education, Science and Technology, Slovenia, under grants P2-0232, L2-7381 and L2-9758. The author would like to thank the Commonwealth Scientific and Industrial Research Organisation (CSIRO), Australia, for providing the MR images used in this study.

References

1. Cobb, J.: Outline for the study of scoliosis. American Academy of Orthopaedic Surgeons Instructional Course Lectures 5, 261–275 (1948)
2. Shea, K., Stevens, P., Nelson, M., Smith, J., Masters, K., Yandow, S.: A comparison of manual versus computer-assisted radiographic measurement: Intraobserver measurement variability for Cobb angles. Spine 23(5), 551–555 (1998)
3. Chockalingam, N., Dangerfield, P., Giakas, G., Cochrane, T., Dorgan, J.: Computer-assisted Cobb measurement of scoliosis. European Spine Journal 11(4), 353–357 (2002)
4. Stokes, I., Aronsson, D.: Computer-assisted algorithms improve eliability of King classification and Cobb angle measurement of scoliosis. Spine 31(6), 665–670 (2006)
5. Bernhardt, M., Bridwell, K.: Segmental analysis of the sagittal plane lignment of the normal thoracic and lumbar spines and thoracolumbar junction. Spine 14(7), 717–721 (1989)
6. Polly, D., Kilkelly, F., McHale, K., Asplund, L., Mulligan, M., Chang, A.: Measurement of lumbar lordosis: Evaluation of intraobserver, interobserver, and technique variability. Spine 21(13), 1530–1535 (1996)

7. Harrison, D., Harrison, D., Cailliet, R., Janik, T., Holland, B.: Radiographic analysis of lumbar lordosis: Centroid, Cobb, TRALL, and Harrison posterior tangent methods. Spine 26(11), E235–E242 (2001)
8. Pinel-Giroux, F.M., Mac-Thiong, J.M., de Guise, J., Berthonnaud, E., Labelle, H.: Computerized assessment of sagittal curvatures of the spine: Comparison between Cobb and tangent circles techniques. Journal of Spinal Disorders & Techniques 19(7), 507–512 (2006)
9. Aaro, S., Dahlborn, M.: Estimation of vertebral rotation and the spinal and rib cage deformity in scoliosis by computer-tomography. Spine 6(5), 460–467 (1981)
10. Ho, E., Upadhyay, S., Chan, F., Hsu, L., Leong, J.: New methods of measuring vertebral rotation from computed tomographic scans: An intraobserver and interobserver study on girls with scoliosis. Spine 18(9), 1173–1177 (1993)
11. Skalli, W., Lavaste, F., Descrimes, J.L.: Quantification of three-dimensional vertebral rotations in scoliosis: What are the true values? Spine 20(5), 546–553 (1995)
12. Krismer, M., Sterzinger, W., Christian, H., Frischhut, B., Bauer, R.: Axial rotation measurement of scoliotic vertebrae by means of computed tomography scans. Spine 21(5), 576–581 (1996)
13. Birchall, D., Hughes, D., Hindle, J., Robinson, L., Williamson, J.: Measurement of vertebral rotation in adolescent idiopathic scoliosis using three-dimensional magnetic resonance imaging. Spine 22(20), 2403–2407 (1997)
14. Hecquet, J., Legaye, J., Duval-Beaupère, G.: Access to a three-dimensional measure of vertebral axial rotation. European Spine Journal 7(3), 206–211 (1998)
15. Kouwenhoven, J.W., Vincken, K., Bartels, L., Castelein, R.: Analysis of preexistent vertebral rotation in the normal spine. Spine 31(13), 1467–1472 (2006)
16. Rogers, B., Haughton, V., Arfanakis, K., Meyerand, E.: Application of image registration to measurement of intervertebral rotation in the lumbar spine. Magnetic Resonance in Medicine 48(6), 1072–1075 (2002)
17. Benameur, S., Mignotte, M., Labelle, H., De Guise, J.: A hierarchical statistical modeling approach for the unsupervised 3-D biplanar reconstruction of the scoliotic spine. IEEE Transactions on Bio-medical Engineering 52(12), 2041–2057 (2005)
18. Adam, C., Askin, G.: Automatic measurement of vertebral rotation in idiopathic scoliosis. Spine 31(3), E80–E83 (2006)
19. Molnár, S., Manó, S., Kiss, L., Csernátony, Z.: Ex vivo and in vitro determination of the axial rotational axis of the human thoracic spine. Spine 31(26), E984–E991 (2006)
20. Petit, Y., Aubin, C.E., Labelle, H.: Spinal shape changes resulting from scoliotic spine surgical instrumentation expressed as intervertebral rotations and centers of rotation. Journal of Biomechanics 37(2), 173–180 (2004)
21. Vrtovec, T., Likar, B., Pernuš, F.: Determination of 3D location and rotation of lumbar vertebrae in CT images by symmetry-based auto-registration. In: Pluim, J., Reinhardt, J. (eds.) Proceedings of the SPIE Medical Imaging 2007: Image Processing Conference. SPIE, vol. 6512 (2007) 65121Q–1
22. Masharawi, Y., Salame, K., Mirovsky, Y., Peleg, S., Dar, G., Steinberg, N., Hershkovitz, I.: Vertebral body shape variation in the thoracic and lumbar spine: Characterization of its asymmetry and wedging. Clinical Anatomy 21(1), 46–54 (2008)
23. Mac-Thiong, J., Labelle, H., Vandal, S., Aubin, C.: Intra-operative tracking of the trunk during surgical correction of scoliosis: A feasibility study. Computer Aided Surgery 5(5), 333–342 (2000)

Coupled Meshfree-BEM Platform for Electrocardiographic Simulation: Modeling and Validations

Linwei Wang[1], Heye Zhang[2], Ken C.L. Wong[1], and Pengcheng Shi[1]

[1] Golisano College of Computing and Information Science
Rochester Institute of Technology, Rochester, New York
maomaowlw@mail.rit.edu
[2] Bioengineering Institute, University of Auckland, Auckland

Abstract. The foremost premise for the success of noninvasive volumetric myocardial transmembrane (TMP) imaging from body surface potential (BSP) recordings is a realistic yet efficient electrocardiographic model which relates volumetric myocardial TMP distributions to BSP distributions. With a view towards the inverse problem, appropriate model simplifications should be emphasized to balance the accuracy of the model with the feasibility of the inversion. In this paper, we present a novel coupled meshfree-BEM platform to represent the combined heart-torso structure and derive the associated TMP-to-BSP models. The numerical accuracy and convergency of the presented approach is verified against analytic solutions on a synthetic geometry. The associated simplifications are justified by comparing models at different level of complexity, which further demonstrates the benefits of homogeneous torso assumption in the inverse problem. Initial simulation experiments on a realistic heart-torso structure further show the physiological plausibility of the presented approach.

1 Introduction

For the success of noninvasive imaging of volumetric myocardial transmembrane potentials (TMPs) from body surface potential (BSP) recordings, the electrocardiographic model is the essential premise to link volumetric myocardial TMP distributions with BSP distributions at any time instant. In order to balance the accuracy of the model with the feasibility of the inversion, particular simplifications should be assumed with a view towards the inverse problem. The plausibility of these simplifications requires sufficient justifications to pave the road for the inverse study.

The common approach to establish the TMP-to-BSP relationship starts from the biodomain theory, where any point in the myocardium is considered to be in either the intra- or extra-cellular space, separated by a theoretical membrane of zero thickness [1]. Usually, the bidomain model is reduced to a boundary element (BE) formulation by ignoring the conductive anisotropy and inhomogeneity in both spaces [2]. As a result, TMP reconstructions have to be confined to heart

T. Dohi, I. Sakuma, and H. Liao (Eds.): MIAR 2008, LNCS 5128, pp. 98–107, 2008.
© Springer-Verlag Berlin Heidelberg 2008

surfaces. In contrast, by considering the electrical anisotropy in both spaces, the finite element (FE) formulation is able to investigate volumetric electrical conduction within the myocardial mass [3]. Nevertheless, the problem size is unnecessarily enlarged by the involvement of myocardial extracellular potential, which is of no direct relevance to the inverse problem. Combining the advantages of above approaches by emphasizing the electrical anisotropy for the active current conduction but neglecting that for passive currents, we could avoid redundant variables and get a formulation particularly beneficial to the inverse purpose.

With regard to the torso representation and its impacts on forward/inverse problems, the consensus has been reached that the geometry is the leading factor compared to material property [4,5]. To reduce model complexity, therefore, it is reasonable to emphasize the accuracy of geometrical modeling and relax unnecessary restrictions on tissue inhomogeneity . The corresponding simplified models should be carefully validated before being used in inverse studies.

Following this spirit, we present a novel coupled meshfree-BEM platform to represent the combined heart-torso structure and construct the TMP-to-BSP model oriented for the inverse problem. The accuracy and convergency of this numerical approach is quantitatively assessed against analytical solutions on a carefully designed synthetic geometry. Models with different levels of complexity are compared, through which the benefits of the homogeneous torso model is justified. The physiological plausibility of the model is then demonstrated by initial simulation experiments on a realistic heart-torso structure customized from MRIs of a specific subject. This study prepares and validates a proper platform of electrocardiographic modeling for the use in inverse studies.

2 Method

2.1 Physical Descriptions of TMP-to-BSP Relationship

Because of the relatively low frequencies (0-100 Hz) in electrocardiograms, the inductive, capacitative and propagation effects can be ignored in biological tissues. The quasi-static approximation of Maxwell's equations, therefore, describes how active cardiac sources determine potential distributions within the torso.

Within the myocardium volume, the bidomain theory [1] defines the distribution of extracellular potentials ϕ_e as:

$$\nabla\cdot((\mathbf{D}_i(\mathbf{r})+\mathbf{D}_e(\mathbf{r}))\nabla\phi_e(\mathbf{r})) = \nabla\cdot(\mathbf{D}_k(\mathbf{r})\nabla\phi_e(\mathbf{r})) = \nabla\cdot(-\mathbf{D}_i(\mathbf{r})\nabla u(\mathbf{r})) \quad \forall \mathbf{r} \in \Omega_h \tag{1}$$

where $\mathbf{r}$ stands for the spatial coordinate, u for TMP and Ω_h for the myocardium volume. $\mathbf{D}_i$ and $\mathbf{D}_e$ are the effective intracellular and extracellular conductivity tensor, and their summations $\mathbf{D}_k$ is termed as the bulk conductivity tensor.

In regions bounded by the heart surface and body surface, potentials ϕ_t are calculated assuming that no other active electrical source exists within the torso:

$$\nabla \cdot (\mathbf{D}_t(\mathbf{r})\nabla\phi_t(\mathbf{r})) = 0 \qquad \forall \mathbf{r} \in \Omega_{t/h} \tag{2}$$

where $\mathbf{D}_t$ is the torso conductivity tensor and $\Omega_{t/h}$ the entire thorax except Ω_h.

With the anisotropic ratio of $\mathbf{D}_k$ being a magnitude smaller than that of $\mathbf{D}_i$, the myocardial electrical anisotropy is predominated by the intracellular domain. Therefore, we only retain the anisotropy of $\mathbf{D}_i$ to reduce model complexity and $\mathbf{D}_k, \mathbf{D}_t$ become scalars σ_k, σ_t. With regard to the conductive inhomogeneity among torso tissues, we propose the use of homogeneous torso model in inverse studies to reduce the size of this problem. To justify such assumption, comparisons should be carried out among formulations with different levels of simplifications on (1) and (2). In this initial study, we consider 2 different simplified formulations.

Formulation 1. Formulation 1 ($F1$) assumes Ω_h and $\Omega_{t/h}$ as homogeneous conductors but preserves their conductivity difference ($\sigma_k \neq \sigma_t$). It reduces (1) and (2) into a Poisson equation (3) and a homogeneous Laplace equation (4) respectively:

$$\sigma_k \nabla^2 \phi_e(\mathbf{r})) = \nabla \cdot (-\mathbf{D}_i(\mathbf{r})\nabla u(\mathbf{r})) \qquad \forall \mathbf{r} \in \Omega_h \qquad (3)$$

$$\sigma_t \nabla^2 \phi_t(\mathbf{r}) = 0 \qquad \forall \mathbf{r} \in \Omega_{t/h} \qquad (4)$$

The associated boundary condition on the heart surface Γ_h is defined to preserve the continuity of potentials and currents on this interface:

$$\phi_e(\mathbf{r}) = \phi_t(\mathbf{r}), \qquad \sigma_k \frac{\partial \phi_e(\mathbf{r})}{\partial n} + \mathbf{D}_i \frac{\partial u(\mathbf{r})}{\partial n} = \sigma_t \frac{\partial \phi_t(\mathbf{r})}{\partial n} \qquad \forall(\mathbf{r}) \in \Gamma_h \qquad (5)$$

Similarly it is assumed that no current (flux) leaves the torso surface Γ_t:

$$\frac{\partial \phi_t(\mathbf{r})}{\partial n} = 0 \qquad \forall \mathbf{r} \in \Gamma_t \qquad (6)$$

where n stands for the outward normal of a surface.

Formulation 2. Formulation ($F2$) assumes $\sigma_k = \sigma_t = \sigma$ to simplify the torso into a homogeneous volume conductor Ω_t. Accordingly, $F1$ (3, 4) is unified into a single Poisson equation describing potential distribution ($\phi(\mathbf{r})$) within Ω_t:

$$\sigma \nabla^2 \phi(\mathbf{r})) = \nabla \cdot (-\mathbf{D}_i(\mathbf{r})\nabla u(\mathbf{r})) \quad \forall \mathbf{r} \in \Omega_t \qquad (7)$$

where Ω_t includes $\Omega_{t/h}$ and Ω_h but without interface in between. Boundary condition (6) still applies on the body surface .

2.2   TMP-to-BSP Model

By coupling the BEM [6] and meshfree method [7], our approach provides a general way to establish TMP-to-BSP relations for torso models at different levels of complexity. In this paper we describe and compare the results for $F1$ and $F2$. Models including more tissue inhomogeneity could be obtained following the same line, but with more redundant variables and increased complexity.

F1. By the *direct method* solution in BEM [6], equation (3) is reformulated into:

$$c(\xi)\phi_e(\xi) + \int_{\Gamma_h} \phi_e(\mathbf{r})q^*(\xi,\mathbf{r})\,\mathrm{d}\Gamma_h - \int_{\Gamma_h} (\frac{\partial\phi_e(\mathbf{r})}{\partial n})\phi^*(\xi,\mathbf{r})\,\mathrm{d}\Gamma_h$$
$$= \int_{\Omega_h} \frac{(\nabla\cdot(\mathbf{D}_i(\mathbf{r})\nabla u(\mathbf{r})))\phi^*(\xi,\mathbf{r})}{\sigma_k}\,\mathrm{d}\Omega_h \qquad (8)$$

where $c(\xi)$ is related to the surface smoothness at any point ξ on Γ_h. $\phi^*(\xi,\mathbf{r})$ and $q^*(\xi,\mathbf{r})$ are the so-called fundamental solution and its normal derivative.

The volume integral on the right hand side (rhs) of (8) is commonly approximated as a summarization of several current dipoles [8]. Instead, we introduce the meshfree strategy into above boundary integral formulation for a simpler yet more direct approximation of the volume integral. With the Green theorem and the integral by part, the rhs of (8) is easily written as:

$$\int_{\Gamma_h} (\frac{\phi^*(\xi,\mathbf{r})}{\sigma_k})\mathbf{D}_i(\mathbf{r})\frac{\partial u(\mathbf{r})}{\partial n}\,\mathrm{d}\Gamma_h - \int_{\Omega_h} (\frac{\nabla\phi^*(\xi,\mathbf{r})}{\sigma_k})\cdot\mathbf{D}_i(\mathbf{r})\nabla u(\mathbf{r})\,\mathrm{d}\Omega_h \qquad (9)$$

By the boundary conditions (5), the first term of (9) is equivalent to:

$$\int_{\Gamma_h} \frac{\phi^*(\xi,\mathbf{r})}{\sigma_k}(\sigma_t\frac{\partial\phi_t(\mathbf{r})}{\partial n} - \sigma_k\frac{\partial\phi_e(\mathbf{r})}{\partial n})\,\mathrm{d}\Omega_h \qquad (10)$$

With equivalent terms on the lhs and rhs eliminated, equation (8) becomes:

$$c(\xi)\phi_e(\xi) + \int_{\Gamma_h} \phi_e(\mathbf{r})q^*(\xi,\mathbf{r})\,\mathrm{d}\Gamma_h - \int_{\Gamma_h} \frac{\sigma_t}{\sigma_k}\phi^*(\xi,\mathbf{r})\frac{\partial\phi_t(\mathbf{r})}{\partial n}\,\mathrm{d}\Gamma_h$$
$$= -\int_{\Omega_h} (\frac{\nabla\phi^*(\xi,\mathbf{r})}{\sigma_k})\cdot\mathbf{D}_i(\mathbf{r})\nabla u(\mathbf{r})\,\mathrm{d}\Omega_h \qquad (11)$$

Applying the BEM [6] to the boundary integral and the meshfree strategy [7] to the volume integral, we get a compact matrix formulation for (11):

$$\mathbf{K}_h\mathbf{\Phi}_e + \mathbf{P}_h\mathbf{Q}_{et} = \mathbf{BU} \qquad (12)$$

where $\mathbf{\Phi}_e, \mathbf{Q}_{et}$ consist of ϕ_e and $\frac{\partial\phi_t}{\partial n}$ from N_h vertices on Γ_h, and $\mathbf{U}$ contains u on M meshfree nodes. $\mathbf{K}_h$ and $\mathbf{P}_h$ are $N_h \times N_h$ matrices constructed by the BEM and $\mathbf{B}$ an $N_h \times M$ matrix from the meshfree method. Similarly, equation (4) could be written in a boundary integral formulation as:

$$c(\xi)\phi_t(\xi) + \int_{\Gamma_{t/h}} \phi_t(\mathbf{r})q^*(\xi,\mathbf{r})\,\mathrm{d}\Gamma_{t/h} = \int_{\Gamma_{t/h}} (\frac{\partial\phi_t(\mathbf{r})}{\partial n})\phi^*(\xi,\mathbf{r})\,\mathrm{d}\Gamma_{t/h} \qquad (13)$$

where $\Gamma_{t/h}$ is the boundary of $\Omega_{t/h}$ and includes Γ_h and Γ_t. Note that, nevertheless, the outward normal direction of Γ_h in $\Gamma_{t/h}$ is opposite to that of Γ_h used in solving (3). By the BEM, (13) becomes:

$$\mathbf{K}_t\mathbf{\Phi}_t + \mathbf{P}_t\mathbf{Q}_t = 0 \qquad (14)$$

where $\mathbf{\Phi}_t = (\mathbf{\Phi}_{te}^T\ \mathbf{\Phi}^T)^T$ and $\mathbf{Q}_t = (\mathbf{Q}_{te}^T\ \mathbf{Q}^T)^T$. $\mathbf{\Phi}_{te}$, $\mathbf{Q}_{te}$ include ϕ_t, $\frac{\partial\phi_t}{\partial n}$ from N_h vertices of Γ_h, and $\mathbf{\Phi}$, $\mathbf{Q}$ consist of ϕ_t, $\frac{\partial\phi_t}{\partial n}$ from N_t vertices of Γ_t.

According to the boundary condition on Γ_h (5), we have:

$$\mathbf{\Phi}_{te} = \mathbf{\Phi}_e \tag{15}$$

$$\mathbf{Q}_{te} = -\mathbf{Q}_{et} \tag{16}$$

The minus in (16), as aforementioned, is caused by the opposite outward normal direction for the boundaries of Ω_h and $\Omega_{t/h}$.

Coupling (12) and (14) on Γ_h by (15,16) and matrix reassembling, we obtain the relation between volumetric myocardial TMPs (**U**) and BSPs (**$\mathbf{\Phi}$**) as:

$$\left(\left(\mathbf{K}_h\ \mathbf{0}\right) + \left(\mathbf{P}_h\ \mathbf{0}\right)\mathbf{P}_t^{-1}\mathbf{K}_t\right)\begin{pmatrix}\mathbf{\Phi}_e\\\mathbf{\Phi}\end{pmatrix} = \mathbf{B}\mathbf{U} \tag{17}$$

In (17), the extracellular potential $\mathbf{\Phi}_e$ is of no direct interests to the inverse problem, though its high dimensionality will largely increase the computational requirement and numerical difficulty of this model.

F2. Following the same line, the *direct method* solution [6] reformulates equation (7) into:

$$c(\xi)\phi(\xi) + \int_{\Gamma_t}\phi(\mathbf{r})q^*(\xi,\mathbf{r})\,d\Gamma_t - \int_{\Gamma_t}(\frac{\partial\phi(\mathbf{r})}{\partial n})\phi^*(\xi,\mathbf{r})\,d\Gamma_t \tag{18}$$

$$= \int_{\Gamma_t}(\frac{\phi^*(\xi,\mathbf{r})}{\sigma})\mathbf{D}_i(\mathbf{r})\frac{\partial u(\mathbf{r})}{\partial n}\,d\Gamma_t - \int_{\Omega_t}(\frac{\nabla\phi^*(\xi,\mathbf{r})}{\sigma})\cdot\mathbf{D}_i(\mathbf{r})\nabla u(\mathbf{r})\,d\Omega_t$$

By boundary condition (6) and the assumption of no active source current leaving Γ_t, the 3rd terms on the lhs and the 1st term on the rhs of (18) are removed. By the BEM and meshfree method, equation (18) links **U** with **$\mathbf{\Phi}$** as::

$$\mathbf{K}\mathbf{\Phi} = \mathbf{B}\mathbf{U} \tag{19}$$

where **K** ($N_t \times N_t$) is constructed from the boundary integral and **B** ($N_t \times M$) from the meshfree method. Since the solution of **$\mathbf{\Phi}$** to (19) given **U** is underdetermined, $\mathbf{A}\mathbf{\Phi} = \mathbf{0}$ is imposed to define the potential integral over Γ_t as zero, where **A** is a $1 \times N_t$ vector. Augmenting **K** into $\mathbf{K}_a$ with **A** and **B** into $\mathbf{B}_a$ with the corresponding all-zero row, we rearrange (19) into:

$$\mathbf{K}_a\mathbf{\Phi} = \mathbf{B}_a\mathbf{U} \tag{20}$$

To avoid the additional computation of solving the linear system of (20) during the inversion, minimal norm (MN) method is applied to get:

$$\mathbf{\Phi} = (\mathbf{K}_a^T\mathbf{K}_a)^{-1}\mathbf{K}_a^T\mathbf{B}_a\mathbf{U} = \mathbf{H}\mathbf{U} \tag{21}$$

where the transfer matrix **H** encodes all the anatomical and electrophysiological information in the patient-specific heart and torso structure. Compared to $F1$, $F2$ seizes primary interests in the inverse problem without involving excessive variables.

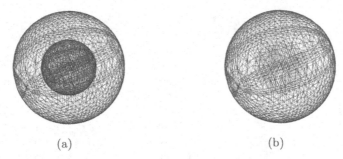

(a)   (b)

Fig. 1. Concentric spheres on coupled meshfree-BEM platform for formulation 1 (a) and formulation 2 (b). In both formulations, the inner sphere is described by a cloud of meshfree points, and the outer sphere by triangulated surface. In addition, the inner spherical surface is discretized into triangular elements in formulation 1.

3   Results

3.1   Analytic Validation and Convergence Analysis

Geometry setup and analytic solutions. By introducing appropriate simplifications into the geometry and fiber structure, it is possible to get analytic solutions for (1, 2). Two concentric spheres are used as an analogue to the heart-torso model. The inner sphere (radius $r \leq R$) has intracellular conductivity tensor $\mathbf{D}_i$ and extracellular conductivity scalar σ_k, while the outer annular region ($R < r \leq 3R$) has isotropic conductivity σ_t. Conductivity values are adopted from [9]. The spatial distribution of TMP is described in the spherical coordinate (r, φ, θ) as:

$$u(r, \varphi, \theta) = -\frac{r}{R} \cos \varphi \tag{22}$$

The solution of Laplace equation (4) can be readily obtained by the separation of variables. To make the Poisson equation (3) analytically solvable, the fiber structure is defined in such a way that the rhs of (3) becomes zero. Firstly, the fiber orientation for any point is assumed as tangential to the spherical surface it lies on, thus defined by the angle α away from the circumferential direction. Secondly, since $\sin^2 \alpha = 0$ is required to satisfy $\nabla \cdot (\mathbf{D}_i \nabla u) = 0$, the fiber orientation is defined as circumferential at any point. With boundary conditions (5) and (6), analytic solutions to (3) and (4) on this synthetic geometry are:

$$\phi_e(r, \varphi, \theta) = \frac{29\sigma_{it}}{29\sigma_k + 52\sigma_t} \frac{r}{R} \cos \varphi \quad (0 \leq r \leq R) \tag{23}$$

$$\phi_t(r, \varphi, \theta) = \frac{54\sigma_{it}}{29\sigma_k + 52\sigma_t} \left(\frac{r}{27R} + \frac{R^2}{2r^2}\right) \cos \varphi \quad (R \leq r \leq 3R)$$

where σ_{i_t} denotes the transverse component of the local conductivity tensor.

Convergence analysis. The coupled meshfree-BEM representation of the concentric spheres for $F1$ and $F2$ are shown in Fig 1. The accuracy of the results are

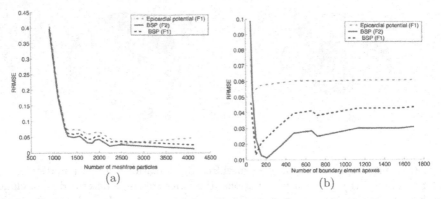

Fig. 2. Convergence analysis. (a) RRMSE of the numeric solutions against analytic solutions with increasing number of meshfree points (900-2200) in the inner sphere. (b) RRMSE of the numeric solutions against analytic solutions with increasing number of vertices (50-1800) on the outer surface. Each figure compares RRMSE of the numeric solutions of BSP computed from $F1$ (dashed blue), epicardial potentials from $F1$ (dash-dotted green) and BSP from $F2$ (solid red).

measured by the relative root mean squared errors (RRMSE) between numerical and analytic solutions. Results for BSPs computed from $F1$, $F2$ and epicardial potentials from $F1$ are analyzed. As we observed, the additional error caused by the assumption of $\sigma_k = \sigma_t$ in $F2$ could be reduced or eliminated by simply varying the nominal value of σ as of intermediate values of σ_k and σ_t. Particularly in this analytic test, $\sigma = (5\sigma_k + 7\sigma_t)/12$ is the exact value to remove this error and used in the following computations.

Fig 2 (a) depicts the convergence of the presented approach against increasing resolution of meshfree representation. The inner surface is represented by 2264 triangles and the outer surface by 3402 triangles. The number of meshfree nodes in the inner sphere increases from around 900 to 2200. As demonstrated, all the RMSEs converge fast towards 5% when the number of meshfree nodes increase up to 1200, and keep steady decreases thereafter. Fig 2 (b) illustrates the convergence of the approach against increasing resolution of BE representation. The number of meshfree points is fixed at a value (1843) which produces small errors while keep reasonable computational efficiency. The number of vertices on the outer surface ranges from 50 to 1800. Even with a very coarse surface representation with about 50 vertices, the RMSE is less that 10%. This shows that in comparison, the resolution of meshfree representation has much more impacts on the model accuracy. Besides, the minimum of all the curves in Fig. 2 (b) might indicate an *optimal* match between the resolution of the meshfree and BE representation.

As shown in both studies, when the additional error caused by $\sigma_k = \sigma_t$ is completely compensated by σ, $F2$ shows higher accuracy than $F1$ because of the larger numeric difficulty in $F1$. In practice, a careful choice of σ based on experimental studies could reduce the error associated with $\sigma_k = \sigma_t$ at no expense of additional computational complexity. The gain of computational reduction

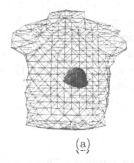
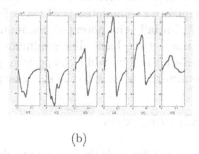

(a)   (b)

Fig. 3. (a), Realistic heart-torso model customized from MRIs of a specific subject. The ventricles are represented by meshfree nodes and the torso by triangulated body surface. (b), Simulated normal QRS morphology of lead $V1$ - $V6$. The potential values are scaled.

and numerical accuracy versus the compensable errors it introduces, therefore, justify the benefits of the homogeneous torso model in inverse problems.

3.2   BSP Maps and ECG Simulations

As an initial demonstration of the physiological plausibility of the TMP-to-BSP model derived from $F2$, simulation studies of normal cardiac activation are performed on a realistic hear-torso model (Fig 3 (a)). MRIs and anatomical locations of the electrodes on the body surface are provided by the PhysioNet Project [10]. Volumetric cardiac electrical activity throughout the heart is simulated by the simple two-variable reaction-diffusion model in [11]. The values for the tissue conductivities are adopted from [9]. Since the ventricular conduction system is absent in current heart model, the first-excited ventricular areas are determined according to the experimental study of [12]. The simulated 6 precordial leads are listed in Fig 3 (b). $V1$ shows a dominant negative defect and $V3 - V6$ display dominant positivity. Besides, R-wave progression is observed that positive R wave increases in amplitude and duration from $V1$ to $V4$. Similarly, the S-wave progression is exhibited as the negative S wave being large in $V1$, larger in $V2$, and then progressively smaller from $V3$ through $V6$. All these features

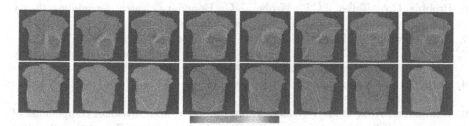

Fig. 4. Simulated temporal sequence of BSP isochrone maps for normal cardiac electrical activation. Top: the front view of the thorax. Bottom: the corresponding back view of the thorax. The color bar encodes BSP values.

agree with the established normal ECG morphology [13]. Fig 4 shows temporal sequence of simulated BSP maps for the ventricular activation. As reported in [14], initially the potential maximum resides on the anterior thorax and the minimum on the back. The minimum then moves over the right shoulder onto the anterior region, while the positive potentials cover the back. In the end, the maximum rotate back to the superior part of the chest.

4   Conclusions

With a view towards the inverse problem, this paper represents a novel coupled meshfree-BEM platform to represent the combined heart-torso model and derive the associated TMP-to-BSP model which directly relate volumetric myocardial TMP distributions to BSP distributions. As demonstrated, by proper simplifications in the presented approach, the computational burden caused by the large-scale TMP-to-BSP modeling is reduced, while the most significant components are preserved to keep the model plausibility. Validated by analytical and simulation studies, the presented platform of electrocardiographic modeling paves the road for the noninvasive imaging of volumetric myocardial TMPs from BSPs.

References

1. Henriquez, C.S.: Simulating the electrical behaviour of cardiac tissue using the bidomain model. Crit. Rev. Biomed. Eng. 21, 1–77 (1993)
2. Fischer, G., Tilg, B., Wach, P., Lafter, G., Rucker, W.: Analytical validation of the bem-application of the bem to the electrocardiographic forward and inverse problem. Comput. Methods Programs Biomed. 55, 99–106 (1998)
3. Fischer, G., Tilg, B., Modre, R., Huiskamp, G.J.M., Fetzer, J., Rucker, W., Wach, P.: A bidomain model based bem-fem coupling formulation for anisotropic cardiac tissue. AMBE 28, 1229–1243 (2000)
4. Brandley, C.P., Pullan, A.J., Hunter, P.J.: Effects of material properties and geometry on electrocardiographic forward simulations. Ann. Biomed. Eng. 28, 721–741 (2000)
5. Cheng, L.K., Bodley, J.M., Pullan, A.J.: The effect of experimental and modeling errors on the electrocardiographic inverse problem. IEEE Trans. Biomed. Eng. (1)
6. Brebbia, C.A., Telles, J.C.F., Wrobel, L.C.: Boundary element techniques: theory and applications in engineering. Springer, Heidelberg (1984)
7. Liu, G.: Meshfree Methods. CRC Press, Boca Raton (2003)
8. Barnard, A.C.L., Duck, I.M., Lynn, M.L.: The application of electromagentic theroy to electrocardiology. Biophys J. 7, 443–462 (1967)
9. Roth, B.J.: Electrical conductivity values used with the bidomain model of cardiac tissue. IEEE Trans. Biomed. Eng. 44(4), 326–328 (1997)
10. Goldberger, A.L., et al.: Physiobank, physiotoolkit, and physionet components of a new research resource for complex physiological signals. Cric. 101, e215–e220 (2000)
11. Aliev, R.R., Panfilov, A.V.: A simple two-variable model of cardiac excitation. Chaos, Solitions & Fractals 7(3), 293–301 (1996)

12. Durrur, D., Dam, R., Freud, G., Janse, M., Meijler, F., Arzbaecher, R.: Total excitation of the isolated human heart. Comp. Methods Appl. Mech. Eng. 41(6), 899–912 (1970)
13. Wagner, G.S.: Marriott's practical electrocardiography. Lippincott williams & wilkins, Philadelphia (2001)
14. Simelius, K.: Modeling cardiac ventricular activation. Int J. Bioelectromagnetism 3, 51–58 (2001)

Source Localization of Subtopographies Decomposed by Radial Basis Functions

Adil Deniz Duru and Ahmet Ademoglu

Biomedical Engineering Institute, Bogazici University
deniz.duru@boun.edu.tr

Abstract. Functional neuroimaging methods give the opportunity of investigating human brain functioning. Mostly used functional neuroimaging techniques include Electroencephalogram (EEG), functional magnetic resonance imaging (fMRI), positron emission tomography (PET) and optical imaging. Among these techniques EEG has the best time resolution, while fMRI has the best spatial resolution. High temporal resolution of EEG is an attractive property for neuroimaging studies. EEG inverse problem is needed to be solved in order to identify the locations and the strength of the electrical sources forming EEG/ERP topographies. Low spatial resolution of the scalp topography causes this localization problem more complicated. In this paper, a spatial preprocessing method, which separates a topography into two or more subtopographies is proposed. The decomposition procedure is based on defining a spatial map with radial basis functions which forms the subtopographies. A simulated data is used to exhibit the advantage of using this decomposition technique prior to EEG source localization. It is shown that the accuracy of the source localization problem is improved by using the subtopographies instead of using the raw topography.

Keywords: Subtopography, radial basis function, source localization.

1 Introduction

EEG is a record of the oscillations of brain electric potential recorded from the electrodes placed on the human scalp. Using these records, very rapid changes in electrical potentials can be measured. Hence, EEG is valuable for studying the timing of brain processes. Spatial distribution of the functional brain activity can be estimated by solving the neuroelectromagnetic inverse problem [1][2][3][4]. This problem has two types of solution; parametric and imaging. In the parametric solutions, brain electrical activity is modelled using a few number of electrical dipoles[5]. On the other hand, imaging type solutions try to estimate the activity using all possible spatial locations distributed in the brain[6]. The brain acitivity which is focal or distributed in space and nonstationary in time, motivated researchers to develop preprocessing methods before they apply source localization algorithms. The problem of identifying the individual EEG components in temporal domain are treated by proposing decomposition methods that involve the time, the frequency, the channel or their various combinations[8][7][9].

T. Dohi, I. Sakuma, and H. Liao (Eds.): MIAR 2008, LNCS 5128, pp. 108–115, 2008.
© Springer-Verlag Berlin Heidelberg 2008

In the spatial domain, EEG topographic maps are analyzed using 2D wavelet decomposition[10].

In this paper, a spatial preprocessing method is proposed prior to source localization algorithm. The method is based on defining the EEG topography with two or more subtopographies. A radial basis function is used to fit the raw topography by solving a non-linear least square optimization problem. This radial basis function formed the first subtopograpy and denoted as approximation while the remaining topography is assigned as the second subtopograpy which is called as detail or residual. Then electrical sources of these subtopographies are estimated by using Multiple Signal Classification algorithm (MUSIC) and standarized Low Resolution Electrical Tomography (sLORETA). The results of the subtopographic localization agreed with the simulation parameters while the localization of raw topographies biased the simulation parameters.

2   EEG Source Localization

EEG source localization problem is formulated in two stages; i)the forward and ii)the inverse problem. Forward problem is to determine the electrical potentials given the source location and strength parameters using a head model. Inverse problem, estimate these parameters from the measurements.

2.1   Forward Problem

Forward problem is defined to compute the electrial potential distribution over the scalp surface based on a head model. The head model is developped using average T1 weighted human brain MR data provided by Montreal Neurology Institute (MNI). Statistical Parameter Mapping software 2005 release (SPM05) which is developed by Wellcome Institute is used for 3D segmentation of the brain, skull and scalp.

The forward problem is solved by the Boundary Element Method (BEM) [12] which is a numerical approximation technique which partitions the surface of a volume conductor into closed triangular meshes. The human head is modelled as three homogeneous conductor layers; the outermost surface being the boundary of the scalp, and the intermediate and the innermost being the one for the skull and the brain, respectively. In order to apply the BEM, a realistic head model is formed and its surfaces are tesselated into triangles using marching cubes algorithm [11] as seen in Fig.2.1.

Finally, 30 channel electrode locations (Fp1, Fp2, F7, F3, Fz, F4, F8, Ft7, Fc3, Fcz, Fc4, Ft8, T7, C3, Cz, C4, T8, Tp7, Cp3, Cpz, Cp4, Tp8, P7, P3, Pz, P4, P8, O1, Oz, O2) are registered to the scalp surface by spline interpolation using the T1 weighted MR data, the inion-nasion and pre-auricular coordinates, and the 10-20 Electrode Placement System.

The forward EEG equation can be written as in Eq.1,

$$V = HJ = HML \tag{1}$$

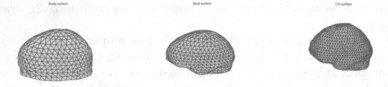

Fig. 1. Scalp, skull and csf surfaces are tessellated with 1000,1000,2000 surfaces respectively

where $V \in \Re^{Nv,1}$ is the electrical potential vector measured by scalp electrodes (N_v is the number of voxels in the brain gray matter volume), $H \in \Re^{Ne,3 \times Nv}$ is the lead field matrix (Ne is the number of electrodes), $J \in \Re^{3 \times Nv}$ is the current density orientation vector, $M \in \Re^{3 \times Nv, Nv}$ contains the normal vectors to the cortical surface at each voxel and $L \in \Re^{Nv,1}$ is the current density amplitude vector.

2.2 Inverse Problem

The inverse problem estimates the source positions and their strength from multichannel EEG data. The solution space for the inverse problem is restricted to the gray matter. A voxel is labeled as a gray matter if it satisfied two conditions: Its probability of being gray matter is higher than that of being white matter and its probability of being gray matter is higher than that of being cerebrospinal fluid (Csf). 3D solution space is sampled with a resolution of $2mm \times 2mm \times 2mm$ and $N_v = 43277$ points are obtained. Two different inverse solutions are implemented based on realistic head model.

As a parametric method, the MUSIC scanning algorithm; this method is based on subdividing the brain tissue into a 3D grid and computing the spatial power spectrum with an eigenbased approach for each voxel element. In order to do this, the transfer function H in Eq.1 has to be computed numerically.

MUSIC algorithm

– Compute the correlation matrix of V.

$$R = \frac{1}{N}(VV^T) \qquad (2)$$

– Eigenvalue decomposition of R

$$R = [\Phi_s \Phi_n] \Lambda [\Phi_s \Phi_n]^T \qquad (3)$$

(Φ_s and Φ_n: signal and noise eigenvector matrices)
(Λ: $\lambda_1 > \lambda_2 > ...\lambda_M$, eigenvalues of R)
– Compute the forward matrix H and its singular value decomposition on each voxel.
$\forall i \in$ Solution space

$$H_i = U_{H_i} S_{H_i} V_{H_i}^T \qquad (4)$$

(U_{H_i} and V_{H_i}: left and right eigenvector matrices)
($\Sigma_{H_i} : \sigma_1 > \sigma_2 > ...\sigma_N$ singular values of H_i)
- Compute the spatial power spectrum Z_i

$$Z_i = \lambda_{min}(\frac{1}{U_{H_i}^T \Phi_n \Phi_n^T U_{H_i}}) \qquad (5)$$

- Find maximum value of Z_j where $1 \le j \le Nv$
  j is the index of the activity.

As an imaging method,

sLORETA. The solution of the regularized, weighted minimum norm problem in Eq.6 is defined as Eq.7 by Pascual-Marqui [13],

$$min(||V - HML||^2 + \alpha L^T WL) \qquad (6)$$

where $W \in \Re^{Nv,Nv}$ is a known symmetric weight matrix and $\alpha > 0$ is the regularization parameter.

$$L = W^{-1}(HM)^T((HM)W^{-1}(HM)^T + C)^\dagger V \qquad (7)$$

where $C \in \Re^{Ne,Ne}$ is the sensor noise covariance matrix.
Computation of weight matrix W is defined in [13] with a simple algorithm.

3   Spatial Decomposition by Radial Basis Function

An RBF is a real-valued function whose value depends only on the distance from the origin, so that $\theta(x) = \theta(||x||)$; or alternatively on the distance from some other point c, called a center, so that $\theta(x,c) = \theta(||x - c||)$. Any function θ that satisfies the property $\theta(x) = \theta(||x||)$ is a radial function.

Two different RBF; a gaussian as in Eq.8 and a morlet function as in Eq.9 kernels are selected to approximate the input image. RBF is fitted to the EEG 2D topography by solving Eq.10 using nonlinear least squares optimization. The mesh images of 2D gaussian and morlet RBFs are seen in Fig.2.

$$V_t(x,y) = \sum_{i=1}^{Nf} a_i e^{-\frac{(x-x_{c_i})^2}{\sigma_{x_{c_i}}^2} - \frac{(y-y_{c_i})^2}{\sigma_{y_{c_i}}^2}}. \qquad (8)$$

$$V_t(x,y) = \sum_{i=1}^{Nf} a_i e^{-\frac{(x-x_{c_i})^2}{\sigma_{x_{c_i}}^2} - \frac{(y-y_{c_i})^2}{\sigma_{y_{c_i}}^2}} cos(k_i(x - x_{c_i}))cos(l_i(y - y_{c_i})). \qquad (9)$$

where V_t is the approximated 2D scalp topography for an instance of time, x_{c_i} and y_{c_i} are coordinates of the center points, N_f is the number of RBFs and a_i is the weighting coefficient of RBF.

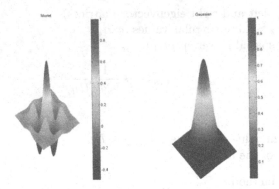

Fig. 2. Mesh images of 2D RBF gaussian kernel and morlet kernel, respectively

The nonlinear least square optimization tries to adjust the parameters of the kernel function V_t using Eq.10

$$\min \|(V_o(x,y) - V_t(x,y)\|$$ (10)

where V_o is the raw 2D scalp topography.

4   Validation of the Method

In order to validate the RBF decomposition method, a simulated multichannel EEG data is generated using BEM. Two stationry radial point sources are assumed; one being superficial while the other being deeper in the brain. Forward problem is solved for these point sources using BEM over the predefined head model given in Fig.2.1 and the topograhies are shown in Fig.3. The inverse problem is solved using both sLORETA and MUSIC for the total topographic

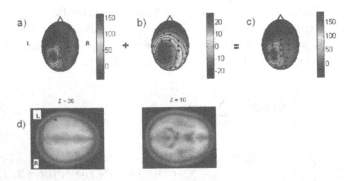

Fig. 3. 2D topography of simulation data for the a)superficial source and b)deeper source. c) Superimposition of these two subtopographies. d)Location of the superficial and deeper source, respectively.

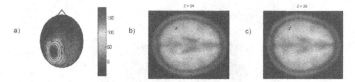

Fig. 4. a)Topography of the simulated superimposed raw data. b)Source localization result of this topography by MUSIC and c)by sLORETA.

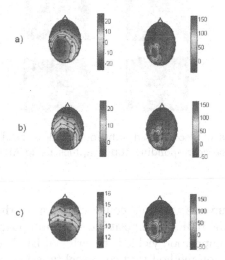

Fig. 5. a) Original raw subtoporaphies. b) Approximation and detail subtopographies decomposed using Morlet RBF and c)Gaussian RBF kernels.

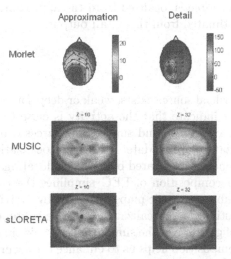

Fig. 6. 2D topographies of decomposed subtopographies based on Morlet RBF. Source localization of the corresponding topographies using MUSIC and sLORETA algorithms.

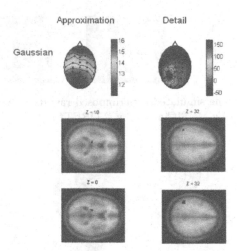

Fig. 7. 2D topographies of decomposed subtopographies based on Gaussian RBF. Source localization of the corresponding topographies using MUSIC and sLORETA algorithms.

activity. Both of the inverse methods could not localize the deeper source as shown in Fig.4. After the RBF decomposition, two suptopographic maps are obtained and their superimposition yielded the original EEG topography. Results of the RBF decomposition method for two kernel functions are shown in Fig.5. When these decomposed topographies are individually localized, it can be observed that the predefined sources can be easily discriminated as shown in Fig.6 and Fig.7 . Superficial source is localized from the approximation output while the deeper source is estimated from the detail output.

5   Conclusion

When a strong or superficial source exists, weak or deep sources remain invisible and localization results indicate that the activity is close to the strong source [14]. In our simulation case, deep and superficial sources can not be separated from the source localization of raw data. Moreover, localization methods interpreted the activity as one source located between the locations of superficial and deep source. Spatial decomposition of EEG simplifies the complexity of scalp topography into two subtopographic maps produced by individual EEG sources prior to their source estimation. Localization of these subtopographies gives us the original source configuration of the simulation. By this simulation it is shown that, spatial RBF decomposition helps us to enhance the accuracy and reliability of the source localization problem.

References

1. Scherg, M., Von Cramon, D.: Evoked dipole source potentials of the human auditory cortex. Electroencephalography and Clinical Neurophysiology 65, 344–360 (1986)
2. Koles, Z.J.: Trends in EEG source localization. Electroencephalography and Clinical Neurophysiology 106, 127–137 (1998)
3. Baillet, S., Mosher, J.C., Leahy, R.M.: Electromagnetic brain mapping. IEEE Signal Processing magazine 1, 14–30 (2001)
4. Michela, C.M., Murraya, M.M., Lantza, G., Gonzaleza, S., Spinellib, L., Grave de Peraltaa, R.: EEG source imaging. Clinical Neurophysiology 115, 2195–2222 (2004)
5. Mosher, J.C., Lewis, P.S., Leahy, R.M.: Multiple Dipole Modeling and Localization from Spatio-Temporal MEG Data. IEEE Trans. On Biomedical Engineering 39(6), 541–557 (1992)
6. Pascual-Marqui, R.D., Michel, C.M., Lehmann, D.: Low resolution electromagnetic tomography: a new method for localizing electrical activity in the brain. Int. J. Psychophysiol. 18, 49–65 (1994)
7. Koenig, T., Marti-Lopez, F., Valdes-Sosa, P.A.: Topographic timefrequency decomposition of the EEG. NeuroImage 14, 383–390 (2001)
8. Gonzalez Andino, S.L., Grave de Peralta Menendez, R., Lantz, C.M., Blank, O., Michel, C.M., Landis, T.: Non-Stationary Distributed Source Approximation: An Alternative to Improve Localization Procedures. Human Brain Mapping 14, 81–95 (2001)
9. Miwakeichi, F., Martinez-Montes, E., Valdes-Sosa, P.A., Nishiyama, N., Mizuhara, H., Yamaguchia, Y.: Decomposing EEG data into space time frequency components using Parallel Factor Analysis. NeuroImage 22, 1035–1045 (2004)
10. Wang, K., Begleiter, H., Porjesz, B.: Spatial enhancement of eventrelated potentials using multiresolution analysis. Brain Topography 10(3), 191–200 (1998)
11. Lorensen, W.E.: Marching Cubes: A High Resolution 3D Surface Construction Algorithm. Computer Graphics 21(4), 163–169 (1987)
12. Hamalainen, S.M., Sarvas, J.: Realistic conductivity geometry model of the human head for interpretation of neuromagnetic data. IEEE Trans. On Biomedical Eng. 36(2), 165–171 (1989)
13. Pascual-Marqui, R.D.: Discrete, 3D distributed, linear imaging methods of electric neuronal activity. Part 1:exact, zero error localization. arXi:0710.3341 [math-ph] (October 17, 2007), http://arxiv.org/pdf/0710.3341
14. Wagner, M., Fuchs, M., Kastner, J.: Evaluation of sLORETA in the Presence of Noise and Multiple Sources 16(4), 277–280 (2004)

Estimation of the Current Density in a Dynamic Heart Model and Visualization of Its Propagation

Liansheng Wang, Pheng Ann Heng, and Wong Tien Tsin

Department of Computer Science and Engineering, The Chinese University of Hong Kong,
Shatin, N.T., Hong Kong
{lswang, pheng, ttwong}@cse.cuhk.edu.hk

Abstract. The inverse approach from MR images to electrical propagation is very novel, but difficult due to complicated processes from electrical excitation to heart contraction. A novel strategy is presented to recover cardiac electrical excitation pattern from medical image sequences and ECG data. We used MRI images to estimate the current density and visualize it on the surface of the heart model. The ECG data also be used to achieve the time synchronization when the propagation of the current density. Experiments are conducted on a set of real time MRI images, also with the real ECG data, and we get favorable results.

Keywords: current density, heart model, ECG, visualization.

1 Introduction

The inverse problem of electrocardiography can be defined as how to determine of the electrical activity of the heart from the imaging sequences and measurements of the body-surface electromagnetic field [1]. Recently, electrocardiographic inverse approaches are becoming of great interests to the research and clinical communities, because the solution to this inverse problem may ultimately improve the ability to detect and treat cardiac diseases early and it has the potentials to describe the patient-specific electrical activity of each myocyte of the heart.

Since the mechanical activities of the myocardium are mainly driven by the cardiac electrical excitation, patient-specific myocardial kinematic measures should, indirectly, reflect the electrical propagation process of the heart. Over the past twenty years, there are many efforts in the medical image computing community devoted to the noninvasive recovery of cardiac motion field from imaging sequences. In general, medical images can directly provide cardiac motion information at some salient landmark points, such as the tag displacements from MR tagging images and the tissue velocities from the MR phase images [15].

This electrical activity, the excitation of the heart, is interdependent with its mechanical activity [2] since the active tension developed in the cardiac muscle is proportional to the excitatory current intensity. Furthermore, in addition to excitation-contraction coupling, there is an evidence that there exists also a feedback

T. Dohi, I. Sakuma, and H. Liao (Eds.): MIAR 2008, LNCS 5128, pp. 116–123, 2008.

pathway, whereby the electrical characteristics of the myocardium are altered by the mechanical state of the tissue, see [3]. However, in spite of these relations, there have been only few attempts to model the combined electromechanical system [2].

Paper [4] has recently proposed a method for estimating both the active (contraction related) and passive (relaxation related) mechanical properties of the heart using dynamic modeling and tagged MR images. Their ultimate goal is to develop a computational framework for estimating the electro-mechanical properties of the heart using a coupled model.

The dense cardiac motion fields, including displacements, velocities and accelerations throughout the myocardium, can then be estimated from those coarse measurements with a priori constraints [5,6,7,8], for which biomechanical models have been the popular choices because of their physics meaningfulness. A recent effort is particularly related to the work [9].

Based on the geometrical structure of the dynamic heart model built from MRI images, our system can calculate the displacement between two points of the deferent time. We employ the FHN (FitzHugh-Nagumo) model to estimate the current density of the heart model from the displacement. Finally we estimate and visualize the propagation of the current on the surface of the dynamic heart model with the ECG data.

2 Forward Model

The model of calculating the electrical fields throughout the body that arise from a cardiac source is called as forward model. In this paper, we introduce the forward model originally came from [4]. The forward problem in electro-cardiology is calculating the electric potential Φ (, t), and magnetic field B (y, t) at a location y on the torso surface at a time t from a given primary current distribution J (y', t) within the heart. We use a piecewise homogeneous torso model consisting of the outer torso, inner torso, lungs, epicardium, and blood masses. Thus, we model the heart as a volume G of $M = 7$ homogeneous layers separated by closed surfaces S_i, $i = 1, ..., M$. Let σ_i^- and σ_i^+ be the conductivities of the layers inside and outside S_i, respectively. Denote by G_i the regions of different conductivities, and by G_{M+1} the region outside the torso, which behaves as an insulator [4]. It has been shown that in the case of a piecewise homogeneous torso model and using quasistatic assumption the electromagnetic field for $y \in G_k$ is given by [10]

$$B(r,t) = B_0(r,t) + \frac{\mu_0}{4\pi} \sum_{i=1}^{M} (\sigma_i^- - \sigma_i^+) \cdot \int_{S_i} \phi(r',t) \frac{(r-r')}{\| r-r' \|^3} \times dS(r'),$$

$$B_0(r,t) = \frac{\mu_0}{4\pi} \int_G \frac{J(r',t) * (r-r')}{\| r-r' \|^3} d^3r'$$

(1)

$$\frac{\sigma_k^- + \sigma_k^+}{2}\phi(r,t) = \phi_0(r)(\sigma_i^- - \sigma_i^+) +$$

$$\frac{1}{4\pi}\sum_{i=1}^{M}(\sigma_i^- - \sigma_i^+)\int_{S_i}\phi(r',t)\frac{(r-r')}{\|r-r'\|^3}\times dS(r'), \tag{2}$$

$$\phi_0(r,t) = \frac{1}{4\pi}\int_G \frac{J(r',t)*(r-r')}{\|r-r'\|^3}d^3r'$$

where μ_0 is the magnetic permeability of the vacuum. To solve the integral equations (1) and (2) we utilize the EFG method, see [11], where the function $\phi(r,t)$ can be locally approximated by locally approximated by

$$\tilde{\phi}(r,t) = \sum_{i=1}^{n_m}v_i(r,r')c_i(r',t) \tag{3}$$

where n_m is the number of mesh basis functions, $\{v_i(r,r')\}$ are basis functions, and $\{c_i(r',t)\}$ are the coefficients. Details of the EFG approximation are given in [11], [12].

3 Parameters Estimation

In this paper, in order to make the calculation stabilized, Tikhonov regularization [13] is applied to this connection with a priori constraint, which is generated from modified FitzHugh-Nagumo model [14]. The classical Tikhonov regularized solution is obtained through minimization of the following equation [16]:

$$\|LJ - B\|^2 + \lambda\|RJ\|^2 \longrightarrow \min \tag{4}$$

Where $\|\cdot\|$ is the Euclidean norm, R is the regularization operator, and λ is a parameter which controls the weight given to the minimization of the side constraint. There are many ways to determine the λ, but we can interpret Tikhonov regularization as a stochastic framework by λ represents the measurement noise variance.

The derivation of the equations is initiated by the concept of lead fields which can be thought as transfer functions between the current sources and the generated magnetic signals [16]. Therefore, the magnetic field values B_i, $i = 1, ..., m$, can be linked to the primary current distribution J_p inside the heart via the lead fields L_i

$$B_i(r_i) = \int_{V'}L_i(r')\cdot J_p(r')dr' \tag{5}$$

where r_i is the location of the ith sensor. The integration volume V' contains all current sources. Discretization of equation (5) produces a matrix formulation

$$B = LJ \tag{6}$$

where vector B_{mx1} contains the magnetic field values and matrix L_{mx3n} is composed of the lead fields. Vector $J_{3nx1} = (J_{1x}, J_{1y}, J_{1z}, J_{2x}, ..., J_{nz})^T$ contains the unknown source strengths.

The main advantage of Tikhonov regularization is that the solution of equation (4) can be expressed in closed form as:

$$J = L_{reg}B = (L^T L + \lambda R^T R)^{-1} L^T B \tag{7}$$

or alternatively

$$J = (R^T R)^{-1} L^T (L(R^T R)^{-1} L^T + \lambda I)^{-1} B \tag{8}$$

provided that the regularization operator R has a full rank $3n$. Both solutions involve the inversion of a $3n \times 3n$ matrix, therefore increasing the computational demands with an increasing number of source points.

Measurements are the instants of depolarization of myofibers calculated from motion field and predictions are the instants of depolarization of myofibers from simulation in equation (8). Since measurement and prediction are the same data, the onsets of electrical excitation in myofibers, L matrix is a identity matrix.

4 Experiments and Results

A computer dynamic heart model has been developed that provides a realistic description of the variation of the human heart surface shape during a single cardiac cycle. The model of heart surface variation was composed on the basis of a set of real time MRI images, applying also physiological knowledge. The initial data comprises a movie of the heart beating: 160 images data set taken at 10 time points for 16 sections of the heart. (Fig. 1 and Fig. 2)

Based on the physical principle, if the displacement between two points at deferent time can be obtained, the force will be computed. In our system, we first get the displacement between two points of deferent time from the geometrical structure of the heart model, and then the myocardial active forces can be calculated using the force equations from the displacement. Because the myocardial active forces are physiologically driven by electrical excitations, we employ the FHN (FitzHugh-Nagumo) model to generate the current density of each point. The propagation of the current is estimated and visualized on the surface of our dynamic heart model with the ECG data. Fig. 3 shows current density images of the dynamic heart model. The arrows in the images are pointed to the propagating directions of the current. [17]

The myocardial active forces are first calculated based on our dynamic heart model. Then we get the current density at each point on the surface of the heart model. From the results, we visualize the propagation of the current on the surface of the dynamic heart which the time synchronization is achieved using the ECG data. Fig. 4 just shows the results of propagation from begin to end. And fig. 5 is the results of the volume variation of the left ventricle and total heart volume.

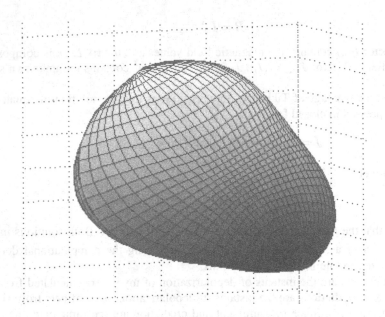

Fig. 1. The shape of the dynamic heart model

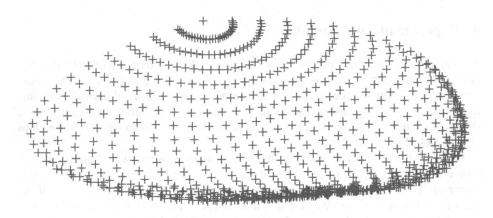

Fig. 2. The structure of the dynamic heart model

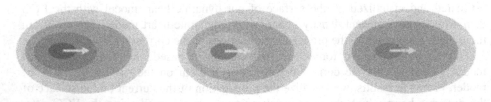

Fig. 3. Current density images of the dynamic heart model, placed close to the anterior surface of the epicardium. The arrows are pointed to the propagating directions of current.

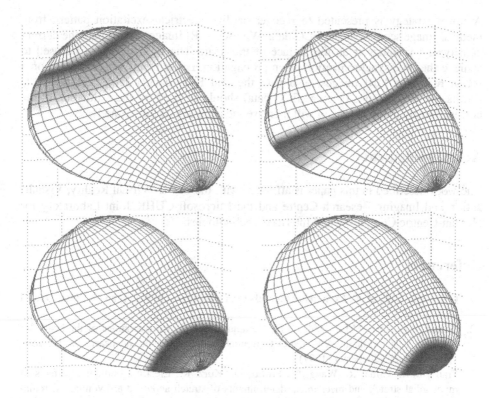

Fig. 4. The results of estimation of the current density in a dynamic heart model and visualization of its propagation. This figure just shows the states of propagation from begin to end.

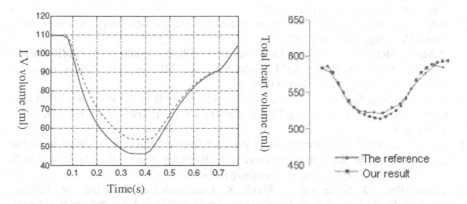

Fig. 5. Volume variation of the left ventricle (left) and total heart volume (right). In the left figure, solid line is for reference, and dashed line is our result.

5   Conclusion

The inverse approach from MR images to electrical propagation is very novel, but difficult due to complicated processes from electrical excitation to heart contraction.

A novel strategy is presented to recover cardiac electrical excitation pattern from medical image sequences and ECG data. We used MRI images to estimate the current density and visualize it on the surface of the heart. The ECG data also be used to achieve the time synchronization when propagation. Experiments are conducted on a set of real time MRI images, also with the real ECG data, and we get favorable results. New constraints (such as ECG data) should be used for the estimation of the current density in the heart and will increase the accuracy of the methods.

Acknowledgment

The work described in this paper is affiliated with the CUHK Virtual Reality, Visualization and Imaging Research Centre and the Microsoft-CUHK Joint Laboratory for Human-Centric Computing and Interface Technologies.

References

1. Gulrajani, R.M., et al.: Comprehenszve Ekctrocar-dzology, ch. 9. Pcrgamon Press, Oxford (1984)
2. Hunter, P.J., Nash, M.P., Sands, G.B.: Computational electro-mechanics of the heart. In: Panfilov, A.V., Holden, A.V. (eds.) Computational Biology of the heart, ch. 12. John Wiley & Sons, Chichester (1997)
3. Franz, M.R., Cima, R., Wang, D., Profitt, D., Kurz, R.: Electrophysiological effects of myocardial stretch and mechanical determinants of stretch-activated arrhythmias. Circulation, 86, 968–978 (November 1992)
4. Jeremic, A., Nehorai, A.: Estimating mechanical properties of the heart using dynamic modeling and magnetic resonance imaging. In: IEEE Int. Conf. Acoust., Speech, Signal Processing, Istanbul, Turkey (June 2000)
5. Prince, J.L., McVeigh, E.R.: Motion estimation form tagged MR image sequences. IEEE Trans. Med. Img. 238–249 (1992)
6. Haber, E., Metaxas, D., Axel, L.: Motion analysis of the right ventricle from MRI images. In: Wells, W.M., Colchester, A.C.F., Delp, S.L. (eds.) MICCAI 1998. LNCS, vol. 1496, pp. 177–188. Springer, Heidelberg (1998)
7. Chandrashekara, R., Mohiaddin, R., Rueckert, D.: Analysis of 3D myocardial motion in tagged MR images using nonrigid image registration. IEEE Trans. Med. Img. 23, 1245–1250 (2004)
8. Wong, C.L., Shi, P.: Finite deformation guided nonlinear filtering for multiframe cardiac motion analysis. In: Barillot, C., Haynor, D.R., Hellier, P. (eds.) MICCAI 2004. LNCS, vol. 3216, pp. 895–902. Springer, Heidelberg (2004)
9. Sanchez-Ortiz, G., Sermesant, M., Rhode, K., Chandrashekara, R., Razavi, R., Hill, D., Rueckert, D.: Localization of abnormal conduction pathways for tachyarrhythmia treatment using tagged MRI. In: Duncan, J.S., Gerig, G. (eds.) MICCAI 2005. LNCS, vol. 3749, pp. 425–433. Springer, Heidelberg (2005)
10. Gcselowitz, D.: IEEE Trans. Magn., vol. 6, pp. 346–347 (1970)
11. Belytschko, T., et al.: Int. J. Numer. Methods Endzology, ch. 9. Pcrgamon Press, Oxford (1984)
12. JcrcmiC, A., et al.: In: Proc. 34th Asalomar Conf. Signals, Syst. Comput., Pacific Grove, CA, pp. 323–327. (2000)

13. MacLeod, R.S., Brooks, D.H.: Recent progress in inverse problems in electrocardiology. IEEE EMBS Magazine 17, 73–83 (1998)
14. Rogers, J., McCulloch, A.: A collation-galerkin finite element model of cardiac action potential propagation. IEEE Trans. BioMed. Eng. 41, 743–756 (1994)
15. Zhang, H., Wong, C.L., Shi, P.: Estimation of Cardiac Electrical Propagation from Medical Image Sequence. In: Larsen, R., Nielsen, M., Sporring, J. (eds.) MICCAI 2006. LNCS, vol. 4191, pp. 528–535. Springer, Heidelberg (2006)
16. Pesola, K., Nenonen, J.: Current density imaging on the epicardial surface of the heart. In: Biomag 2000, Espoo, August 13-17, pp. 835–838 (2000)
17. Luo, G., Heng, P.A.: LV Shape and Motion: B-Spline Based Deformable Model and Sequential Motion Decomposition. IEEE Transactions on Information Technology in Biomedicine 9(3), 430–446 (2005)

Identification of Atrophy Patterns in Alzheimer's Disease Based on SVM Feature Selection and Anatomical Parcellation

Lilia Mesrob[1,2,3], Benoit Magnin[2,3,4], Olivier Colliot[3,5], Marie Sarazin[2,6],
Valérie Hahn-Barma[6], Bruno Dubois[2,6,7,8], Patrick Gallinari[1,8],
Stéphane Lehéricy[2,3,8,9,10], Serge Kinkingnéhun[2,3,11], and Habib Benali[3,4,8]

[1] LIP6, Paris, France
[2] INSERM U610, Paris, France
[3] IFR-49, SHFJ, Orsay, France
[4] INSERM U678, Paris, France
[5] CNRS UPR640-LENA, Paris, France
[6] Research and Resource Memory Centre, Groupe Hospitalier Pitié-Salpêtrière, Paris, France
[7] IFR-70, Groupe Hospitalier Pitié-Salpêtrière, Paris, France
[8] UPMC Univ Paris 06, Paris, France
[9] Department of Neuroradiology, Groupe Hospitalier Pitié-Salpêtrière, Paris, France
[10] Center for NeuroImaging Research – CENIR, Paris, France
[11] e(ye)BRAIN, Paris, France

Abstract. In this paper, we propose a fully automated method to individually classify patients with Alzheimer's disease (AD) and elderly control subjects based on anatomical magnetic resonance imaging (MRI). Our approach relies on the identification of gray matter (GM) atrophy patterns using whole-brain parcellation into anatomical regions and the extraction of GM characteristics in these regions. Discriminative features are identified using a feature selection algorithm and used in a Support Vector Machine (SVM) for individual classification. We compare two different types of parcellations corresponding to two different levels of anatomical details. We validate our approach with two distinct groups of subjects: an initial cohort of 16 AD patients and 15 elderly controls and a second cohort of 17 AD patients and 13 controls. We used the first cohort for training and region selection and the second cohort for testing and obtained high classification accuracy (90%).

1 Introduction

Due to aging of the population, Alzheimer's disease (AD) is increasingly becoming a crucial public health issue [1]. Early detection and diagnosis of AD is an important task which would enable more effective treatment of patients with currently available medication such as cholinesterase inhibitors. AD is characterized by progressive gray matter (GM) loss which occurs presymptomatically in some neuroanatomical structures [2]. Thus, magnetic resonance imaging (MRI) measurements, primarily in the GM, could be sensitive markers of the disease and assist early diagnosis.

T. Dohi, I. Sakuma, and H. Liao (Eds.): MIAR 2008, LNCS 5128, pp. 124–132, 2008.
© Springer-Verlag Berlin Heidelberg 2008

MRI studies in AD have demonstrated that volumetry of medial temporal lobe (MTL) anatomical structures, such as the hippocampus, the amygdala and the entorhinal cortex can be useful in the diagnosis of AD [2],[3],[4],[5],[6]. However, in AD, even though atrophy starts in the MTL, it is not confined to these regions and patients present with a distributed spatial pattern of atrophy. Moreover, MTL atrophy is not specific of AD and is also present in other forms of dementia. There has thus recently been a growing interest for high-dimensional classification methods that can combine information from anatomical regions distributed over the whole brain to discriminate between individual subjects [7],[8],[9].

In this paper, we propose a method to automatically discriminate between patients with AD and elderly control subjects based on Support Vector Machine (SVM) [10] classification from whole brain anatomical MRI. Our approach is based on a parcellation of the MRI into different regions in which tissue characteristics are estimated [11]. We introduce a feature selection approach which aim is to identify regions contributing to the pattern of atrophy of AD. We compare two different types of parcellations corresponding to two different levels of details. Moreover, we introduce a bootstrap procedure in order to obtain more robust estimates of the classification results. We validate our approach in two distinct cohorts of subjects composed of AD patients and elderly healthy controls matched for age and gender.

2 Method

Our approach is composed of the following steps. Individual MR images are first parcellated into anatomical regions of interest (ROI) using registration with a labeled template (Section 2.1). In addition to a standard parcellation based on the Automated Anatomical Labeling (AAL) [12], we also propose a refined parcellation which corresponds to a more specific level of anatomical details (Section 2.2). Tissue characteristics of gray matter (GM), white matter (WM) and cerebrospinal fluid (CSF) are then extracted separately in each of these ROI (Section 2.3). The most discriminative regions are then identified using a multivariate feature selection step (Section 2.4). Individual subjects are finally classified using a non-linear SVM (Section 2.5). Robust estimates of classification results are obtained using a bootstrap approach.

2.1 Brain Parcellation into 90 Regions Using AAL

The first parcellation that we propose relies on the AAL introduced by Tzourio-Mazoyer et al. [12]. MR images were automatically parcellated into 90 anatomical ROI using the spatial normalization module of SPM2 (Statistical Parametric Mapping, University College London, UK). The 90 anatomical regions correspond to all cortical structures included in the AAL atlas except the cerebellum. In the first step, the MRI of each subject was warped to the Montreal Neurological Institute (MNI) standard space applying 16-parameters affine registration followed by nonlinear deformations (linear combination of cosine transform basis functions). The SPM2 default parameters were used. Then, the inverse transformation was applied to warp the anatomical atlas AAL to the individual's space resulting in the parcellation of the original MRI into 90 regions.

2.2 Refined Brain Parcellation into 487 Regions

The AAL atlas provides an anatomical driven parcellation. However, certain structures are very large compared to others. Early AD is characterized by local alterations in some sensitive regions such as the hippocampus and medial temporal lobe. These early changes, relatively well identified in group voxel-based analyses, could go undetected when extracting parameters from a too large region. The effect of the local damage is then "diluted" and is not revealed at the scale of the whole region. It is thus of interest to assess whether a refined parcellation would provide increased sensitivity to subtle alterations.

To address this issue, we propose a refinement of the AAL atlas with the two following constraints: 1) the volume of the new regions should not be less than that of the smallest structure in the AAL, namely the amygdala, (250 voxels with voxel size=2x2x2mm^3) and 2) the presence of the three brain tissues (GM, WM and CSF) should be preserved in the new structures. The first constraint led to the subdivision of 80 from the 90 ROI into 477 smaller regions. Thus, the new atlas contained 487 ROI (Fig. 1). The second constraint was necessary to ensure good separation of the Gaussian models, i.e. the correct parameter extraction (see Section 2.3). To that purpose, we aimed at subdividing the regions following the axis that was approximately orthogonal to the cortical surface. Anatomical structures in the anterior and posterior portions of the brain were divided in sub regions following the inferosuperior direction, whereas structures in the superior and lateral portions were parcellated following the anteroposterior direction.

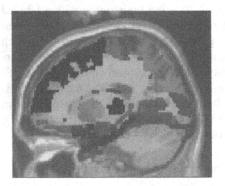 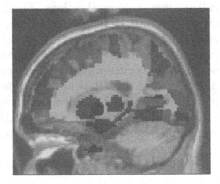

Fig. 1. Regions of AAL parcellation (left panel) and refined parcellation (right panel) illustrated on the same sagittal slice of the MNI MRI single-subject brain

2.3 Parameter Extraction

Local tissue parameter extraction was performed in each ROI using a Gaussian Mixture Model (GMM) where Gaussians describe the voxel intensity distribution of the three brain tissues: GM, WM and CSF [11]. The first Gaussian corresponds to the CSF, the second to the GM and the third to the WM. This Gaussian mixture can be represented as:

$$\alpha_1 * N(\mu_1, \sigma_1^2) + \alpha_2 * N(\mu_2, \sigma_2^2) + \alpha_3 * N(\mu_3, \sigma_3^2), \text{ where } \alpha_1 + \alpha_2 + \alpha_3 = 1$$

where α_i is the weight coefficient, μ_i the mean, and σ_i the standard deviation of each Gaussian.

These parameters were estimated with the Expectation Maximization (EM) algorithm. The weighted ratio $\alpha_{2*}\mu_2/\sigma_2$ between the mean and the standard deviation of the GM Gaussian was used for the subjects' classification. The feature vector for each subject was thus constituted by the weighted ratio for each of the 90 regions.

As an example, voxel intensity histograms in the left hippocampus of a control subject as well as the separation of the Gaussian models are shown in Fig. 2. The histograms correspond to the hippocampal region of the original 90 ROI parcellation and to one of the three hippocampal sub-regions of the new 487 ROI parcellation.

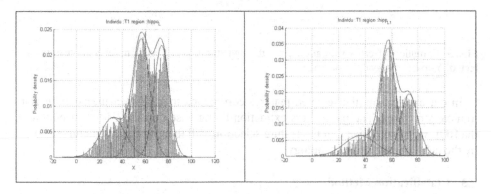

Fig. 2. Voxel intensity histograms and separation of Gaussian models in the left hippocampus of a control subject. Left panel: in the hippocampal region of the original 90 ROI parcellation. Right panel: in one of the three hippocampal sub-regions of the new 487 ROI parcellation. X-axis: voxel intensity, Y-axis: probability density.

2.4 Feature Selection

The aim of this step is to identify the most relevant features (or parameters) for the classification. The SVM-Recursive Feature Elimination (SVM-RFE) [13] algorithm estimates at each step the features' weights (using linear SVM) and retrieves the features with the least weights keeping in the end the most relevant features. In order to determine the optimal number of features to select, we applied recursively the SVM-RFE eliminating at each iteration only one feature and calculating the classification accuracy of the selected ones. To obtain a more robust feature selection, we embedded a bootstrap with 500 resamplings in this procedure. To this purpose, we drew without replacement approximately 75% of each group to obtain a training set. The remaining 25% were used as a test set. The procedure was repeated 500 times. We thus obtained the correct classification rate for the 500 drawings. Thus, for each level corresponding to the number of selected features, the eliminated feature was the most frequently chosen one within the different resamplings and the cross-validation (CV) error was estimated as the mean of the 500 samples' CV errors. The level with the least CV error gave the optimal number of features and the set of the selected features (Fig. 3).

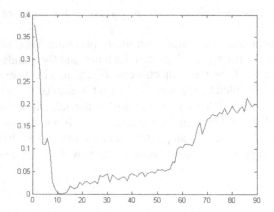

Fig. 3. Evolution of cross-validation error through iterations. X-axis: number of features selected, Y-axis: cross-validation error.

In our application, the selected features correspond to MRI measurements in anatomical structures. The parameters extraction being based on the GM distribution in the ROI, we hypothesize that the feature selection will identify brain structures altered by the neurodegenerative pathology.

2.5 Classification Method

Subjects' classification was performed using nonlinear SVM [10] with RBF (radial basis function) kernel. To obtain robust estimates of the classification accuracy, a bootstrap with 5000 resamplings was added in the learning and cross-validation steps. Bootstrap is a generalization of the leave one out (LOO) method. The large number of samples insures that every subject's data have participated in the cross-validation step. Accuracy was evaluated for every subset of data and global accuracy was evaluated as the mean of the 5000 resamplings.

3   Experiments and Results

3.1   Validation Data

The validation of the algorithm was performed using two different cohorts. The initial cohort (Cohort 1) included 15 AD patients (mean age±standard deviation (SD)=70.2±6, mini-mental score (MMS)=23.6±2.5, five males, ten females) and 16 elderly healthy controls (age=71.0±4, MMS=29.0±1, six males, ten females). A second cohort (Cohort 2) included 17 AD patients (age=74.5±5, MMS=23.6±2, five males, twelve females) and 13 controls (age=70.0±7, MMS=28.3±1.4, four males, nine females). Patients were recruited at the Research and Resource Memory Center of the Pitié-Salpêtrière hospital. The local ethics committee approved the study and written informed consent was obtained from all participants. In each subject, a T1-weighted volume MRI scan was acquired using the spoiled gradient echo sequence (SPGR) (TR/TE/flip angle: 23ms/5ms/35°, 256×256 matrix; voxel size=0.859x0.859x1.5mm^3) on a 1.5T scanner (General Electric, Milwaukee, WI, USA).

3.2 Cross-Validation Results with Initial Cohort

The SVM-RFE algorithm identified 12 regions from the original 90 ROI atlas and 43 regions from the refined 487 ROI atlas as being the most relevant for the discrimination. Selected regions included (but not only) the hippocampus, the parahippocampal gyrus, the precuneus, the calcarine, the posterior cingulate gyrus, the inferior and the polar temporal regions (Fig. 4).

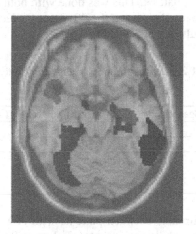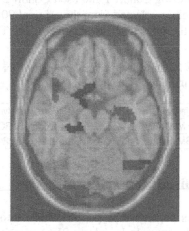

Fig. 4. Some selected regions from the AAL atlas (left panel) and from the refined atlas (right panel) illustrated on the same axial slice of the MNI MRI single-subject brain

The following classification experiments were performed:

- to assess the added value of our local tissue segmentation method, we compared the results obtained with the features extracted from the EM algorithm ($\alpha*\mu/\sigma$ in each region) to those obtained with the mean GM concentration in each region i.e. the mean probability of the voxels to belong to the GM given by the standard tissue segmentation procedure in SPM2;
- we compared the results obtained using the original 90 ROI parcellation to those obtained using the refined 487 ROI parcellation;
- we compared the results obtained using all regions to those obtained using only the regions selected by the SVM-RFE algorithm.

Results are summarized in Table 1.

Table 1. Classification results obtained for Cohort 1 with different MRI measurements, different number of features and different types of parcellations

MRI measurement	Nb features	Parcellation type	Specificity (%)	Sensitivity (%)	Accuracy (%)
GM concentration	90	Original 90 ROI	66.1	65.8	66.0
GM $\alpha*\mu/\sigma$	90	Original 90 ROI	74.3	78.7	76.5
GM $\alpha*\mu/\sigma$	12	Original 90 ROI	98.8	99.0	98.9
GM $\alpha*\mu/\sigma$	487	Refined 487 ROI	66.0	53.6	59.8
GM $\alpha*\mu/\sigma$	43	Refined 487 ROI	99.8	99.9	99.9

3.3 Evaluation on Data from Another Cohort

In Cohort 1, feature selection allowed achieving very good classification results (close to 100%). However, it is unclear whether the selected regions are representative of the atrophy distribution in AD or if they are specific to this particular group of subjects. In other words, it is necessary to assess the generalization ability of the feature selection step. To that purpose, we used the regions selected from Cohort 1, trained the SVM using Cohort 1 and used Cohort 2 as a test dataset. This was done with both the 12 regions selected from the original 90 ROI parcellation and the 43 regions selected from the refined 487 ROI parcellation. The results are presented in Table 2.

Table 2. Classification results obtained for Cohort 2 when performing feature selection and SVM training on Cohort 1

MRI measurement	Nb features	Parcellation type	Specificity (%)	Sensitivity (%)	Accuracy (%)
GM α*μ/σ	12	Original 90 ROI	96.0	84.3	90.2
GM α*μ/σ	43	Refined 487 ROI	62.3	85.9	74.1

4 Discussion and Conclusion

In this paper, we proposed a method to discriminate between patients with AD and elderly controls based on SVM classification, whole-brain anatomical parcellation and multivariate feature selection.

In order to derive an index of local brain atrophy, we estimated tissue characteristics in each of the parcelled regions. This index provided a good discrimination between patients and controls, indicating that it is a sensitive marker of early AD. In particular, it proved superior to a standard measurement of GM concentration (76.5% instead of 66%).

We introduced a feature selection approach based on the SVM-RFE algorithm. Though the selection was data driven and not based on prior knowledge, selected regions comprised structures such as the hippocampus, the parahippocampal gyrus, the precuneus and the temporal lobes which are known to be early altered in the degenerative disease. The feature selection provided increased classification accuracy on Cohort 1 (98.9% instead of 76.5%). It should be noted that the added value of the feature selection step might be accentuated by the fact that the subjects groups were relatively small. Importantly, results showed a good generalization ability of this feature selection step as a high classification accuracy was maintained when using a different cohort for validation (90.2%) while using the regions selected from the initial one. This suggests that the selected regions are representative of the pattern of atrophy in AD.

We proposed a refined brain parcellation which aim was to divide the large regions of the AAL atlas into smaller sub regions while preserving the presence of the three brain tissues. Our purpose was to assess whether a refined parcellation would allow detecting more subtle alterations of the gray matter. While this refined parcellation provided good classification results on Cohort 1 (when combined with the feature selection step), this was not the case for the inter-cohort validation where the classification accuracy dropped to 74%. This seems to indicate that the selected regions of the refined atlas do not have good generalization ability and are rather specific of the cohort which has been used for selection.

We chose to keep two separated cohorts in order to provide a completely unbiased evaluation of the classification. However, this resulted into smaller validation groups. Future validations on larger groups of participants are required to confirm the results of the present study.

Recently, several groups have used SVM classification to discriminate between patients with AD and elderly controls based on whole-brain anatomical MRI. Klöppel et al. [7] achieved 92%-95% accuracy on AD patients with average MMS of about 16 but the result dropped to 81% when considering more early patients (mean MMS equal to 23.5). Vemuri et al. [8] obtained about 89% accuracy when combining MR data with demographical and genetic information (median MMS between 20 and 22). Fan et al. [9] achieved 94% accuracy between AD patients and controls (mean MMS equal to 23). Our best inter-cohort validation results reached 90.2% accuracy.

In conclusion, we have introduced a method to automatically discriminate between patients with AD and elderly controls. Using separate learning and test datasets, we obtained high classification accuracy. This new approach has potential to become a useful tool to assist in the early diagnosis of AD.

References

1. Ferri, C.P., Prince, M., Brayne, C., Brodaty, H., Fratiglioni, L., Ganguli, M., Hall, K., Hasegawa, K., Hendrie, H., Huang, Y., Jorm, A., Mathers, C., Menezes, P.L., Rimmer, E., Scazufca, M.: Global prevalence of dementia: a Delphi consensus study. Lancet 336, 2112–2117 (2005)
2. Fox, N.C., Warrington, E.K., Freeborough, P.A., Hartikainen, P., Kennedy, A.M., Stevens, J.M.: Presymptomatic hippocampal atrophy in Alzheimer's disease. A longitudinal MRI study. Brain. 119, 2001–2007 (1996)
3. Jack, C.R.J., Petersen, R.C., Xu, Y.C., O'Brien, P.C., Smith, G.E., Ivnik, R.J.: Prediction of AD with MRI-based hippocampal volume in mild cognitive impairment. Neurology 52, 1397–1403 (1999)
4. Dickerson, B.C., Goncharova, I., Sullivan, M.P., Forchetti, C., Wilson, R.S., Bennett, D.A., Beckett, L.A., de Toledo-Morrell, L.: MRI-derived entorhinal and hippocampal atrophy in incipient and very mild Alzheimer's disease. Neurobiol. Aging. 22, 747–754 (2001)
5. Visser, P.J., Verhey, F.R., Hofman, P.A., Scheltens, P., Jolles, J.: Medial temporal lobe atrophy predicts Alzheimer's disease in patients with minor cognitive impairment. J. Neurol. Neurosurg. Psychiatry 72, 491–497 (2002)
6. Du, A.T., Schuff, N., Kramer, J.H., Ganzer, S., Zhu, X.P., Jagust, W.J.: Higher atrophy rate of entorhinal cortex than hippocampus in AD. Neurology 62, 422–427 (2004)
7. Klöppel, S., Stonnington, C.M., Chu, C., Draganski, B., Scahill, R., Rohrer, J.D., Fox, N.C., Jack, C.R.J., Ashburner, J., Frackowiak, R.S.J.: Automatic classification of MR scans in Alzheimer's disease. Brain (in press)
8. Vemuri, P., Gunter, J.L., Senjem, M.L., Whitwell, J.L., Kantarci, K., Knopman, D., Boeve, B.F., Peterson, R.C., Jack, C.R.J.: Alzheimer's Disease Diagnosis in Individual Subjects using Structural MR Images: Validation Studies. NeuroImage 39, 1186–1197 (2008)

9. Fan, Y., Batmanghelich, N., Clark, C.M., Davatzikos, C.: Spatial patterns of brain atrophy in MCI patients, identified via high-dimensional pattern classification, predict subsequent cognitive decline. NeuroImage 39, 1731–1743 (2008)
10. Cortes, C., Vapnik, V.: Support-vector networks. Mach. Learn. 20(3), 273–297 (1995)
11. Magnin, B., Kinkingnehun, S., Pelegrini-Issac, M., Colliot, O., Sarazin, M., Dubois, B., Lehericy, S., Benali, H.: Support-Vector-Machine Based Classification of Alzheimer Disease from whole brain anatomical MRI (unpublished data, 2008)
12. Tzourio-Mazoyer, N., Landeau, B., Papathanassiou, D., Crivello, F., Etard, O., Delcroix, N.: Automated anatomical labelling of activations in SPM using a macroscopic anatomical parcellation of the MNI MRI single subject brain. NeuroImage 15, 273–289 (2002)
13. Guyon, I.: Gene selection for cancer classification using support vector machines. Mach. Learn. 46, 389–422 (2002)

A Surface-Based Fractal Information Dimension Method for Cortical Complexity Analysis

Yuanchao Zhang[1,2], Jiefeng Jiang[2], Lei Lin[1,2], Feng Shi[2], Yuan Zhou[2], Chunshui Yu[3], Kuncheng Li[3], and Tianzi Jiang[2]

[1] Department of Mathematics, Zhejiang University, Hangzhou 310027,
People's Republic of China
[2] National Laboratory of Pattern Recognition, Institute of Automation, Chinese Academy of Sciences, Beijing 100080, People's Republic of China
jiangtz@nlpr.ia.ac.cn
[3] Department of Radiology, Xuanwu Hospital of Capital Medical University, Beijing 100053, People's Republic of China

Abstract. In this paper, we proposed a new surface-based fractal information dimension (FID) method to quantify the cortical complexity. Unlike the traditional box-counting method to measure the capacity dimension, our method is a surface-based fractal information dimension method, which incorporates surface area into the probability calculation and thus encapsulates more information of the original cortical surfaces. The accuracy of the algorithm was validated via experiments on phantoms. With the proposed method, we studied the abnormalities of the cortical complexity of the early blind (EB; n=15), compared with matched controls (n=15). We found significantly increased FIDs in the left occipital lobe and decreased FIDs in the right frontal and right parietal lobe in early blind compared with controls. The results demonstrated the potential of the proposed method for identifying cortical abnormalities.

Keywords: Fractal Dimension; Blind; Information Dimension; Occipital Lobe; Cortical Complexity; Cortical Surface.

1 Introduction

The human cortical surface is a highly complex structure with rich cortical convolutions. In order to better understand the cortical surface, several methods have been developed to quantify the complexity of cortical surface in recent years. For example, Zilles et al. [1] proposed a gyrification index which was defined by the ratio of the inner contours of the brain to its outer contours. Luders et al. [2] developed a curvature-based approach to estimate local gyrification on the cortical surface. Thompson et al. [3] presented a surface-based fractal analysis based on parametric meshes. Free et al. [4] presented a three-dimensional fractal analysis method and applied it to the white matter surface. Schaer et al. [5] developed a surface-based approach to quantify local cortical gyrification. Among these methods, fractal dimension (FD) has been widely used to describe the geometrical property of complex objects in biology and

T. Dohi, I. Sakuma, and H. Liao (Eds.): MIAR 2008, LNCS 5128, pp. 133–141, 2008.

medicine. The fractal, first proposed by Mandlebrot [27], has been widely used to describe self-similar structures to which it is difficult to apply shape analysis in a usual way. The shape complexity of a fractal is measured by its fractal dimension: the more complex an object, the greater its FD value. Fractal dimension is a very compact quantitative measure of the morphological complexity, condensing all the details into a single numeric value. It may help us investigate normal maturation [7], abnormal brain development [8], and neurodegenerative processes [6].

Most of the previous fractal analysis methods were voxel-based. Compared with voxel-based method, cortical surface is a direct reflection of cortical folding and provides more accurate details of the cerebral cortex. The surface-based fractal analysis method proposed by Thompson was based on a three-dimensional parametric mesh [3], it has been used to to investigate cortical complexity profile in a lot of studies, such as normal children [11], gender difference [9], first-episode schizophrenia [10], Williams Syndrome [12]. However, their method needs tremendous human intervention to delineate the sulci. Im et al. used the surface-based box-counting dimension to study the relationship between the cortical complexity and cortical thickness, sulcal depth, folding area [28]. Their box-counting algorithm misses some boxes that intersect the reconstructed cortical surfaces (Fig. 3), thus it greatly harms the accuracy of the obtained FD. In this paper, we proposed a new surface-based fractal analysis method which is able to measure the cortical folding complexity. This method incorporated surface area into the probability calculation to obtain the fractal information dimension. The accuracy of our method is validated via experiments on phantoms. In addition, our method was automatic and easy to implement.

The blind provides a unique model to investigate whether lack of visual experience will lead to functional and structural reorganization of the human brain. In previous studies, Noppeney et al. [13] reported that the early blind exhibit gray and white matter decreased in early visual areas and the optic radiation relative to sighted controls. In addition, they also observed white matter increases in the sensory-motor system, which may reflect experience-dependent plasticity in the spared modalities. Pan et al. [14] also found that the early blind (EB) exhibits significantly reduced WM volumes in the optic tract, optic radiation and significant GM losses in the early visual cortex on early blind Chinese adults. As an illustration, our surface-based fractal information dimension method was applied in detecting the abnormalities of the cortical complexity of EB.

2 Materials and Method

2.1 Subjects

A total of 15 individuals with early-onset blindness (blind before 1 year old, mean age 22.2; 8 males and 7 females) and 15 sighted controls (mean age 22.3; 8 males and 7 females) were included in the study. All subjects were right-handed. The blind subjects were recruited from the Special Education College of Beijing Union University and studied in accord with local ethical committee guidelines.

2.2 MRI Acquisition

3D structural MR images of each participant's brain were obtained by a 3.0 Tesla MR scanner (Trio system; Siemens Magnetom scanner, Erlangen, Germany) with magnetization prepared rapid acquisition gradient echo (MP-RAGE). T1 weighted scans were obtained in 176 axial slices according to the following protocol: TR=2000ms, TE=2.6ms, Nex=1, Slice thickness=1mm, Flip Angle=15°, matrix=256 × 224, 1 × 1 mm^2 in-plane resolution.

2.3 Pre-processing

Each scan was processed to get the pial surface using *FreeSurfer* [15][16], In brief, the preprocessing stage contained four steps. First, intensity nonuniformity correction and normalization to stereotaxic space using linear transformation were applied to the input image. Second, the voxels of the brain were segmented into GM, WM, cerebrospinal fluid (CSF) and background. Third, tessellations of the GM/WM boundary, boundary smoothing and automated topological correction were performed to obtain the initial surface. Fourth, the obtained surface was used as the initial value for the deformable model to reconstruct the pial surface. Then each pial surface was separated into four lobes, namely, frontal lobe, occipital lobe, parietal lobe and temporal lobe. The interfaces of GM/CSF were checked manually to assure the accuracy of the segmentation.

2.4 Fractal Information Dimension Estimation

Let F be any non-empty bounded subset of R^n, cubes with edge r are used to cover F. Let $N(r)$ be the total number of points of F and $Nb(r)$ be the total number of boxes needed to cover F. If the ith cube contains $N_i(r)$ points, the probability that a point of F fall into the ith cube is:

$$P_i(r) = N_i(r) / N(r).$$ (1)

For each cube size r, the information capacity is defined by

$$I(r) = -\sum_{i=1}^{Nb(r)} P_i(r) \ln P_i(r) ,$$ (2)

and the FID is defined by equation:

$$FID_F = \lim_{r \to 0} \frac{I(r)}{-\ln r} .$$ (3)

Because in fact the cube size r can not be arbitrarily small, the limit maybe can not be reached. So linear fitting method is used to get an estimation of theoretical value of the FID, i.e. $lnI(r)$ is fitted with $-lnr$. The fitted slope is the fractal information dimension (FID) estimation of F. In our surface-base FID method, F is a 2-D surface which is represented by triangles. Assuming the density is the same at every point of F, the number of points on the surface is proportional to the area. Thus the probability $P_i(r)$ can also be defined by

$$P_i(r) = A_i(r) / A(r) , \qquad (4)$$

where $A(r)$ is the total area of F and $A_i(r)$ is the area of the part of F which lies inside the ith cube.

In the implementation of the method, bounding box of the given surface mesh F was obtained. A 3D mesh with cube size r was overlaid onto the bounding box to cover F. The information capacity $I(r)$ was calculated. This step was repeated several times and the FID was obtained by using linear regression. To test the accuracy of our method, we constructed three regular geometrical objects as well as two well-known fractals using VTK (http://www.vtk.org) and measured their dimension. (1) a 100×100 plane (Fig. 1,a).(2) a 100×100×100 cube surface (Fig. 1,b). (3) a spherical surface with radius 50 (Fig.1,c). (4) 4th, 5th, 6th iteration Sierpinski carpets with initial square edge 100 (Fig.1, d) (5) 9th, 10th, 11th iteration Sierpinski gaskets with initial triangle edge 100 (Fig.1, e). For comparison, we also calculated the FDs of the five typical phantoms using the box counting method in [28].

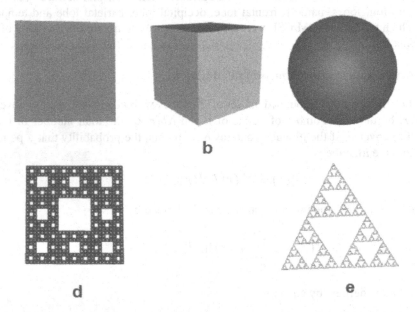

Fig. 1. Constructed phantoms. (a) plane, (b) cube surface. (c) spherical surface. (d) 6th iteration Sierpinski carpet. (e) 9th iteration Sierpinski gasket.

As regard to the selection of the range of cube size r, we chose the average edge length of the surface mesh F to be the smallest cube size, the step length was chosen to be the cube size r, and the largest cube size was chosen to be 13 times of average edge length of F.

The FID of each lobe was evaluated by using our surface-based fractal information dimension method. Unpaired two-sample t-tests were used to test for statistically significant differences in FIDs for each lobe. The level of significance for the results was set at $p<0.05$.

3 Result

We listed the phantom results of FD obtained by using box-counting method in [28] and our FIDs (Table 1). For the real data, the plot of linear fitting was shown in Fig. 2 for one subject, from which a FID of 2.208 was estimated. The adjusted r^2 value for this regression was 0.999. We found that early blind had greater FID than control subjects in the left occipital lobe, and that the early blind subjects had smaller FID than normal subjects in the right frontal lobe and right parietal lobe. The tested p-value was

Table 1. Fractal information dimension of phantoms

Object	FD	Our FID	Theoretic Value
Plane	1.982	1.995	2
Cube surface	2.033	2.042	2
Spherical surface	1.859	2.002	2
4th iteration Sierpinski Carpet	1.828	1.8708	1.893
5th iteration Sierpinski Carpet	1.857	1.8828	1.893
6th iteration Sierpinski Carpet	1.881	1.8844	1.893
9th iteration Sierpinski Gasket	1.548	1.609	1.585
10th iteration Sierpinski Gasket	1.552	1.598	1.585
11th iteration Sierpinski Gasket	1.553	1.5943	1.585

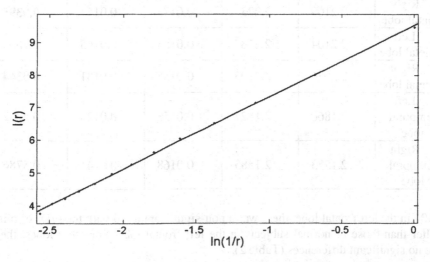

Fig. 2. Plot of linear fitting for one subject, the adjusted r^2 value for this regression is 0.999

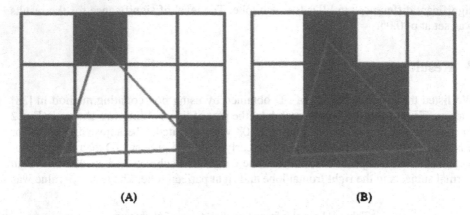

(A)   **(B)**

Fig. 3. Comparison between the box-counting algorithm in [28] (A) and our algorithm (B)

Table 2. Fractal information dimension (FID) of four lobes of real data

Lobe	Mean FID of Early Blind	Mean FID of Control	SD of Early Blind	SD of Control	P Value
Left occipital lobe	2.2170	2.2026	0.0210	0.0125	**0.0303**
Right occipital lobe	2.2263	2.2170	0.0139	0.0193	0.1444
Left frontal lobe	2.2161	2.2256	0.0123	0.0131	0.0501
Right frontal lobe	2.2109	2.2237	0.0173	0.0151	**0.0395**
Left parietal lobe	2.2104	2.2187	0.0153	0.0165	0.1600
Right parietal lobe	2.2076	2.2193	0.0155	0.0131	**0.0344**
Left temporal lobe	2.1860	2.1827	0.0158	0.0123	0.5282
Right temporal lobe	2.1553	2.1585	0.0168	0.0141	0.5786

0.0501 in the left frontal lobe, there was a non-significant trend with the FIDs of blind smaller than those of normal subjects in the left frontal lobe. For other lobes, there were no significant differences (Table 2).

4 Discussion and Conclusions

A surface-based fractal information dimension method is presented in this paper. Many research studies have adopted fractal analysis to explore the morphological properties of the human brain using segmented MR images [4][8][17][18][19][20][21] [26]. In these studies, the FD of WM, GM and WM/GM surface were computed, mostly by the box-counting method. In order to eliminate the influence of thickness and give a more compact description of the shape, some researchers computed the skeletons of the cerebral cortex [7][22] from the segmented MR images and then used box-counting to obtain the FD. The above cited works calculated the skeletons slice by slice. Zhang et al. [6] applied a 3D skeletonization algorithm to WM, and then analyzed the FD of the skeletons. However, voxel-based methods have two major drawbacks: they cannot preserve the topology of cortical surface (e.g. the skeletons and surfaces may include holes); nor can discrete voxels accurately present a continuous structure. Surface-based method can overcome these two drawbacks and extracted surface provides more accurate details of the cerebral cortex than a segmented MRI image. The first surface-based fractal analysis method proposed in [3] by reparametrizing the surface mesh to obtain the fractal dimension needs tremendous human intervention to delineate the sulci [3]. Compared with their method, our method is an automatic one which does not need extra human intervention.

As we can see from Table 2, the obtained FIDs of the phantoms were very close to their theoretical values. In comparison with the box-counting method in [28], our method was more accurate. In fact, the cortex surface is composed of many triangles, we need to count the boxes occupied by one or more triangles. However, as stated in the "fractal dimension" section in [28], "the number of grid boxes occupied by one or more vertices of cortical surface, N(r) is counted". This strategy is flawed in theory. Take Fig. 3 as an example. Just considering those boxes occupied by triangle vertices will miss some boxes occupied by the triangle. This flaw is responsible for the failure of the method to estimate the FD of a sphere, which we can see in Table 2. Our method overcomes the drawback.

By applying our method in detecting abnormal cortical regions in EB, we have found that there were significant structural abnormalities in EB. Although the abnormalities are likely to reflect the disturbances in the processes of brain development, the mechanism of cortical folding is still unknown. Previous study on enucleated monkeys showed increased convolution in occipital lobe [23], which is consistent with our increased FIDs of the occipital lobe. The decreased FIDs of EB in the right frontal and right parietal lobe may be due to the increased connectivity between the occipital lobe and frontal lobe [24] as well as the increased connectivity between the occipital lobe and parietal lobe [25] respectively.

Acknowledgement

This work was partially supported by the Natural Science Foundation of China, Grant Nos. 30425004, 30570509 and 60121302, and the National Key Basic Research and Development Program (973) Grant No. 2003CB716100.

References

1. Zilles, K., Armstrong, E., Schleicher, A., Kretschmann, H.J.: The Human Pattern of Gyrification in the Cerebral Cortex. Anatomy and Embryology 179, 173–179 (1988)
2. Luders, E., Thompson, P.M., Narr, K.L., Toga, A.W., Janckeb, L., Gaser, C.: A Curvature-Based Approach to Estimate Local Gyrification on the Cortical Surface. Neuroimage 29, 1224–1230 (2006)
3. Thompson, P.M., Schwartz, C., Lin, R.T., Khan, A.A., Toga, A.W.: Three-Dimensional Statistical Analysis of Sulcal Variability in the Human Brain. Journal of Neuroscience 16(13), 4261–4274 (1996)
4. Free, S.L., Sisodiya, S.M., Cook, M.J., Fish, D.R., Shorvon, S.D.: Three-Dimensional Fractal Analysis of the White Matter Surface from Magnetic Resonance Images of the Human Brain. Cerebral Cortex 6(6), 830–836 (1996)
5. Schaer, M., Cuadra, M.B., Tamarit, L., Lazeyras, F., Eliez, S., Thiran, J.P.: A Surface-based Approach to Quantify Local Cortical Gyrification. IEEE Trans. On Medical Imaging 27(2), 161–170 (2008)
6. Zhang, L., Liu, J.Z., Dean, D., Sahgal, V., Yue, G.H.: A Three-Dimensional Fractal Analysis Method for Quantifying White Matter Structure in Human Brain. Journal of Neuroscience Methods 150(2), 242–253 (2006)
7. Lee, J.M., Yoon, U., Kim, J.J., Kim, I.Y., Lee, D.S., Kwon, J.S., Kim, S.I.: Analysis of the Hemispheric Asymmetry Using Fractal Dimension of a Skeletonized Cerebral Surface. IEEE Trans. on Biomedical Imaging 51, 1494–1498 (2004)
8. Esteban, F.J., Sepulcre, J., de Mendizábal, N.V., Goñi, J., Navas, J., de Miras, J.R., Bejarano, B., Masdeu, J.C., Villoslada, P.: Fractal Dimension and White Matter Changes in Multiple Sclerosis. Neuroimage 36(3), 543–549 (2007)
9. Luders, E., Narr, K.L., Thompson, P.M., Rex, D.E., Jancke, L., Steinmetz, H.: Gender Differences in Cortical Complexity. Nat. Neurosci. 7, 799–800 (2004)
10. Narr, K.L., Bilder, R.M., Kim, S., Thompson, P.M., Szeszko, P., Robinson, D., Luders, E., Toga, A.W.: Abnormal Gyral Complexity in First-Episode Schizophrenia. Biol. Psychiatry 55(8), 859–867 (2004)
11. Blanton, R.E., Levitt, J.G., Thompson, P.M., Narr, K.L., Capetillo-Cunliffe, L., Nobel, A.: Mapping Cortical Asymmetry and Complexity Patterns in Normal Children. Psychiatry Res. 107, 29–43 (2001)
12. Thompson, P.M., Lee, A.D., Dutton, R.A., Geaga, J.A., Hayashi, K.M., Eckert, M.A.: Abnormal Cortical Complexity and Thickness Profiles Mapped in Williams Syndrome. J. Neurosci. 25, 4146–4158 (2005)
13. Noppeney, U., Friston, K., Ashburner, J., Frackowiak, R., Price, C.: Early Visual Deprivation Induces Structural Plasticity in Gray and White Matter. Current Biology 15(13), R488–R490 (2005)
14. Pan, W.J., Wu, G.Y., Li, C.X., Lin, F.C., Sun, J.M., Lei, H.: Progressive Atrophy in the Optic Pathway and Visual Cortex of Early Blind Chinese Adults: A Voxel-Based Morphometry Magnetic Resonance Imaging Study. Neuroimage 37(1), 212–220 (2007)
15. Dale, A.M., Fischl, B., Sereno, M.I.: Sereno: Cortical surface-based analysis. I. Segmentation and surface reconstruction. Neuroimage 9, 179–194 (1999)
16. Fischl, B., Sereno, M.I., Dale, A.M.: Cortical Surface-Based Analysis. II: Inflation, Flattening, and a Surface-Based Coordinate System. Neuroimage 9, 195–207 (1999)
17. Bullmore, E., Brammer, M., Harvey, I., Persaud, R., Murray, R., Ron, M.: Fractal Analysis of the Boundary between White Matter and Cerebral Cortex in Magnetic Resonance Images: a Controlled Study of Schizophrenic and Manic-Depressive Patients. Psychol. Med. 24(3), 771–781 (1994)

18. Cook, M.J., Free, S.L., Manford, M.R., Fish, D.R., Shorvon, S.D., Stevens, J.M.: Fractal Description of Cerebral Cortical Patterns in Frontal Lobe Epilepsy. Eur Neurol. 35(6), 327–335 (1995)
19. Kiselev, V.G., Hahn, K.R., Auer, D.P.: Is the Brain Cortex a Fractal? Neuroimage 20(3), 1765–1774 (2003)
20. Takahashi, T., Murata, T., Omori, M., Kosaka, H., Takahashi, K., Yonekura, Y., Wada, Y.: Quantitative Evaluation of Age-Related White Matter Microstructural Changes on MRI by Multifractal Analysis. Journal of the Neurological Sciences 225(1-2), 33–37 (2004)
21. Zhang, L., Dean, D., Liu, J., Sahgal, V., Wang, X., Yue, G.: Quantifying Degeneration of White Matter in Normal Aging Using Fractal Dimension. Neurobiology of Aging 28(10), 1543–1555 (2006)
22. Ha, T.H., Yoon, U., Lee, K.J., Shin, Y.W., Lee, J.M., Kim, I.Y., Ha, K.S., Kim, S.I., Kwon, J.S.: Fractal Dimension of Cerebral Cortical Surface in Schizophrenia and Obsessive–Compulsive Disorder. Neurosci. Lett. 384(1-2), 172–176 (2005)
23. Dehay, C., Giroud, P., Berland, M., Killackey, H., Kennedy, H.: Contribution of Thalamic Input to the Specification of Cytoarchitectonic Cortical Fields in the Primate: Effects of Bilateral Enucleation in the Fetal Monkey on the Boundaries, Dimensions, and Gyrification of Striate and Extrastriate Cortex. Journal of Comparative Neurology 367(1), 70–89 (1996)
24. Liu, Y., Yu, C.S., Liang, M., Li, J., Tian, L.X., Zhou, Y., Qin, W., Li, K.C., Jiang, T.Z.: Whole Brain Functional Connectivity in the Early Blind. Brain 130, 2085–2096 (2007)
25. Wittenberg, G.F., Werhahn, K.J., Wassermann, E.M., Herscovitch, P., Cohen, L.G.: Functional Connectivity between Somatosensory and Visual Cortex in Early Blind Humans. European Journal of Neuroscience 20, 1923–1927 (2004)
26. Kedzia, A., Rybaczuk, M., Dymecki, J.: Fractal Estimation of the Senile Brain Atrophy. Neuropathol. 35(4), 237–240 (1997)
27. Mandlebrot, B.B.: The Fractal Geometry of Nature. W.H. Freeman, New York (1982)
28. Im, K., Lee, J.M., Yoon, U., Shin, Y.W., Hong, S.B., Kim, I.Y., Kwon, J.S., Kim, S.I.: Fractal Dimension in Human Cortical Surface:Multiple Regression Analysis with Cortical Thickness, Sulcal Depth, and Folding Area. Human Brain Mapping 27, 994–1003 (2006)

Wavelet-Based Compression and Segmentation of Hyperspectral Images in Surgery

Hamed Akbari[1], Yukio Kosugi[1],
Kazuyuki Kojima[2], and Naofumi Tanaka[2]

[1] Tokyo Institute of Technology, Yokohama 226-8502, Japan
[2] Tokyo Medical and Dental University, Tokyo, Japan
{d05akbari,kosugi}@pms.titech.ac.jp

Abstract. Considering the anatomical variations and unpredictable nature of surgeries, visibility during surgery is very important especially to correctly diagnose problems. Hyperspectral imaging has developed as a compact imaging and spectroscopic tool that can be used for different applications including medical diagnostics. This paper presents the application of hyperspectral imaging as a visual supporting tool to detect different organs and tissues during surgeries. It will be useful for finding ectopic tissues and diagnosis of tissue abnormalities. The high-dimensional data were compressed using wavelet transform and classified using artificial neural networks. The performance of this method is evaluated for the detection of the spleen, colon, small intestine, urinary bladder, and peritoneum in a surgery on a pig.

Keywords: Hyperspectral Image, Multi-Dimensional Image, Segmentation, Medical Imaging.

1   Introduction

Medicine is no longer limited to the human eyes or to the visual spectrum. Various modalities and technologies can now be used to extend human vision. Hyperspectral imaging technology has been developed from a complex technique in satellite or aircraft systems and evolved into a compact tool in imaging and spectroscopy that can be used in medical diagnostics. This technology is capable to capture both the spatial and spectral information of an object in one snapshot. In fact, the imaging system produces several narrow band images in different wavelengths. Compared to conventional color cameras and other filter based imaging systems; this system produces full contiguous spectral data with spectral and spatial information. Fig. 1 shows a schematic view of a hyperspectral image and a spectral graph. It enables different wavelength selections in computer, and can simultaneously cover a broad spectral range. Hyperspectral imaging has already been commercialized in the medical field with the Oxyvu, launched by HyperMed Inc., is an example of a commercialized product based

T. Dohi, I. Sakuma, and H. Liao (Eds.): MIAR 2008, LNCS 5128, pp. 142–149, 2008.

on hyperspectral imaging [1]. Hyperspectral imaging was developed to possibly provide quantitative information regarding the spatial tissue oxygen saturation in patients with peripheral vascular disease [2]. This technique has been used to predict healing and track its progress in foot ulcers of diabetic patients [3]. Hyperspectral imaging may provide reliable data in near real-time with a convenient device for the surgeon in the operating room. It shows promise for increasing sensitivity of detection of residual tumor over current surgical tissue sampling techniques [4]. Hyperspectral imaging endoscope is used for the early detection of dysplasia and cancer in lung epithelia [5]. This technique is used as a visual supporting tool to enhance the regions covered with a layer of blood during surgeries [6].

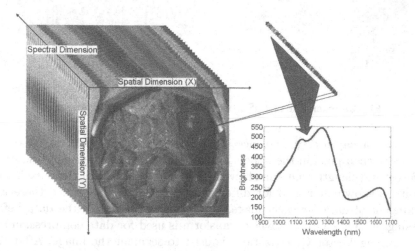

Fig. 1. On the left, a schematic view of a hyperspectral image of pig's abdomen is shown. On the right, the spectral graph of one pixel from the spleen is shown. The graph dipictes the brightness for each wavelength in that pixel.

In this research, using hyperspectral images, a library of spectral signatures for abdominal organs have been created. Using these signatures, the abdominal view through a large incision is segmented. This technique can be useful for finding ectopic tissues and diagnosis of tissue abnormalities, particularly those that were not predicted. This technique may circumvent the need for decisional biopsies as the information can be visually displaced. The surgical hyperspectral data are captured during a surgery on a pig. Wavelet transform is used as the compression method and the artificial neural networks is used for classification.

2   Material and Methods

To capture the hyperspectral image data, ImSpector N17E manufactured by Spectral Imaging Ltd., Oulu, Finland, is used. ImSpector is a direct sight imaging spectrograph that can be quickly combined with a broad range of industrial and scientific monochrome area cameras to form a spectral camera. The N17E model has the spectral range 900 - 1700 nm, Dispersion 110 nm/mm, and Spectral resolution 5 nm (with 30 μm slit). Fig. 2 shows a schematic view of the ImSpector. The light sources are two 500 W halogen lamps with a white diffuser screen. The two sources provide approximately uniform illumination on the subject. Also, the camera has been calibrated and fixed on the frame. The distance between the lens and the abdomen is constant. Therefore, the illumination can be considered to be constant in our study.

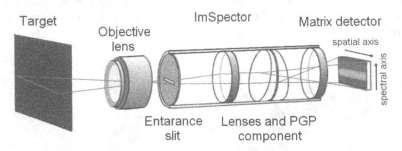

Fig. 2. Schematic of ImSpector hyperspectral imaging sensor

The camera captures a sequence of images in different spectral bands. In other words, each pixel in the hyperspectral image has a sequence of brightness in different wavelength that can show the spectral signature of that pixel. This signature is shown in Fig. 3 for different abdominal organs. Since there is a large amount of data for each image, it is better to compress the data before processing. In this study, a wavelet transform is used for data compression and LVQ (Learning Vector Quantization) is used to segment the image. After this step majority of pixels were detected, although there were some pixels which were lost because of glare. Most of these pixels were located at the mid portion of organs. For solving this problem, we have applied image fill function and region growing as post processing steps.

2.1 Wavelet Compression

Wavelet compression is a form of data compression well suited for signal compression. Wavelet compression can be perfect, lossless data compression, or a certain loss of quality is accepted with lossy data compression. This means that the transient elements of a signal data can be represented by a smaller amount of data than would be the case if some other transform, such as the more widespread discrete cosine transform, had been used. The first step in this technique is a wavelet transform. This produces as many coefficients as there are data in the signal. In this stage, it is only a transform and there is no compression yet. These coefficients can then be compressed more easily because the information is statistically concentrated in just a few coefficients. The compression features of a given wavelet basis are primarily linked to the relative scarceness of the wavelet domain representation for the signal. The notion behind compression is based on

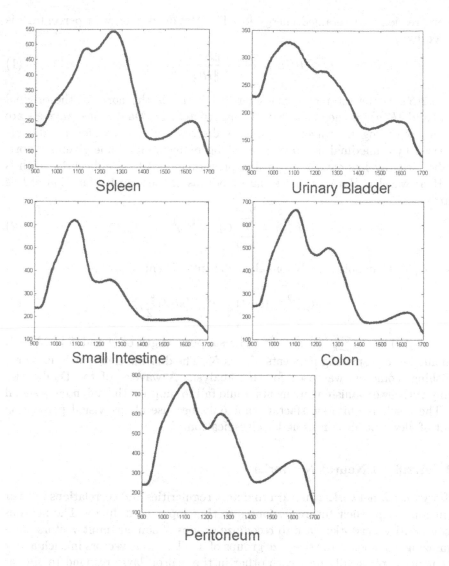

Fig. 3. Spectral signatures, the horizontal axis shows different wavelengths in nanometer, the vertical axis shows the brightness

the concept that the regular signal component can be accurately approximated using a small number of approximation coefficients and some of the detail coefficients [7]. The compression procedure contains following steps: Decompose choosing the db3 wavelet (Daubechies-3) and the level 3 (i.e. 1/8 compression). Compute the wavelet decomposition of the signal S at level 3. Threshold detail coefficients for each level from 1 to 3 are calculated. A threshold is selected and the threshold is applied to the detail coefficients. The compression approach consists of taking the wavelet expansion of the signal and keeping the largest absolute value coefficients. The threshold is set based on balancing the amount of compression and retained energy [8]. The Retained energy in percentage is defined by:

$$RSE = 100 \times \frac{\|X(n)\|^2}{\|R(n)\|^2} \tag{1}$$

where RSE is the retained signal energy, $\|X(n)\|$ is the norm of the original signal and $\|R(n)\|$ is the norm of the reconstructed one. Daubechies wavelets are a family of orthogonal wavelets defining a discrete wavelet transform and characterized by a maximal number of vanishing moments for some given support. Daubechies wavelets have no explicit expression except for Daubechi1, which is the Haar wavelet. However, the square modulus of the transfer function of h is clear:

$$P(y) = \sum_{k=0}^{N-1} C_k^{N-1+k} y^k \tag{2}$$

where C_k^{N-1+k} denotes the binomial coefficients. Then:

$$|m_0(\omega)|^2 = (cos^2(\frac{\omega}{2}))^N P(sin^2(\frac{\omega}{2})) \tag{3}$$

where $m_0(\omega) = \frac{1}{\sqrt{2}} \sum_{k=0}^{2N-1} h_k e^{-ik\omega}$. The support length of ψ and ϕ is $2N - 1$. The number of vanishing moments of ψ is N. The db3 wavelet, which has three vanishing moments, was used for this analysis. A wavelet of the Daubechies family with fewer vanishing moments would fail to suppress the polynomial signal [9]. The result is quite satisfactory, not only because of the visual perception point of view but also on using for classification.

2.2   Artificial Neural Networks

Self-organizing networks can learn to detect regularities and correlations in their input and adapt their future responses to that input accordingly. The neurons of competitive networks learn to recognize groups of similar input vectors. Self-organizing maps learn to recognize groups of similar input vectors in such a way that neurons physically near each other in the neuron layer respond to similar input vectors. Learning vector quantization (LVQ) is a method for training competitive layers in a supervised manner. A competitive layer automatically learns to classify input vectors. However, the classes that the competitive layer finds are dependent only on the distance between input vectors. If two input vectors are very similar, the competitive layer probably will put them in the same class. There is no mechanism in a strictly competitive layer design to say whether or not any two input vectors are in the same class or different classes. LVQ networks, on the other hand, learn to classify input vectors into target classes chosen by the user. Learning vector quantization is a supervised nearest-neighbor pattern classifier based on competitive learning. An LVQ network has a first competitive layer and a second linear layer. The competitive layer learns to classify input vectors in much the same way as the competitive layers of Self-Organizing and

Learn. The linear layer transforms the competitive layer's classes into target classifications defined by the user [10]. Here we have input vectors of sixteen elements (the wavelet-based compressed pixel signature), and each input vector is to be assigned to one of seven classes (spleen, peritoneum, urinary bladder, small intestine, colon, background, and ambiguous regions). For preparing a set of input/target pairs for training for first step, we capture 100 pixels data from each region in the surgical hyperspectral images. Twelve subclasses are supposed for seven classes. The classifier has been trained with a subset of manually labeled samples for 250 epochs and then it has been applied on other hyperspectral images.

2.3   Post Processing

Now for detecting missed pixels that are detected as ambiguous regions, the image is reprocessed using the image fill function. It labels pixels which are surrounded by one organ pixel as a part of that organ. After this step, some pixels which were lost because of glare are detected. As the second step in post processing, to determine the boundaries of each organ, a region growing method is applied. It expands each region in the boundary until it finds a neighbor pixel that is labeled as another organ. The sequence in which organ growing is carried out follows this priority string: colon, small intestine, peritoneum, spleen, and urinary bladder. Fig. 4 shows a segmented image using the method.

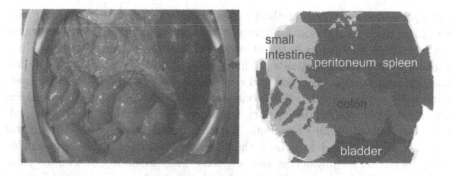

Fig. 4. The RGB image is shown on the left side. Using method described, the segmented image can be viewed on the right side. Spleen is shown in red, peritoneum in pink, urinary bladder in blue, colon in green, and small intestine in yellow.

3   Experimental Results

The experiment was done on a pig. The pig went under a general anesthesia and a large incision was created on the pig's abdomen and internal organs were explored. Vital signs were evaluated during the surgery to assure a constant oxygen delivery to the organs. Seven hyperspectral images were captured. The images are 683×240 pixels and 320 wavelength bands. The performance of the method was evaluated for detection of the spleen, peritoneum, urinary bladder, small intestine, and colon. The evaluation was performed for the quality of detection in respect to hand-created maps. The hand-created maps are used as the reference maps in calculating the detection rates of our method. Performance criteria for organ or tissue detection are false negative rate (FNR) and false positive rate (FPR), which are calculated for each organ. When a pixel is not detected as an organ or tissue pixel, the detection is a false negative if the pixel is a pixel of that organ on the hand-created map. FNR for an organ is defined as the number of false negative pixels divided by the total number of the organ pixels on the hand-created map. When a pixel is detected as an organ pixel, the detection is a false positive if the pixel is not the organ pixel on the hand-created map. FPR is defined as the number of false positive divided by the total number of non-organ pixels on the hand-created map. The numerical results on FPR and FNR for each organ are given in Table 1.

Table 1. Evaluation results

Organs	Spleen	Urinary Bladder	Peritoneum	Colon	Small Intestine
FPR	0.5%	1.3%	6.3%	1.2%	12.3%
FNR	1.3%	1.4%	7.1%	15%	2.7%

4   Conclusion

This paper proposed a new method of hyperspectral imagery as a visual supporting tool during surgeries. Additionally, spectral signatures of various organs or tissues, whose signatures have not been analyzed earlier, are presented. Furthermore, as timesaving methods are much desired during surgeries, a fast data processing technique is proposed and evaluated. Powerful algorithms to generate the data will be useful for surgeons and medical technicians, as timesaving methods are much desired during surgeries. In this study, we proposed and evaluated a fast data processing technique. Large quantities of data in hyperspectral images can be processed to extend the range of wavelengths and can provide useful information for physicians and surgeons. This previously unseen information can be precisely processed and analyzed and displayed in a visual format. This extension of the surgeon's vision would be a significant breakthrough. Hyperspectral imaging allows physicians or surgeons to survey and examine a vast area less invasively without actually removing tissue. Advantage of this concept is the ability to both spatially and spectrally determine the differences among variant tissues or organs in surgery. The image-processing algorithm can incorporate detailed classification procedures that would be used for region extraction and identification of organs or tissues. Applying this technology to surgery will allow a novel exploration of anatomy and pathology, and may offer hope as a new tool for early cancer detection.

References

1. Cancio, L.C., Batchinsky, A.I., Mansfield, J.R., Panasyuk, S., Hetz, K., Martini, D., Jordan, B.S., Tracey, B., Freeman, J.E.: Hyperspectral Imaging: A New Approach to the Diagnosis of Hemorrhagic Shock. J. Trauma-Injury Infect. Crit. Care 60(5), 1087–1095 (2006)
2. Kellicut, D.C., Weiswasser, J.M., Arora, S., Freeman, J.E., Lew, R.A., Shuman, C., Mansfield, J.R., Sidawy, A.N.: Emerging Technology: Hyperspectral Imaging. Perspectives in Vascular Surgery and Endovascular Therapy 16(1), 53–57 (2004)
3. Khaodhiar, L., Dinh, T., Schomacker, K.T., Panasyuk, S.V., Freeman, J.E., Lew, R., Vo, T., Panasyuk, A.A., Lima, C., Giurini, J.M., Lyons, T.E., Veves, A.: The Use of Medical Hyperspectral Technology to Evaluate Microcirculatory Changes in Diabetic Foot Ulcers and to Predict Clinical Outcomes. Diabetes Care 30(4), 903–910 (2007)
4. Freeman, J.E., Panasyuk, S., Rogers, A.E., Yang, S., Lew, R.: Advantages of Intraoperative Medical Hyperspectral Imaging (MHSI) for The Evaluation of The Breast Cancer Resection Bed for Residual Tumor. J. Clin. Oncol. 23(16S), 709 (2005)
5. Lindsley, E.H., Wachman, E.S., Farkas, D.L.: The hyperspectral imaging endoscope: a new tool for in vivo cancer detection. In: Proceedings of the SPIE, vol. 5322, pp. 75–82 (2004)
6. Monteiro, S.T., Kosugi, Y., Watanabe, E.: Towards a Surgical Tool Using Hyperspectral Imagery as Visual Aid. In: Proc. AMI-ARCS 2004, France, pp. 97–103 (2004)
7. Chui, C.K.: Wavelets: a tutorial in theory and applications. Academic Press Professional, Inc., San Diego (1993)
8. Karam, J., Saad, R.: The Effect of Different Compression Schemes on Speech Signals. International Journal of Biomedical Sciences 1(1), 230–234 (2006)
9. Daubechies, I.: Ten lectures on wavelets. Society for Industrial and Applied Mathematics. Philadelphia (1992)
10. Kohonen, T.: Self-Organization and Associative Memory. Springer, Berlin (1987)

A Novel Level Set Based Shape Prior Method for Liver Segmentation from MRI Images

Kan Cheng[1], Lixu Gu[1,*], Jianghua Wu[1], Wei Li[1], and Jianrong Xu[2,*]

[1] Department of Software, Shanghai Jiaotong University,
800 Dongchuan Road, Shanghai 200240, China
[2] Shanghai Renji Hospital, Shanghai
gu-lx@cs.sjtu.edu.cn

Abstract. Liver segmentation in MR Image is the first step of our automated liver perfusion analysis project. Traditional Level Set methods and active contours were often used to segment the liver, but the results were not always promising due to noise and the low gradient response on the liver boundary. In this paper we propose a novel level set based variational approach that incorporates shape prior knowledge into the improved Chan-Vese's model [1] which can overcome the leakage and over-segmentation problems. The experiments are taken on abdomen MRI series and the results reveal that our improved level set based shape prior method can segment liver shape precisely and a refined liver perfusion curve without respiration affection can be achieved.

Keywords: Liver Segmentation, Level Set, Shape Prior.

1 Introduction

Medical image segmentation is a fundamental research topic, for which numerous approaches have been proposed during the past several decades. Among them, level set methods, which were first introduced by Osher and Sethian[2] for capturing moving fronts, plays an important role. They model the propagating curve as a specific level set of a higher dimensional surface. So as time progresses, the surface can change to take on the desired shape.

In 1989, D.Mumford and J.Shah gave the famous Mumford-Shah's functional which was discussed comprehensively in [3,4]. In this approach, the segmentation problem is to find a piecewise smooth function which approximates the image and also prohibit the excessive length of the boundaries between any two contiguous regions. Later in 2001, Chan and Vese proposed a new model that combines the Mumford-Shah's functional and level set methods, which can handle curves, surfaces with topological changes conveniently. Besides this, Kass, Witkins and Terzopoulos [5] introduced the classic snake model for segmenting objects in images.

However, all of these models above fail to segment objects from images when the objects are occluded by other objects or some parts of them are in low gray contrasts

---

* Corresponding authors.

T. Dohi, I. Sakuma, and H. Liao (Eds.): MIAR 2008, LNCS 5128, pp. 150–159, 2008.

or even missing, because they are all gray intensity based. Actually, these situations always happen in our abdomen MRI images. Therefore, making use of the prior shape information makes sense. In recent years, there has been much effort in trying to integrate prior shape knowledge into level set based segmentation. For example, In [6], Cremers et al. introduced statistical shape knowledge into the Mumford-Shah's functional. In [7], Cremers et al. incorporates a level set based shape term into Chan-Vese's segmentation model [1].

But in our practical experiment, we found that these models still have some defects. They do not allow for the translation, rotation and scaling of the prior shapes. The prior shapes have to be placed exactly at the locations of the desired objects, with exactly the same poses and scales, which is too ideal to be met in real applications.

In this paper, a novel shape prior segmentation approach based on Chan-Vese's model [1] is proposed. It not only allows translation, rotation and scaling of prior shapes, but also performs object supervision before segmentation to achieve better segmentation result and high performance. Moreover, some statistical methods are introduced to get a suitable initial prior shape.

The outline of this paper is as follows: In section 2, a brief review of level set and CV model will be discussed. In section 3, we will detail our novel variational model. In section 4, our method will be validated in several experiments. Finally we conclude the paper in section 5.

2 Level Set and CV Model

Firstly we want to declare that although this work is built on the region-based level set scheme introduced by Chan and Vese, other data-driven level set schemes should also be employed. Essentially, the level set method is a moving interface problem. Its main idea is to embed the propagating curve as the zero level set of a higher dimensional function, such as the signed distance to the interface. For example, given an object $\Omega \subset R^2$, which is assumed to be closed and bounded, and $\partial\Omega$ is its boundary. We define the function as follows:

$$\phi(x, y, t = 0) = \pm d \tag{1}$$

Where d is the distance from (x,y) to $\partial\Omega$ at t = 0, and the plus (minus) sign is chosen if the point (x,y) is outside (inside) the subset Ω.

In [1], Chan and Vese propose to generate a segmentation of an input image f(x) by minimizing the functional:

$$E_{cv}(c_1, c_2, \phi) = \int_\Omega \left\{ (u - c_1)^2 H(\phi) + (u - c_2)^2 (1 - H(\phi)) + \mu |\nabla H(\phi)| \right\} dx \tag{2}$$

Where: $u: \Omega \to R^2$ is an image defined on Ω, c_1 and c_2 are two scalar variables. Hence, H denotes the Heaviside function. The last term in (4) $\int_\Omega |\nabla H(\phi)|$ measures the length of the zero-crossing of ϕ, and $\mu > 0$ is a parameter that describes how large the length of the boundaries is permitted. The Euler-Lagrange equation for this formula is implemented by gradient descent:

$$\frac{\partial \phi}{\partial t} = \delta(\phi)\left[\mu div(\frac{\nabla \phi}{|\nabla \phi|}) - (u - c_1)^2 + (u - c_2)^2\right] = 0 \tag{3}$$

c_1 and c_2 are updated in alternation with the level set evolution to take on the mean gray value of the input image u in the regions defined by $\phi > 0$ and $\phi < 0$ respectively:

3 The Improved Model

3.1 Feature Image

In the MR images of liver, due to the liver movement and the blood flow, part of the boundary is usually not clear and intensity inhomogeneity exists, where the CV model does not work well. Consequently, borrowing the idea of Xianhua Duan, Deshen Xia in [8], we here introduce the feature image according to the object intensity, which brings in better result and less iterations. The feature image function can be described as below:

$$f = |u - m|^p \tag{4}$$

Here u is the input image, and m represents the intensity of the manually defined seed point. The scalar variable p has a value range from 0.001 to 2.5, which can has different values in different images. We choose this manual contrast enhancing method because it's simple but can meet our requirement well. To make it shown as a binary image, we need to normalize it:

$$f = 255 * \frac{f - \min(f)}{\max(f) - \min(f)} \tag{5}$$

Where min(f) is the minimal intensity value of image f which is obtained from functional (4), and max(f) is the maximal intensity value. Functional (5) encourages enhancing gradient where the boundary is not very clear, with which the number of iterations can be reduced.

Figure 1(a) is an example of MRI liver image, showing relatively low gray contrast when Figure 1(b) shows the feature image we got by formula (5).

3.2 Labeling Function and Initial Result

The proposed model requires an initial segmentation result which could be achieved by implementation of CV model. However, because of the low quality of liver MRI, there are some flaws such as leakage and over segmenting, which are shown in Fig.2.

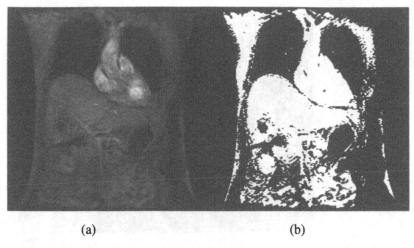

(a)   (b)

Fig. 1. (a) is a MRI image of liver with low gray contrast and (b) is the feature image we got by functional (12). Here we make p = 1.0, and set seed point at (137, 73). From the images above, the gradient has been enhanced, and the intensity inhomogeneity of target region has been reduced.

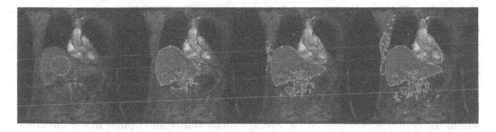

Fig. 2. Active contours procedure. The propagation starts from left to right.

To solve these problems, the labeling function L is introduced. We define L(x, y) = 1 if point (x, y) is in the target region; while in the region we are not interested, set L(x, y) = -1. From formula (3) we can get the iterative function of ϕ, and then define that in each step of curve evolution, the function ϕ only works when L > 0. Consequently, a better initial result for matching can be obtained (Fig.3).

3.3 Getting Initial Shape Model

To complete our variational model, a suitable shape model as prior knowledge is needed. We choose to use some statistical methods to get the initial shape model, 30 abdomen MRI images were segmented manually by experienced radiologists, the initial shape model can be achieved by follow steps:

At first, 20 points on the contour of the 1st image are chosen as the feature points which can represent the segmentation contour. Therefore we use registration method to find the corresponding 20 points on the 2nd, 3rd ... 30th images to get 20 groups of points.

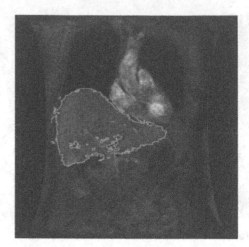

Fig. 3. Initial segmentation result with labeling function, where most extra parts are removed

In the second step, we target at finding a coordinate with the highest probability in each group, where the Mean Shift [9], a classical method to find the densest region in distribution of identical sample points, is employed. After the initial point x is chosen, the Mean Shift vector of point x can be defined as:

$$M_h(x) \equiv \frac{1}{k} \sum_{x_i \in s_h} (x_i - x) \qquad (6)$$

Here s_h is a circle with center point x and radius h, k is the number of points falling within the region s_h. Obviously, the average mean shift should point in the direction of most rapid increase of the probability density function, and have a length proportional to the magnitude of the gradient. Therefore in each iteration, point x is moved a step along the Mean Shift vector direction, and the Mean Shift Vector of the new coordinate will be recalculated. After enough iterations, s_h will finally converge to the densest region, and the final center point will be what we want. The Mean Shift vector moving process is show in (Fig.4) below.

Consequently, a most probable point position is calculated in each group, so 20 feature points are achieved. Afterwards we use cubic spline curve algorithm to outline the contour, which is treated as the initial shape model contour.

3.4 Training of Shape Model

In [7], Cremers et al. incorporates a level set based shape term into Chan-Vese's segmentation model. But in real applications, we found that their model has a shortcoming which cannot be overlooked. Their model does not allow for the translation, rotation and scaling of the prior shapes. In fact, the prior shapes usually cannot be exactly located on target objects, with the same poses and scales. Therefore, we propose that

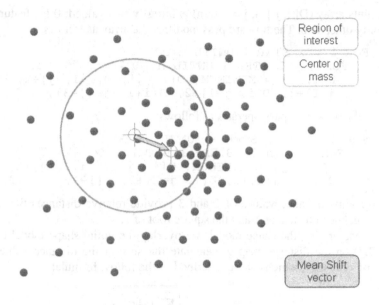

Fig. 4. The Mean Shift Vector movement

we can match the shape models to the initial segmentation results, which can regular-ize their positions, poses and scales. This key step allows affine transformation of the prior shapes.

The gradient descent method is employed in object matching. Firstly, we define the transformation of shape model as rigid-body transformation, which means our trans-formation matrix only includes translation, rotation and scaling parameters.

$$
\begin{bmatrix} x \\ y \\ 1 \end{bmatrix} * \begin{bmatrix} s_x\cos\theta & -s_y\sin\theta & x_c(1-s_x\cos\theta)+y_cs_y\sin\theta+t_x \\ s_x\sin\theta & s_y\cos\theta & y_c(1-s_y\cos\theta)-x_cs_x\sin\theta+t_y \\ 0 & 0 & 1 \end{bmatrix} = \begin{bmatrix} x' \\ y' \\ 1 \end{bmatrix} \tag{7}
$$

Here (x_c,y_c) is the central coordinates, s_x and s_y are the scale parameters in the x axis and y axis respectively. Moreover, θ represents the shape model turn angle; t_x and t_y are the translation parameters.

Thereafter, we need a distance map which is formed by assigning each pixel a value to the nearest edge pixel. In our application, the CV model's evolving result (Fig 3) is naturally a signed distance map. However, because of the low quality of our MRI image series, it is always difficult to distinguish liver's boundary region with others, which makes our signed distance map noisy.

To solve this problem, we choose to remove the noise part in our initial segmenta-tion result (Fig 3), and then recalculate the distance map. We define the points on the contour of that image (green curve) as feature points. The distance values can be de-termined in two passes through the image by a process known as "chamfering". The image points array (D[i, j] i, j = 1 to n) is initially two valued: 0 for feature points and infinity otherwise. The forward pass modifies the array as follows:

```
FOR i = 2 STEP 1 UNTIL n DO
    FOR j = 2 STEP 1 UNTIL n DO
        D[i, j] = MINIMUM( D[i, j], D[i-1, j]+2, D[i-1,
        j-1]+3, D[i, j-1]+2, D[i+1, j-1]+3);
```

Similarly, the backward pass operates as follows:

```
FOR i = (n-1) STEP -1 UNTIL 1 DO
    FOR j = (n-1) STEP -1 UNTIL 1 DO
        D[i, j] = MINIMUM( D[i, j], D[i+1, j]+2,
        D[i+1, j+1]+3, D[i, j+1]+2, D[i-1, j+1]+3);
```

The incremental distance values of 2 and 3 provide relative distances that approximate the Euclidean distances 1 and the square root of 2.

After transforming the shape model, we overlap the initial shape model (obtained in step 3.3) on the distance map to calculate the sum of the distance values as the measure of similarity, which can be described as the follow formula:

$$F(t_x, t_y, \theta, s_x, s_y) = \sqrt{\frac{\sum_{i=1}^{N} D^2(p_i)}{N}} \tag{8}$$

Where the meanings of shape parameters t_x, t_y, θ, s_x and s_y have been explained in functional (7), p_i represents the ith point which was overlapped by the shape model contour, and N is the total number of this kind of points. In addition, $D(p_i)$ is the distance value of p_i, which can be looked up in the distance map.

At each step of the curve evolution, we seek to estimate the shape parameters by gradient descent method, with the target of finding the proper t_x, t_y, θ, s_x and s_y so that $F(t_x, t_y, \theta, s_x, s_y)$ is minimized. Consequently, the transformation functional (7) can be used to get the final shape model curve.

3.5 Shape Prior Segmentation

To cope with the problem of unsuccessfully segmentation on low quality images, prior shape knowledge is introduced into the level set scheme. The basic idea is to extend the image-based cost functional by a shape energy which favors certain contour formations:

$$E_{total}(\phi) = E_{cv}(c_1, c_2, \phi) + \alpha E_{shape}(\phi) \ (\alpha > 0) \tag{9}$$

The shape comparison term should reflect the difference between two shapes. Therefore we choose to borrow the idea of Tony Chan and Wei Zhu in [10], and define it as follows:

$$E_{shape}(\phi, \psi) = \int (H(\phi) - H(\psi))^2 dx \tag{10}$$

Here, H(x) is the Heaviside function, φ is the signed distance function (SDF) mentioned in (1), and ψ is the SDF of final shape model obtained in step 3.4. With combination of formula (9) and (10), the liver can be segmented with shape prior knowledge successfully.

4 Experiment Result

To evaluate our novel method, a series of 2D 256* 256 abdomen MRI images are used in experiment, which are taken with a GE Genesis Signa HiSpeed CT/I system at the Shanghai First People's Hospital, and the parameters are: slick thickness 15.0, repetition time 4.7, echo time 1.2, magnetic field strength 15000, flip angle 60 degrees.

The experiments are performed on a PC with Pentium D 2.8Ghz, 1G RAM. We will show the result with two images. One is the abdomen MRI (Fig.5), and the other is the same image with some missing parts (Fig.6). The initial prior shape is a similar but not exactly fit liver. In addition, the parameters chosen are: $\mu = 0.1$, $\varepsilon = 1$, $a = 1$, $\nabla t = 0.1$.

Compare the experiment result below to result segmented by CV model (Fig.2), it shows that if the low-level segmentation criterion is violated due to unfavorable lighting conditions, background clutter or partial occlusion of the objects of interest, then the purely image-based segmentation scheme such as CV model will fail to converge to the desired segmentation result. However, our novel method can deal with it and end up with a satisfied result, besides, different positions and poses of prior shapes are also allowed.

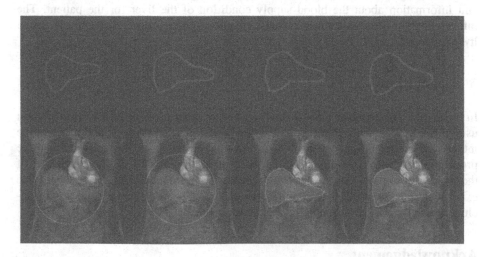

Fig. 5. The first row is the evolution of prior shape training, and the last image in the first row is the final prior shape. With the help of that shape, the second row shows the process of active contour evolution and our segmentation result.

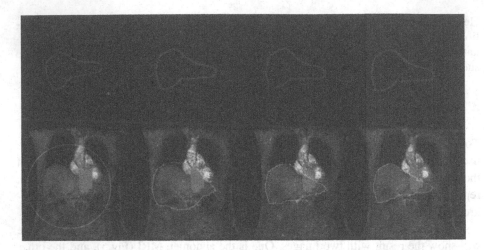

Fig. 6. The first row is the evolution of prior shape training, and the last image in the first row is the final prior shape. With the help of that shape, the second row shows the process of active contour evolution and our segmentation result. In this segmentation, even there are some missing parts, the result is still reliable.

The segmented liver shape we got here can be used as input of the liver perfusion mechanism in our lab. For certain illnesses related to the liver, the blood flow to the liver has to be studied. By injecting a contrast agent into the patients' body while taking MRI images in fixed time intervals, the concentration of the contrast agent can be studied while it flows through the patients' body. A short time after the injection the contrast agent reaches the liver and the MRI images at that time can reveal important information about the blood supply condition of the liver for the patient. The information can lead to a more accurate diagnosis. The overall procedure is called liver perfusion.

5 Conclusion

In this paper, we introduce a novel level set based variational model for segmentation using prior shapes, which helps us detect the liver perfusion position and measure the intensity. Feature image was employed to get better result and faster speed, and we propose a new measure which help to perform the training of given shapes. All of these make our model permits translation, scaling and rotation of the prior shape. The experiment results reveal that even if some part of the given image is missing or occluded, we can still get a reliable segmentation result.

Acknowledgement

This research is partially supported by the Chinese National Natural Science Foundation under Grant No. 30770608, Chinese National 863 research foundation under

Grand No. 2007AA01Z312 and the National Fundamental Research Program (973) under Grant No. 2006CB504801 and 2007CB512701.

References

1. Chan, T., Vese, L.: Active contours without edges. IEEE Transaction on Image Processing 10(2), 266–277 (2001)
2. Osher, S., Sethian, J.A.: Fronts propagating with curvature dependent speed: algorithms based on Hamilton-Jacobi formulations. J. Comp. Phys. 79, 12–49 (1988)
3. Mumford, D., Shah, J.: Optimal approximation by piecewise smooth functions and associated variational problems. Comm. Pure Appl. Math. 42, 577–685 (1989)
4. Morel, J., Solimini, S.: Variational methods in image segmentation. Birkhauser, Boston (1995)
5. Kass, M., Witkin, A., Terzopoulos, D.: Snakes: active contourmodels. Int'l J. Comp. Vis. 1, 321–331 (1987)
6. Cremers, D., Tischhauser, F., Weickert, J., Schnorr, C.: Diffusion snakes: introducing statistical shape knowledge into the mumford-shah functional. Int. J. of Computer Vision 50(3), 295–313 (2002)
7. Cremers, D., Sochen, N., Schnorr, C.: Towards recognition-based variational segmentation using shape priors and dynamic labeling. In: Griffin, L.D., Lillholm, M. (eds.) Scale-Space 2003. LNCS, vol. 2695, pp. 388–400. Springer, Heidelberg (2003)
8. Duan, X., Xia, D.: Cardiac MRI Segmentation by Using Level Set Method with Priors Shape Information Based on Object Supervision. Journal of Jiangsu University of Science and Technology (2006)
9. Comaniciu, D., Meer, P.: Mean Shift: a robust approach toward feature space analysis (2002)
10. Chan, T., Zhu, W.: Level Set Based Shape Prior Segmentation. In: Proceedings of the 2005 IEEE Computer Society Conference on Computer Vision and Pattern Recognition, vol. 2 (2005)

Statistical Shape Space Analysis Based on Level Sets

Nina Kozic[1], Miguel Á. González Ballester[1], Moritz Tannast[2],
Lutz P. Nolte[1], and Mauricio Reyes[1]

[1] MEM Research Center, Institute for Surgical Technology and Biomechanics,
University of Bern, Switzerland
[2] Department of Orthopaedic Surgery,
Inselspital University of Bern, Switzerland

Abstract. A framework for optimisation of specific criteria across the
shape variability found in a population is proposed. The method is based
on level set segmentation in the parametric space defined by Principal
Component Analysis (PCA). The efficient narrow band evolution of the
level set allows to search for the instances only in the neighborhood of the
zero level set and not in the whole shape space. We are able to optimise
any given criterion not to provide a single best fitting instance in the
shape space, but rather to provide a group of instances that meet the
criterion. This effectively defines a partition in the shape space, which
can have any topology. The method works for data of any dimension,
determined by the number of principal components retained. Results are
shown on the application to shape analysis of human femora.

1 Introduction

Statistical shape analysis techniques enjoy a remarkable popularity in the medical image analysis community. Its flagship, the Active Shape Model (ASM),
proposed by Cootes et al. [1] provides a method to study the structure of a
population of point data sets or meshes, decomposing the variability encountered across the population in a compact representation. This decomposition is
obtained via PCA [2].

Statistical shape models have been extensively used for image segmentation [1]
and shape estimation from sparse sets of landmarks, e.g. for image-free computer
assisted surgery [3]. In all these cases, the aim is to find the instance in the
statistical shape model that best approximates the input data, subject to some
regularisation constraints [3].

Optimisation in shape space of more complex criteria based on clinically
meaningful shape measures related to anatomical locations has not been fully
explored. Sierra et al. [4] formulate a minimisation process based on Lagrange
multipliers to incorporate such additional constraints, and then optimise this criterion based on a gradient descent algorithm starting from the mean of the shape
distribution. This is used in their application to generation of virtual anatomical models for surgery simulation, instantiated by specifying clinical parameters

T. Dohi, I. Sakuma, and H. Liao (Eds.): MIAR 2008, LNCS 5128, pp. 160–167, 2008.
© Springer-Verlag Berlin Heidelberg 2008

that depend non-linearly on the shape coefficients. However, their optimisation will only converge to a local minimum, which will not necessarily be the instance of the shape space that best meets the constraints.

Further, existing works aim at finding a single instance from the statistical shape model as the solution to their problem. In certain cases, it may be interesting to find *all* instances of the shape model that meet a certain criterion. For example, one may be interested in estimating which range of the population falls within a given anatomical criterion, thus establishing a partition of the shape space into "valid" and "invalid" shapes. To our knowledge, this is the first work that addresses this problem.

In this paper, we propose a method for global optimisation of shape constraints that effectively finds all instances in the PCA shape space that meet a given criterion. Our method is based on level set segmentation in the parametric shape space defined by PCA. Using the high dimensionality of level sets will allow for the segmentation of the space of any dimension, determined by the number of principal components retained. Moreover, the ability to represent the space with complex topologies can be used to identify disconnected subsets of the shape space that meet the criterion.

To avoid confusion, it should be mentioned that the combination of statistical shape models and level sets has been presented in previous works [5]. However, these works are of very different nature to ours, as they deal with the construction of statistical models of shapes represented by level sets (usually derived from distance maps). This is fundamentally different to the work presented in this paper.

Section 2 will briefly introduce the basic concepts behind statistical shape models based on PCA. Section 3 will present the level set formulation employed in our framework. In section 4 the key idea of this paper is introduced, that is, the use of level set segmentation in PCA shape space. Section 5 deals with initialisation and computationally efficient optimisation. In section 6 we illustrate our method by an application to anatomical studies. Finally, discussion and conclusions are provided in section 7.

2   Principal Component Analysis

PCA is a multivariate factor analysis technique aiming at finding a low-dimensional manifold in the space of the data, such that the distance between the data and its projection on the manifold is small [2]. PCA is the best, in the mean-square error sense, linear dimension reduction technique.

Given a set of training data $\{t_1, t_2, ..., t_N\}$ in a given orthonormal basis of $\mathcal{R}^D$, PCA finds a new orthonormal basis $\{u_1, ..., u_D\}$ with its axes ordered. This new basis is rotated such that the first axis is oriented along the direction in which the data has its highest variance. The second axis is oriented along the direction of maximal variance in the data, orthogonal to the first axis. Similarly, subsequent axes are oriented so as to account for as much as possible of the variance in the data, subject to the constraint that they must be orthogonal to the preceding axes. Consequently, these axes have associated decreasing "indices" λ_d, $d = 1, ..., D$, corresponding to the variance of the data set when projected on the axes. The *principal components* are the set of new ordered basis vectors.

The way to find the principal components is to compute the sample covariance matrix of the data set, S, and then find its eigenstructure

$$SU = U\Lambda$$

U is a $D \times D$ matrix which has the unit length eigenvectors $u_1, ..., u_D$ as its columns, and Λ is a diagonal matrix with the corresponding eigenvalues $\lambda_1, ..., \lambda_D$. The eigenvectors are the principal components and the eigenvalues their corresponding projected variances.

3 Level Set Segmentation

Segmentation techniques based on active contours, or deformable models, have been widely used in image processing for different medical applications [6,7]. The idea behind active contours is to extract the boundaries of homogeneous regions within the image, while keeping the model smooth during deformation. A particular instatiation of this paradigm is that of active contours based on level sets [8,9,10,11,12].

Let us consider a parameterized closed surface $C(s) : S = [0, 1]^{D-1} \rightarrow \mathcal{R}^D$ defined in a bounded region $\Omega \in \mathcal{R}^D$. In order to segment the observed image $\mu : \Omega \rightarrow \mathcal{R}$ we propose to minimize the following energy functional:

$$E(C) = a \int_\omega (\mu - M)\,dx + b \int_S |C'|\,ds, \tag{1}$$

where $\omega \subset \Omega$ and $C = \partial\omega$ is the region inside the curve. The first term represents the boundary force that attracts the evolving curve towards a predefined segmentation constraint $M = const$, while the second term regulates the smoothness of the curvature. a and b are scalar weights.

The proposed energy functional is not easy to solve because of the unknown set of complex contours C and unidentified image topologies. The segmentation algorithm developed in this work is based on the implicit representation of deformable models implemented within the framework of level sets. This implicit representation for evolving curves, introduced by Osher and Sethian [13], allows automatic change of topologies without re-parametrization. Using the level set formulation, the boundary contour $C = \partial\omega$ can be modelled as a zero level set of a Lipschitz function ϕ, defined on the entire image domain Ω as: $\phi(x) > 0$ $inside C = \omega$, $\phi(x) = 0$ on $C = \partial\omega$ and $\phi(x) < 0$ $outside C = \Omega \setminus \omega$.

Having the Heaviside function $H(\phi)$ defined on the whole image domain and its corresponding Dirac function $\delta(\phi) = \frac{d}{d\phi}H(\phi)$, we can replace the unknown variable C by the level set function $\phi(x)$ as:

$$E(\phi) = a \int_\Omega (\mu - M)\,H(\phi)\,dx + b \int_\Omega \delta(\phi)\,|\nabla(\phi)|\,dx, \tag{2}$$

where the curvature value $|C(\phi = 0)| = \int_\Omega \delta(\phi)\,|\nabla(\phi)|\,dx$ is estimated directly from the level set function [14]. By minimizing the energy functional with respect to ϕ we get a model associated Euler-Lagrange equation for boundary flow:

$$\frac{\partial \phi}{\partial t} = a\,(\mu - M)\,\delta(\phi) + b\,div(\frac{\nabla\phi}{|\nabla\phi|})\,\delta(\phi). \tag{3}$$

4 Optimisation in PCA Shape Space Using Level Sets

Let us consider the shape space defined by the weighted linear combination of the first $L \leq D$ eigenvectors $\boldsymbol{u}_1, ..., \boldsymbol{u}_L$ of the PCA decomposition of a set of training shapes in $\mathcal{R}^D$. Each element $m \in \mathcal{R}^D$ in this shape space is defined by a set of coefficients $\alpha_1, ..., \alpha_L$:

$$m = \overline{m} + \sum_{i=1}^{L} \alpha_i \sqrt{\lambda_i}\,\boldsymbol{u}_i, \tag{4}$$

where $\lambda_1, ..., \lambda_L$ are the eigenvalues corresponding to each principal component, and $\overline{m}$ is the arithmetic mean of the training sets (Figure 1).

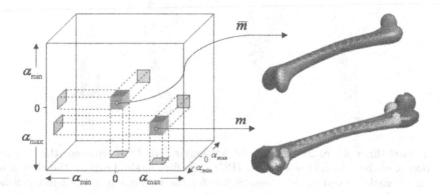

Fig. 1. Shape space defined by the three first principal components. The center element (labelled in the figure $\overline{m}$) corresponds to the mean of the population. Each element in this shape space is formed by a linear combination of the principal components, in this case $m = \overline{m} + \alpha_1\sqrt{\lambda_1}\boldsymbol{u}_1 + \alpha_2\sqrt{\lambda_2}\boldsymbol{u}_2 + \alpha_3\sqrt{\lambda_3}\boldsymbol{u}_3$.

Now let us consider a scalar mapping $\mathcal{M} : A = [\alpha_{min}, \alpha_{max}]^L \rightarrow \mathcal{R}$. This mapping represents a clinically meaningful anatomical criterion derived from the shapes in the PCA shape space. We now would like to find all instances in the shape space that meet a certain criterion dependent on the scalar measure M. This problem is approached as a segmentation in the space defined by the mapping $\mathcal{M}$ defined above, and solved using the level sets framework described in section 3. Thus, adopting the nomenclature of the previous section, $\mu = \mathcal{M}$ will be the L-dimensional "image" μ to be segmented, defined in the domain of shape coefficients $\Omega = A$. An illustrative example is shown in section 6; the following section addresses computational efficiency.

5   Computational Issues

In order to decrease the computational complexity of the standard level set method we apply a *narrow band level set* approach, which uses only the points close to the evolving front at every time step [15,16]. First we initialize a thin band around the zero-level set, that contains the neighboring points with distance to the zero-level less than d_{max} and we update the level set only on these points, instead of re-calculating it for each grid point. As the zero-level set corresponding to the front evolves, we must ensure that it stays within the band. We re-initialize the band when the front is close to the edge of the domain, using the current zero-level set as the initial surface.

We initialize our level set function using *automatic seed initialization* and then iteratively evolve the curve toward the segmented region by minimizing the energy functional. The seed initialization consists of partitioning the data image μ into N L-dimensional windows $W_{n,n=1..N}$ of predefined size. Then we initialize the corresponding circular signed distance on each L-dimensional window W_n.

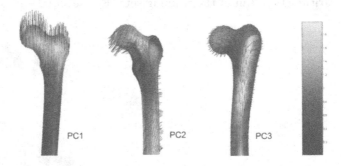

Fig. 2. First three modes of variation for left femur. The lines represent the positive direction of of the principal component (PC). The first mode describes the change of the femur length, second mode is responsible for the inclination of the femoral head and the third mode describes a deformation of the posterior part of the femoral head and a slight torsion and curvature of the central region.

6   Results

We present results obtained from a training set of 30 surface models extracted from CT data. These models represent complete left human femurs. Correspondences across data sets were established with a spherical harmonic (SPHARM) based shape representation method [17]. These correspondences are further optimized via a Minimum Description Length (MDL) optimization [18]. The average shape was computed by simple averaging of corresponding landmarks across the data sets. The remaining variation was analyzed by PCA (Figure 2).

We retain the first three principal components u_1, u_2 and u_3, which account for 89.22% of shape variability in the population. This will allow us to explain and visualize each step of the method as 3D images, although it can be applicable to data of any dimension. The shape space is thus built by sampling the space of shape coefficients, generating the corresponding shape, and then computing the mapping M to obtain the measure of interest. In this case, we use the range $-3 \leq \alpha_i \leq 3$ for every shape coefficient. This accounts for 99.7% of the shape variability encompassed in each principal component.

The clinical measure of interest $\mathcal{M}$ in our example, defined as:

$$FIA(\alpha_1, \alpha_2, \alpha_3) = \frac{1}{F}|ang(\overline{m}) - ang(m)|, \tag{5}$$

represents the difference between the angle of femoral stem implant and the angle of femoral inclination (FI) of the generated instance mesh, where F is normalization factor. Femoral inclination is defined as frontal plane alignment of femoral head and neck relative to shaft, and is commonly employed in clinical practice as a descriptive parameter (Figure 3). In normal adults, the neck of the femur forms an angle of from $126°$ to $128°$ with the shaft and any big variation from this value results in hip deformations [19].

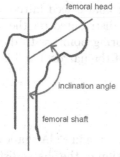
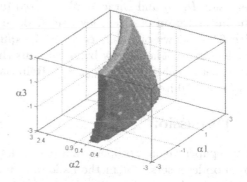

Fig. 3. Femoral inclination angle is chosen to fit the Omnifit EON femoral stem implant designed by Stryker with offset $127°$

Fig. 4. Automatic 3D level set segmentation gives the spectrum of shapes that have femoral inclination $127° \pm 2.5°$

We generate our scalar 3D map by computing FIA values, and the obtained range of femoral inclination angles from $125.5°$ to $145.6°$ correlates well with previous studies [20]. We compute the set of bones that have $127°$ neck angles, as designed for Omnifit EON femoral stem implant by Stryker Orthopaedics. As discussed in the previous section, we do not need to explicitly compute M for every point in the shape space, but only in a narrow band around the zero level set. The segmented area represents the range of parametric values that generate femur shapes that have a similar range of the femoral inclination $127° \pm 2.5°$ (Figure 4).

It can be seen in Figure 5 that the second principle component mostly affects the value of the femoral inclination and that the spectrum of segmented shapes moves toward the greater variation of the first and third principle component.

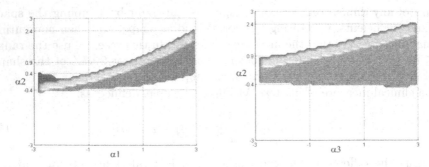

Fig. 5. 2D maps are showing the segmented spectrum of shapes and its high dependance on the second principle component

These results can also be of high importance in the field of femoral stem design, and can lead to choosing the representative parameters that would yield to the implant shape that best fits the populations.

In our numerical experiments, we use the Cauchy distribution to approximate Heaviside $H_\varepsilon(\phi)$ and Dirac $\delta_\varepsilon(\phi) = H'_\varepsilon(\phi)$ functions: $H_\varepsilon(\phi) = \frac{1}{2}(1 + \frac{2}{\pi}atan(\phi))$. The initialization of a zero level set is done using automatic seed initialization with 64 windows of radius equal to 4, equidistantly distributed on the shape space domain. The narrow band contains the neighboring points with distance to the zero-level less than $d_{max} = 4$. Reinitialization of the narrow band is done after every 10 iterations.

7   Discussion

In this paper we have proposed a framework for optimisation in PCA shape space based on level sets. The method allows to find a partition of the shape distribution into regions that meet / do not meet a given criterion. Illustrative results have been shown for anatomical analysis of femur bone. Although the example has been elaborated for 3D maps (i.e. taking only 3 principal components), the method is applicable to maps of any dimension and topology.

To our knowledge, this is the first research into the problem of finding all instances in a shape distribution meeting a given criterion. The practical use of such a concept is of extreme importance in the study of the anatomical evidence of a pathology, or the morphologic features in implant design. Ongoing work includes the application of the proposed method to bone implant fitting assessment taking into account shape and biomechanical properties of a combined shape and intensity statistical bone model.

References

1. Cootes, T.F., Taylor, C.J., Cooper, D.H., Graham, J.: Active shape models - their training and applications. Comp. Vis. Image Underst. 61(2) (1995)
2. Bishop, C.: Neural Networks for Pattern Recognition. Oxford University Press, Oxford (1995)

3. Rajamani, K.T., Styner, M.A., Talib, H., Zheng, G., Nolte, L.P., González, M.A.: Statistical deformable bone models for robust 3d surface extrapolation from sparse data. Medical Image Analysis 11(2), 99–109 (2007)

4. Sierra, R., Zsemlye, G., Szekely, G., Bajka, M.: Generation of variable anatomical models for surgical training simulators. Medical Image Analysis 10(2), 275–285 (2006)

5. Leventon, M., Grimson, W.E.L., Faugeras, O., Wells, W.M.: Level set based segmentation with intensity and curvature priors. In: Procedings of IEEE Workshop on Mathematical Methods in Biomedical Image Analysis (2000)

6. Kass, M., Witkin, A., Terzopoulos, D.: Snakes: Active contour models. International Journal of Computer Visualisation 1, 321–331 (1980)

7. McInerney, T., Terzopoulos, D.: Deformable models in medical images analysis: a survey. Medical Image Analysis 1(2), 91–108 (1996)

8. Mumford, D., Shah, J.: Optimal approximation by piecewise smooth functions and associated variational problems. Communications on Pure and Applied Mathematics 42, 577–685 (1989)

9. Chan, T.F., Vese, L.A.: Active contours without edges. IEEE Transactions on Image Processing 10, 266–277 (2001)

10. Chen, X.F., Guan, Z.C.: Image segmentation based on Mumford-Shah functional. Journal of Zhejiang University SCIENCE 5, 123–128 (2004)

11. Tsai, A., Yezzi, A., Willsky, A.S.: Curve evolution implementation of the Mumford-Shah functional for image segmentation - denoising, interpolation, and magnification. IEEE Trans. on Image Processing 10, 1169–1186 (2001)

12. Zhao, H.-K., Chan, T., Merriman, B., Osher, S.: A variational level set approach to multiphase motion. J. of Computational Physics 127, 179–195 (1996)

13. Osher, S., Sethian, J.A.: Fronts propagating with curvature-dependent speed: Algorithms based on Hamilton-Jacobi formulation. Journal of Computational Physics 79, 12–49 (1988)

14. Evans, L.C., Gariepy, R.F.: Measure Theory and Fine Properties of Functions. CRC Press, Boca Raton (1992)

15. Adalsteinsson, D., Sethian, J.A.: A fast level set method for propagating interfaces. Journal of Computational Physics 118, 269–277 (1995)

16. Li, C., Xu, C., Konwar, K.M., Fox, M.D.: Fast distance preserving level set evolution for medical image segmentation. In: Proceedings of ICARCV (2006)

17. Brechbühler, C., Gerig, G., Kübler, O.: Parametrization of closed surfaces for 3-d shape description. Comp. Vis. Image Underst. 61, 154–170 (1995)

18. Davies, R.H., Twining, C.J., Cootes, T.F., Waterton, J.C., Taylor, C.J.: A minimum description length approach to statistical shape modelling. IEEE Transactions on Medical Imaging 21(5), 525–537 (2002)

19. Platzer, W., Kahle, W., Frotscher, M.: Color Atlas and Textbook of Human Anatomy: Locomotor System. Thieme Medical Publishers (2004)

20. Tannast, M., Kubiak-Langer, M., Langlotz, F., Puls, M., Murphy, S.B., Siebenrock, K.: Noninvasive three-dimensional assessment of femoroacetabular impingement. Journal of Orthopaedic Research 25, 122–131 (2007)

Statistical Piecewise Assembled Model (SPAM) for the Representation of Highly Deformable Medical Organs

Jun Feng[1,2], Peng Du[2], and Horace H.S. Ip[2,3]

[1] School of Information and Technology, Northwest University, 710069 Xi'an China
[2] Image Computing Group, City University of Hong Kong, Kowloon Hong Kong
[3] Centre for Innovative Applications of Internet And Multimedia Technologies (*AIMtech*),
City University of Hong Kong, Hong Kong
{feng@cs, pengdu2@student, cship}@cityu.edu.hk

Abstract. We propose a novel Statistical Piecewise Assembled Model (SPAM) to address the open problem of small sample size encountered when applying Point Distribution Models (PDM) in 3-D medical data analysis. Specifically, in our SPAM, the Statistical Frame Model (SFM) constructed from the salient landmarks characterizes the global topological variability of the structure. Then the landmarks are employed to partition a complex object surface into piecewise segments. After that, the Statistical deformable Piecewise surface segment Models (SPMs) are established to define the fine details of local surface shape variations. The hierarchical nature of SPAM enables it to generate much more variation modes than conventional statistical models given a very small sample size training set. The experimental results demonstrate that SPAM can achieve more accuracy rates for model representation compared with traditional Active Shape Model (ASM) and Multi-resolution ASM.

Keywords: Statistical Deformable Model; Point Distribution Model; Organ Representation.

1 Introduction

Model based shape matching is a fundamental problem in computer vision. As one of the important branches of Statistical Deformable Model (SDM), Cootes' Active Shape Model (ASM) provided a promising framework to constrain the allowable deformations of shapes by a Point Distribution Model (PDM) built from a set of landmarks [1]. However, the extension of ASM for three dimensional medical organs are hampered by the following challenges: (i) the labeling process of landmarks is very time-consuming and tedious; (ii) the number of landmark points used for the model construction is limited by the sample size of the object, especially for highly deformable medical organs, and (iii) point correspondence of the landmarks among the samples is hard to be defined, particularly for soft tissue organs. To address the small sample size problem, one possible approach as proposed by Cootes is to combine ASM with finite element method (FEM) to enable the generation of sufficient

T. Dohi, I. Sakuma, and H. Liao (Eds.): MIAR 2008, LNCS 5128, pp. 168–176, 2008.
© Springer-Verlag Berlin Heidelberg 2008

vibrational modes for the ASM construction [2]. However, the associated computations in 3-D space are very expensive.

3-D statistical deformable models (SDM) have flourished in recent years due to the great demand for medical data segmentation and reconstruction. Brett proposed an algorithm to establish the corresponding matching between faceted surfaces for automatic landmark generation [3]. Kelemen carried out Principal Component Analysis (PCA) on spherical harmonic parameters rather than the spatial coordinates of sets of points [4]. Frangi proposed an automatic construction scheme for multiple-object such as left and right ventricles [5]. Kaus presented a three-dimensional PDM from segmented images. Corresponding surface landmarks are established by adapting a triangulated learning shape to segmented volumetric images of the remaining shapes [6]. More recently, a novel Bridging Scheme for Model Building (BSMB) was proposed which can construct 3-D PDM from a set of binary images automatically [7]. In their work, the correspondence is carried out from the template to the sample via the "bridge", through which better accuracy can be achieved.

However, since all of the above SDMs belong to global-based deformable templates, they cannot provide topological flexibility like the local-based free-formed models. Furthermore, not much work has been done to address the small sample size problem for statistical shape models. As a result, the subspace of "allowable shapes" spanned by the relatively few eigenvectors limits the ability of a PDM to follow the finer details of a complex shape. In 2006, Feng and Ip proposed a Multi-Resolution Integrated Model [8], which can capture the major variations of the organ shapes from a small sample size of the training set. However, since the low resolution models are generated by simple sub-sampling, high curvature surface points may be filtered out, and cannot be recalled in the subsequent process of model upgrading.

In this paper, we propose a novel scheme for 3-D SDM called *Statistical Piecewise Assembled Model* (SPAM) to address the small sample size problem encountered in biomedical object reconstruction. Specifically, SPAM consists of a Statistical Frame Model (SFM) and a set of Statistical Piecewise surface segment Models (SPMs). The former characterizes the global topological variability of the structure, while the latter defines the fine details of the local surface shape variation. The significance of SPAM is that its hierarchical nature enables it to generate much more variation modes than conventional SDM given a very small sample size training set.

The rest of the paper is organized as follows. Section 2 presents the construction of SFM and SPMs. Section 3 describes the process of SPAM based model fitting. Section 4 demonstrates the experimental results and evaluations. The paper is concluded in section 5.

2 The SPAM Model

The SPAM model is consisted of a global statistical deformable model (called the Statistical Frame Model or SFM) that describes the global variation modes of a medial organ, and a set of statistical deformable surface segment models (called Statistical Piecewise Models or SPMs) that describe the local variation modes of the organ surface. During the model construction process of SPAM, we first independently build the SFM and a set of SPMs, then "assemble" them to form the complete SPAM.

2.1 Statistical Frame Model (SFM)

Frequently, for many medical applications, especially for highly deformable organs, the eigen-modes derived from a small sample size training set cannot accurately capture and characterize the major variations of all surface points of the organ shapes. Particularly, for significantly deformable anatomies, noise coming from individuals would dominate over important variable components. To capture the major variations from the limited samples, we propose to generate an architectural frame of the organ surface based on a small number of salient feature points (landmarks) on the anatomy surface. This Statistical Frame Model (SFM) of the surface therefore represents the coarse structure of the biomedical object and provides the architecture to "assemble" the statistical deformable surface segments in the later process.

Given a set of 3D shape samples S_i ($i = 1, \ldots, N$), a Frame Model FM_i of S_i is defined as the set of n landmark points on the surface of S_i such that $FM_i = (x_{i1}, y_{i1}, z_{i1}, \ldots, x_{ik}, y_{ik}, z_{ik}, \ldots, x_{in}, y_{in}, z_{in})^T$ (see the first column of Fig.1). The set of FM_i ($i = 1, \ldots$, N) obtained from the shape sample set are regarded as training shapes for constructing SFM of the shape. Since the landmarks are typically points on the shape that have the most salient surface features such as high curvature points or points with distinctive visual features. The point correspondence among the set of FM_i can be easily established using well-known descriptors such as geometrics invariant [9]. To construct the SFM, given the correspondence between the landmarks, the set of FMs are first normalized by general 3-D alignment algorithm [10] and a Principal Component Analysis (PCA) is then applied to obtain the major eigen-modes of the corresponding landmark points in the training set.

Specifically, the mean shape of FMs is calculated by: $\overline{FM} = \dfrac{1}{N}\sum_{i=1}^{N} FM_i$ and the deviations of the landmarks with respect to those for the mean shape are obtained

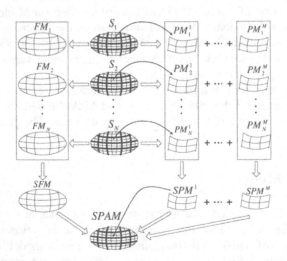

Fig. 1. A scheme for the construction of SPAM. Refer to the text for detail explanation.

by: $dFM_i = FM_i - \overline{FM}$. Then $3n \times 3n$ covariance matrix S_{FM} can be calculated from: $S_{FM} = \dfrac{1}{N} \sum\limits_{i=1}^{N} dFM_i dFM_i^T$. So the principal axes of the deviations are described by $(\varphi_{FM}^1 \mid \varphi_{FM}^2 \mid ... \mid \varphi_{FM}^{3n})$, the unit eigenvectors of S_{FM} such that $S_{FM} \phi_{FM}^k = \lambda_{FM}^k \phi_{FM}^k$ ($k =$ $1, \ldots, 3n$), where λ_{FM}^k is the kth largest eigenvalue of S_{FM} and $(\phi_{FM}^k)^T \phi_{FM}^k = 1$. In this way, a shape in the training set can be approximated using the mean frame shape and a weighted sum of these deviations obtained from the first t_{FM} modes, i.e.

$FM = \overline{FM} + \Phi_{FM} \Omega_{FM}$ where $\Phi_{FM} = (\varphi_{FM}^1 \mid \varphi_{FM}^2 \mid ... \mid \varphi_{FM}^{t_{FM}})$ is the matrix of the first t_{FM} eigenvectors, and $\Omega_{FM} = (\omega_{FM}^1 \mid \omega_{FM}^2 \mid ... \mid \omega_{FM}^{t_{FM}})^T$ is a vector of weights. The constraints of ω_{FM}^k ($k = 1, \ldots, t_{FM}$) can be made such that the Mahalanobis distance (D_m) from the mean is less than a suitable threshold, D_{max}: $D_m^2 = \sum\limits_{k=1}^{t_{FM}} \left(\dfrac{(\omega_{FM}^k)^2}{\lambda_{FM}^k} \right) \leq D_{max}^2$.

Therefore, the SFM characterizes the coarse structure as well as major variations of a class of anatomy. Since the number of the landmarks will not be too large, a small size sample set is able to capture all the major modes of the deformations across the individuals.

2.2 Statistical Piecewise Models (SPMs)

Based on the landmarks of a medical organ, a set of piecewise surface segments can be derived from the organ surface sample. Specifically, each piece of surface segment, PM, is defined by four adjacent landmarks. Similar to the construction of a SFM, corresponding surface segments obtained from a set of organ surface samples can be used to construct a Statistical Piecewise Model (SPM) for a given surface segment. Before applying PCA to the set of surface segment samples, we first align the four corners of the surface segment to the four corresponding landmarks on the organ surface. Specifically, given two groups of points: $S(P_k)$ and $S'(P_k')$, where $P_k = (x_k, y_k, z_k)$, $P_k' = (x_k', y_k', z_k')$, ($k = 1, \ldots, 4$), which can be represented as:

$$S = \begin{bmatrix} x_1 & x_2 & x_3 & x_4 \\ y_1 & y_2 & y_3 & y_4 \\ z_1 & z_2 & z_3 & z_4 \\ 1 & 1 & 1 & 1 \end{bmatrix} \qquad S' = \begin{bmatrix} x_1' & x_2' & x_3' & x_4' \\ y_1' & y_2' & y_3' & y_4' \\ z_1' & z_2' & z_3' & z_4' \\ 1 & 1 & 1 & 1 \end{bmatrix}$$

the overlap of S and S' can be achieved by multiplying S with a transformation matrix T, where $T = (S' \cdot S^T) \cdot (S \cdot S^T)^{-1}$. As a result, the corner points of SPM keep stable during deformation.

Suppose the organ surface is partitioned into M pieces of surface segments with n_j ($j = 1, \ldots, M$) points for the jth surface segment (see the right part of Fig.1). Then the jth Piecewise Model can be represented as $PM^j = \overline{PM^j} + \Phi_{PM^j} \Omega_{PM^j}$, where $\Phi_{PM^j} = (\varphi_{PM^j}^1 \mid \varphi_{PM^j}^2 \mid ... \mid \varphi_{PM^j}^{t_{PM^j}})$ is the matrix of the first t_{PM^j} eigenvectors, and

$\Omega_{PM^j} = (\omega^1_{PM^j} \mid \omega^2_{PM^j} \mid ... \mid \omega^{t_{PM^j}}_{PM^j})^T$ is a vector of weights to adjust the shape variations of PM^j while constraining it be to similar to those in the training set. This way, each SPM describes the fine variation modes of a surface segment of the medical organ (see Fig. 1).

2.3 Assembling SFM and SPMs to Form SPAM

The SPAM of a highly deformable medical organ is formed by assembling the set of M Statistical Piecewise Models (SPMs) over the Statistical Frame Model (SFM) of the organ (see the bottom part of Fig. 1). A major challenge of SPAM is to ensure the geometric continuity at the boundaries of the various statistical piecewise models during deformation. Since the SPMs of the surface segments are constructed separately, the corresponding surface segments will therefore deform independent of each other. Consequently, discontinuities or disconnections may occur at the boundaries of adjacent segments. To ensure the integrity and consistency of SPAM, a preliminary match between SPMs and SFM are achieved by performing affine transformations on SPMs in such a way that the corner points of SPMs and corresponding feature points of SFM overlap with each other.

The hierarchical nature of SPAM enables it to generate much more variation modes than conventional statistical models given a very small size training set. Theoretically, the variation modes of SPAM would be $t_{FM} \times t_{PM^1} \times t_{PM^2} ... \times t_{PM^M}$.

3 SPAM Based Model Fitting

In this section, we propose a hierarchical deformation scheme for fitting the SPAM model of the organ to a new organ sample X. The general idea of fitting SPAM to X is that we first fit Statistical Frame Model of the SPAM to X in order to achieve a global coarse fitting, then fit the set of Statistical Piecewise Models of the SPAM to X independently to achieve local surface fitting.

Initially, the set of landmarks of X is identified based on their shape descriptors [11] or texture descriptors [12]. Since the landmarks are highly distinctive or salient features on the organ surface, many point correspondence algorithms (eg. [9]) can be applied to match them to those on SPAM. Based on the correspondences of landmarks of X and $\overline{FM}$, a transformation $\wp_{FM}$ can be defined, and an approximate alignment between X and $\overline{FM}$ can be achieved in the least-squares error sense. Then a set of weights of the variation modes are calculated by $\Omega^X_{FM} = (\Phi_{FM})^{-1}(X_{FM} - \wp_{FM}(\overline{FM}))$. Since Φ_{FM} is the positive definite matrix of the eigenvectors, we have $(\Phi_{FM})^{-1} = (\Phi_{FM})^T$. Therefore, the Frame Model (FM) of the surface of X can be approximately represented as $X_{FM} = \wp_{FM}(\overline{FM}) + \Phi_{FM}\Omega^X_{FM}$.

From X_{FM}, the SPMs can be guided to their initial locations that are close to the corresponding surface segments of X. The fine deformation (fitting) of the surface is carried out segments by segments. The fitting processes of SPMs are similar to that of SFM. Therefore, each surface segment can be represented as

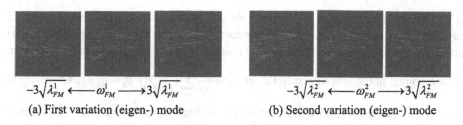

$$-3\sqrt{\lambda_{FM}^1} \longleftarrow \omega_{FM}^1 \longrightarrow 3\sqrt{\lambda_{FM}^1} \qquad\qquad -3\sqrt{\lambda_{FM}^2} \longleftarrow \omega_{FM}^2 \longrightarrow 3\sqrt{\lambda_{FM}^2}$$

(a) First variation (eigen-) mode   (b) Second variation (eigen-) mode

Fig. 2. First two variation modes of SFM

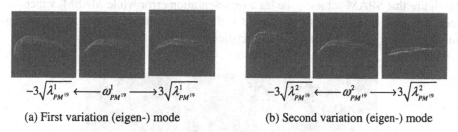

$$-3\sqrt{\lambda_{PM^{19}}^1} \longleftarrow \omega_{PM^{19}}^1 \longrightarrow 3\sqrt{\lambda_{PM^{19}}^1} \qquad -3\sqrt{\lambda_{PM^{19}}^2} \longleftarrow \omega_{PM^{19}}^2 \longrightarrow 3\sqrt{\lambda_{PM^{19}}^2}$$

(a) First variation (eigen-) mode   (b) Second variation (eigen-) mode

Fig. 3. Deformation modes of a SPM^j ($j = 19$)

$X_{PM^j} = \wp_{PM^j}(\overline{PM^j}) + \Phi_{PM^j}\Omega_{PM^j}^X$, and the whole surface of X can be represented by assembling X_{FM} with X_{PM^j} ($j = 1, \ldots, M$).

4 Experiments and Results

We demonstrate the feasibility of SPAM and validate our approach on the liver organ which is a typical soft-tissue organ in the human anatomy. Liver is a highly deformable organ, and is highly variable among individuals. In our experiments, we use only 12 liver samples ($N = 12$), with 1472 points for each surface. We compare SPAM with conventional ASM and a Multi-resolution ASM (MASM) [8]. For this experiment, the SFM consists of 60 landmark points ($n = 60$) identified on the liver surface and 55 surface segments are extracted accordingly ($M = 55$). Fig.2 shows the mean Frame Model ($\overline{FM}$) and the 1st (Fig.2 a) and 2nd (Fig.2 b) largest variation modes of the resulting SFM. Fig. 3 gives the mean Piecewise Model ($\overline{PM^j}$, $j = 19$) and the first (Fig. 3a) and second (Fig.3b) largest deformation modes of one of SPMs to show that SPMs can indeed capture the detail variations of the local surface shapes. Furthermore, we assemble all the piecewise models (PMs) with respect to the SFM. In Fig. 4, we show the first and second largest deformation modes of one of the SPMs after assembled over SFM. We can observe that the corner points of the PM (which are also the landmarks) have been kept fixed during the segment deformation, which ensures the connectivity and consistency of the resulting *Statistical Piecewise Assembled Model*. We further illustrate the assembling result of several PMs on the SFM in Fig. 5.

To evaluate and compare the accuracy of SPAM, traditional ASM and MASM, 12 leave-one-out experiments have been conducted. The accuracy rates are designed to reflect the representational accuracy of a model in terms of the mean distance between surface points(in the unit of pixel), i.e. $error = \dfrac{1}{M}\sum_{j=1}^{M}(\dfrac{1}{n_j}\sum_{k=1}^{n_j}\| p_k^j - q_k^j \|)$, where p_k^j is the kth point of the jth surface segment on a model built from 11 surface samples, and q_k^j is the corresponding point of p_k^j on the remaining surface sample. Figure 6 depicts the respective error rates comparison of the three methods. We can observe from the figure that SPAM achieves the least representation error while MASM, which has been designed specifically to emphasize surface smoothness rather than representational accuracy, gives the largest representation error.

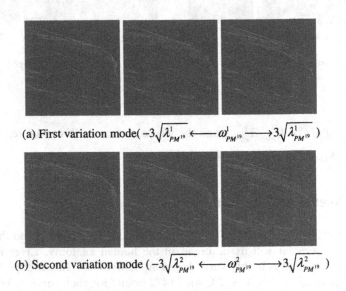

(a) First variation mode($-3\sqrt{\lambda_{PM^{19}}^1} \longleftarrow \omega_{PM^{19}}^1 \longrightarrow 3\sqrt{\lambda_{PM^{19}}^1}$)

(b) Second variation mode ($-3\sqrt{\lambda_{PM^{19}}^2} \longleftarrow \omega_{PM^{19}}^2 \longrightarrow 3\sqrt{\lambda_{PM^{19}}^2}$)

Fig. 4. Assembling a SPM over SFM

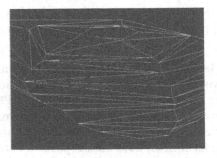

Fig. 5. Result of assembling several PMs over the SFM

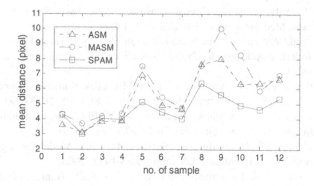

Fig. 6. Comparison of shape representational error rates of ASM, MASM and SPAM

5 Conclusion

In this paper, we propose a novel *Statistical Piecewise Assembled Model* (SPAM) to address the open problem of small sample size encountered when applying Point Distribution Models (PDM) for 3-D medical organ analysis. SPAM consists of a Statistical Frame Model (SFM) that serves to provide a framework for partitioning a complex deformable object surface into a set of statistical piecewise surface segment models (SPMs) that describe the detail local surface deformability of the organ. We have shown that the hierarchical nature of SPAM enables it to generate much more variation modes than conventional statistical deformable models from a very small sample size training set. Our *Statistical Piecewise Assembled Model* (SPAM) provides a powerful and compact way to describe the geometry as well as the deformability of complex medical and biomedical objects and is a promising tool for 3D medical reconstruction, segmentation, registration as well as morphological analysis. In addition, the global as well as local shape parameters derived from SPAM can be applied to 3-D model classification and retrieval.

Acknowledgement

This work is jointly supported by Research Grants Council of Hong Kong SAR, China [Project no.Cityu113706] and China Postdoctoral Science Foundation funded project [no. 20070421126].

References

1. Cootes, T.F., Taylor, C.J., et al.: Active Shape Models-Their Training and Applications. Computer Vision and Image Understanding 61(1), 38–59 (1995)
2. Cootes, T.F., Taylor, C.J.: Combining point distribution models with shape models based on finite element analysis. Image and Vision Computing 13(5), 403–409 (1995)
3. Brett, A.D., Hill, A., et al.: A Method of 3-D Surface Correspondence for Automated Landmark Generation. In: 8th British Machine Vision Conference, pp. 709–718 (1997)

4. Kelemen, A., Szekely, G., et al.: Three-dimensional Model-based Segmentation of Brain MRI. IEEE Trans. Med. Imaging 18(10), 828–839 (1999)
5. Frangi, A.F., et al.: Automatic Construction of Multiple-Object Three-Dimensional Statistical Shape Models: Application to Cardiac Modeling. IEEE Trans. Med. Imaging 21(9), 1151–1166 (2002)
6. Kaus, M.R., Pekar, V., et al.: Automated 3-D PDM construction from segmented images using deformable models. IEEE Trans. Med. Imaging 22(8), 1005–1013 (2003)
7. Zhao, Z.E., Teoh, E.K.: A new scheme for automated 3D PDM construction using deformable models. Image and Vision Computing 26(2), 275–288 (2008)
8. Feng, J., Ip, H.H.S.: MistO: A Multi-Resolution deformable Model for segmentation of Soft-Tissue organs. In: ICIP, Atlanta, USA, pp. 1909–1912 (2006)
9. Rivilin, E., Weiss, I.: Local Invariants For Recognition. IEEE Trans. on Pattern Anal. & Mach. Intell. 17(3), 226–238 (1995)
10. Besl, P.J., Mckay, N.D.: A Method for Registration of 3D Shapes. IEEE Trans. on Pattern Anal. & Mach. Intell. 14(2), 239–256 (1992)
11. Feng, J., Ip, H.H.S., et al.: Robust Point Correspondence Matching and Similarity Measuring for 3D Models by Relative Angle-Context Distributions. Image and Vision Computing (September 15, 2007)
12. Cootes, T.F., Taylor, C.J.: Using grey-level models to improve active shape model search. In: Proceedings of the 12th ICPR, vol. 1, pp. 63–67 (1994)

Amygdala Surface Modeling with Weighted Spherical Harmonics

Moo K. Chung[1,2], Brendon M. Nacewicz[2], Shubing Wang[1],
Kim M. Dalton[2], Seth Pollak[3], and Richard J. Davidson[2,3]

[1] Department of Statistics, Biostatistics and Medical Informatics
[2] Waisman Laboratory for Brain Imaging and Behavior
[3] Department of Psychology and Psychiatry
University of Wisconsin, Madison, WI 53706, USA
mkchung@wisc.edu

Abstract. Although there are numerous publications on amygdala volumetry, so far there has not been many studies on modeling local amygdala surface shape variations in a rigorous framework. This paper present a systematic framework for modeling local amygdala shape. Using a novel surface flattening technique, we obtain a smooth mapping from the amygdala surface to a sphere. Then taking the spherical coordinates as a reference frame, amygdala surfaces are parameterized as a weighted linear combination of smooth basis functions using the recently developed weighted spherical harmonic representation. This new representation is used for parameterizing, smoothing and nonlinearly registering a group of amygdala surfaces. The methodology has been applied in detecting abnormal local shape variations in 23 autistic subjects compared against 24 normal controls. We did not detect any statistically significant abnormal amygdala shape variations in autistic subjects. The complete amygdala surface modeling codes used in this study is available at http://www.stat.wisc.edu/~mchung/research/amygdala.

1 Introduction

Amygdala is an important brain substructure that has been implicated in abnormal functional impairment in autism [7] [14]. Since the abnormal structure might be the cause of the functional impairment, there have been many studies on amygdala volumetry in autism. However, most amygdala volumetry results are somewhat inconsistent [2] [16] [10] [14]. The previous studies traced the amygdalae manually and by counting the number of voxels within the region of interest (ROI), the total volume of the amygdalae were estimated. The limitation of the traditional ROI-based volumetry is that it can not determine if the volume difference is spread all over the ROI or localized within specific regions of the ROI.

In this paper, we present a new framework for addressing the problem of local amygdala shape analysis using the recently developed *weighted spherical harmonic representation* [5]. The weighted spherical harmonic representation

T. Dohi, I. Sakuma, and H. Liao (Eds.): MIAR 2008, LNCS 5128, pp. 177–184, 2008.

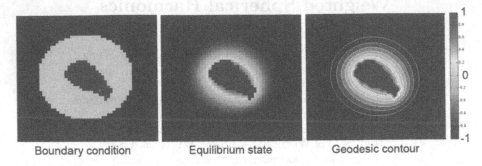

Fig. 1. The diffusion equation with a heat source (amygdala) and a heat sink (enclosing sphere). After sufficient number of iterations, the equilibrium state is reached. By tracing the geodesic path from the heat source to the heat sink using the geodesic contour, we obtain a smooth spherical mapping.

formulates surface parameterization, filtering and nonlinear surface registration in a unified Hilbert space framework. Since the proposed method requires a surface flattening to a sphere, we have developed a new and very fast surface flattening technique based on the equilibrium state of heat diffusion. By tracing the geodesic path of heat equilibrium state from a heat source (amygdala) to a heat sink (sphere), we obtain a smooth spherical mapping. Solving an isotropic heat equation in a 3D image volume is computationally trivial, so our proposed method offers a much simpler numerical implementation than previous surface flattening techniques such as conformal mappings [1] [9] [11], quasi-isometric mappings [17] and area preserving mappings [4]. These flattening methods are not trivial to implement and computationally insensitive. Once we obtain the weighted spherical harmonic representation of amygdalae, the group difference between 23 autistic and 24 control subjects is statistically tested using the Hotelling's T^2 statistic on the estimated surface coordinates.

2   Methods

High resolution anatomical magnetic resonance images (MRI) were obtained using a 3-Tesla GE SIGNA scanner with a quadrature head coil. Details on image acquisition parameters are given in [14]. MRIs are reoriented to the pathological plane [6] for optimal comparison with anatomical atlases. Manual segmentation was done by an expert and the reliability of the manual segmentation was validated by two raters on 10 amygdale resulting in interclass correlation of 0.95 and the intersection over the union of 0.84 [14]. Once binary segmentation is obtained, the marching cubes algorithm was used to extract the boundary of amygdale. Afterwards, we we flattened the amaygada surfaces using the proposed method.

2.1   Surface Flattening Via Diffusion

Given an amygdala binary segmentation $\mathcal{M}_a$, we put a larger sphere $\mathcal{M}_s$ that encloses the amygala (Figure 1 left). The amygdala is assigned the value 1 while the enclosing sphere is assigned the value -1, i.e.

$$f(\mathcal{M}_a, \sigma) = 1 \text{ and } f(\mathcal{M}_s, \sigma) = -1$$

for all σ. The parameter σ denotes the diffusion time. The amygdala and the sphere serve as a heat source and a heat sink respectively. Then we solve an isotropic diffusion equation

$$\frac{\partial f}{\partial \sigma} = \Delta f \tag{1}$$

with the given boundary condition. Δ is the 3D Laplacian. After sufficiently enough time, the solution reaches the heat equilibrium state where the additional diffusion does not make any change in the heat distribution (Figure 1 middle). The heat equilibrium state can be also obtained by letting $\frac{\partial f}{\partial \sigma} = 0$ and solving for the Laplace equation

$$\Delta f = 0$$

with the same boundary condition. The resulting equilibrium state is given in Figure 1 (middle).

Once we obtained the equilibrium state, we trace the geodesic path from the heat source to the heat sink for every mesh vertices on the isosurface of the amygdala. The trajectory of the geodesic path provides a smooth mapping from the amygdala surface to the sphere. The geodesic path can be traced by following the gradient of the equilibrium state but this requires solving an additional system of differential equations. So we have avoided using the equilibrium gradient. Instead we have constructed numerous geodesic contours that correspond to the level set of the equilibrium state (Figure 1 right). Then the geodesic path is constructed by finding the shortest distance from one contour to the next and connecting them together. This is done in an iterative fashion as shown in Figure 2, where five contours corresponding to the values 0.6, 0.2, -0.2, -0.6, -1.0 are used to flatten the amygdala surface. Once we obtained the spherical mapping, we can project the Euler angles (θ, φ) onto the amygdala surface (Figure 3) and the Euler angles serve as the underlying parameterization for the weighted spherical harmonic modeling.

2.2   Weighted Spherical Harmonics

Since the technical detail and numerical implementation for the weighted spherical harmonic modeling is given in [5], we will only briefly describe the basic idea here. The *weighted spherical harmonic representation* fixes the Gibbs phenomenon (ringing effects) associated with the traditional Fourier descriptors and spherical harmonic representation [4] [8] [9] [12] [15] by weighting the series expansion with exponential weights. The exponential weights make the representation converges faster and reduces the amount of wiggling. If surface coordinates

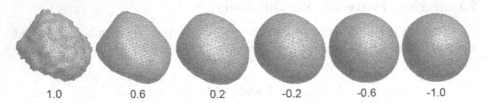

Fig. 2. Amygala surface flattening process following the geodesic path of the equilibrium state of heat diffusion. The numbers corresponds to the geodesic contours. For simple shapes like amygda, 5 to 10 contours are sufficient for tracing the geodesic path.

are abruptly changing or their derivatives are discontinuous, the Gibbs phenomenon will severely distort the surface shape as shown in Figure 4, where a cube is reconstructed with both the traditional ($k = 42, \sigma = 0$) and the new weighted spherical harmonics ($k = 42, \sigma = 0.001$). The weighted version has less ringing effects.

From the surface flattening, the mesh coordinates for the amygdala surface ∂M_a can be parameterized by the Euler angles $\theta \in [0, \pi], \varphi \in [0, 2\pi)$ associated with the unit sphere as

$$p(\theta, \varphi) = (p_1(\theta, \varphi), p_2(\theta, \varphi), p_2(\theta, \varphi))'.$$

See Figure 3 for how the Euler angles are used to parameterize the amygdala surface. The weighted spherical harmonic representation of the coordinates is then given by

$$p(\theta, \varphi) = \sum_{l=0}^{k} \sum_{m=-l}^{l} e^{-l(l+1)\sigma} f_{lm} Y_{lm}(\theta, \varphi),$$

where

$$f_{lm} = \int_{\theta=0}^{\pi} \int_{\varphi=0}^{2\pi} p(\theta, \varphi) Y_{lm}(\theta, \varphi) \sin \theta d\theta d\varphi.$$

are the Fourier coefficient vectors and Y_{lm} are spherical harmonics of degree l and order m. The coefficients f_{lm} are estimated by one degree at a time in the least squares fashion using the recently developed *iterative residual fitting* algorithm. We have used the 15-th degree representation for this study (Figure 5).

Once amgydala surfaces are represented with the weighted spherical harmonics, the *spherical harmonic correspondence* can be used to nonlinearly align all 47 amygdale surfaces. The technical details on the spherical harmonic correspondence is given in [5]. The average left and right amygdala templates are constructed by averaging the Fourier coefficients of all 24 control subjects. The smooth surfaces in Figure 6 are the constructed average templates. The template surfaces serve as the reference coordinates for projecting the subsequent statistical parametric maps.

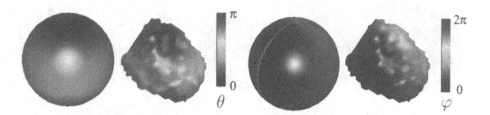

Fig. 3. Amygdala surface parameterization using the Euler angles (θ, φ). The point $\theta = 0$ corresponds to the north pole of a unit sphere. The parameterization is needed for the weighted spherical harmonic modeling.

2.3   Comparing Two Groups of Surfaces

Let i be the group index and j be the subject index. Let n_i be the sample size in the i-th group. For convenience, let the first group to be normal controls ($n_1 = 24$) and the second group to be autistic ($n_2 = 23$). We propose the following stochastic model on the weighted spherical harmonics. For surface coordinates $p_{ij} = (p_{ij}^1, p_{ij}^2, p_{ij}^3)'$, we model

$$p_{ij}(\theta, \varphi) = \sum_{l=0}^{k} \sum_{m=-l}^{l} e^{-l(l+1)\sigma} \mu_{lm}^{ij} Y_{lm}(\theta, \varphi) + \Sigma^{1/2}(\theta, \varphi) \epsilon_{ij}(\theta, \varphi),$$

where μ_{lm}^{ij} are unknown Fourier coefficient vectors, Σ is the covariance matrix, which allows the spatial dependence among p_{i1}, p_{i2}, p_{i3}, and ϵ_{ij} are independent and identically distributed Gaussian random vector field. A similar stochastic modeling approach has been used in [13] where the canonical expansion of a Gaussian random field is used to model deformation vector fields. Then we test the following null H_0 and alternate H_1 hypotheses:

$$H_0 : \sum_{l=0}^{k} \sum_{m=-l}^{l} e^{-l(l+1)\sigma} \mu_{lm}^{1j} Y_{lm}(\theta, \varphi) = \sum_{l=0}^{k} \sum_{m=-l}^{l} e^{-l(l+1)\sigma} \mu_{lm}^{2j} Y_{lm}(\theta, \varphi)$$

vs.

$$H_1 : \sum_{l=0}^{k} \sum_{m=-l}^{l} e^{-l(l+1)\sigma} \mu_{lm}^{1j} Y_{lm}(\theta, \varphi) \neq \sum_{l=0}^{k} \sum_{m=-l}^{l} e^{-l(l+1)\sigma} \mu_{lm}^{2j} Y_{lm}(\theta, \varphi).$$

The unknown group mean for the i-th group is estimated by

$$\bar{p}_i = \frac{1}{n_i} \sum_{j=1}^{n_i} p_{ij}.$$

The group mean difference vector $\bar{p}_2 - \bar{p}_1$ is shown as white arrows in Figure 6. The group difference is only shown in the regions with P-value < 0.01 for better visualization. The direction of white arrows is where the mean control surface

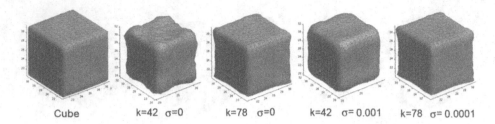

Cube   k=42 σ=0   k=78 σ=0   k=42 σ= 0.001   k=78 σ= 0.0001

Fig. 4. The severe Gibbs phenomenon shown in the traditional spherical harmonic model of a cube ($\sigma = 0$) for degrees $k = 42, 78$. The weighted versions can reduce the Gibbs phenomenon in the representation by introducing small weights corresponding to $\sigma = 0.001, 0.0001$.

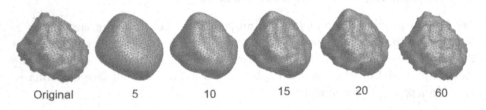

Original   5   10   15   20   60

Fig. 5. The spherical harmonic modeling of a left amygdala surface with various degrees. We have chosen degree 15 representation in this study.

should be moved to match with the mean amygdala surface. The significance of the group difference can be tested using the Hotelling's T^2 statistic given by

$$H(\theta, \varphi) = \frac{n_1 n_2 (n_1 + n_2 - 4)}{3(n_1 + n_2)(n_1 + n_2 - 2)} (\bar{p}_2 - \bar{p}_1)' \widehat{\Sigma}^{-1} (\bar{p}_2 - \bar{p}_1),$$

where

$$\widehat{\Sigma} = \frac{1}{n_1 + n_2 - 2} \left[\sum_{j=1}^{n_1} (p_{1j} - \bar{p}_1)(p_{1j} - \bar{p}_1)' + \sum_{j=1}^{n_2} (p_{2j} - \bar{p}_1)(p_{2j} - \bar{p}_2)' \right].$$

$H(\theta, \varphi)$ is distributed as a F-statistic with 3 and $n_1 + n_2 - 4$ degrees of freedom.

3 Results

The volumes for control subjects ($n_1 = 24$) are left 1883 ± 176mm^3, right 1874 ± 172mm^3. The volumes for autistic subjects ($n_2 = 23$) are left 1859 ± 182mm^3, right 1862 ± 181mm^3. The volume difference between the groups are not statistically significant (P-value $= 0.64$ for left and 0.81 for right).

From the ROI-based volumetry, it is not clear if the local shape difference is still present within amygdala. So we have performed the Hotelling's T^2 test the average surface template at each mesh vertex. The resulting P-value is given in

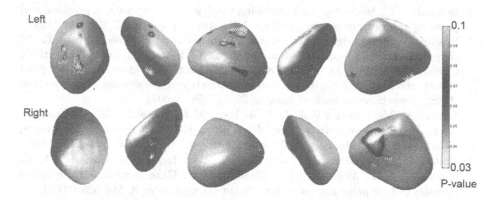

Fig. 6. The P-value of Hotelling's T^2 statistic projected onto the average amydala template constructed from 24 control subjects. The white arrows show the direction where the average control surface should move to match the average autistic surface.

Figure 6. The minimum P-value is 0.03 for both the left and the right amygdale. Although, at a fixed point, this is sufficiently low P-value to be taken as a significant signal, the result will not pass the multiple comparison correction based on the random field theory [18] or false discovery rate (FDR) [3]. So we conclude that there is no abnormal local amygdala shape difference in autism.

4   Conclusions

The paper developed a unified framework for quantifying a population of amygdala surfaces. Our main contribution is the new amygdala surface flattening technique that utilizes the idea of the geodesic path of heat equilibrium. The proposed flattening technique is simple enough to be applied to various applications. Using the spherical mapping established from the new flattening technique, we have applied the recently developed weighted spherical harmonic representation to parameterize, to register amygdala surfaces, and to detect local shape difference. We found no statistically significant local amygdala shape difference between autism and control. The complete compute codes used for this study is available at http://www.stat.wisc.edu/~mchung/research/amygdala.

References

1. Angenent, S., Hacker, S., Tannenbaum, A., Kikinis, R.: On the laplace-beltrami operator and brain surface flattening. IEEE Transactions on Medical Imaging 18, 700–711 (1999)
2. Aylward, E.H., Minshew, N.J., Goldstein, G., Honeycutt, N.A., Augustine, A.M., Yates, K.O., Bartra, P.E., Pearlson, G.D.: Mri volumes of amygdala and hippocampus in nonmentally retarded autistic adolescents and adults. Neurology 53, 2145–2150 (1999)

184   M.K. Chung et al.

3. Benjamini, Y., Hochberg, Y.: Controlling the false discovery rate: a practical and powerful approach to multiple testing. J. R. Stat. Soc, Ser. B 57, 289–300 (1995)
4. Brechbuhler, C., Gerig, G., Kubler, O.: Parametrization of closed surfaces for 3d shape description. Computer Vision and Image Understanding 61, 154–170 (1995)
5. Chung, M.K., Shen, L., Dalton, K.M., Evans, A.C., Davidson, R.J.: Weighted fourier representation and its application to quantifying the amount of gray matter. IEEE transactions on medical imaging 26, 566–581 (2007)
6. Convit, A., McHugh, P., Wolf, O.T., de Leon, M.J., Bobinkski, M., De Santi, S., Roche, A., Tsui, W.: Mri volume of the amygdala: a reliable method allowing separation from the hippocampal formation. Psychiatry Res. 90, 113–123 (1999)
7. Dalton, K.M., Nacewicz, B.M., Johnstone, T., Schaefer, H.S., Gernsbacher, M.A., Goldsmith, H.H., Alexander, A.L., Davidson, R.J.: Gaze fixation and the neural circuitry of face processing in autism. Nature Neuroscience 8, 519–526 (2005)
8. Gerig, G., Styner, M., Jones, D., Weinberger, D., Lieberman, J.: Shape analysis of brain ventricles using spharm. In: MMBIA, pp. 171–178 (2001)
9. Gu, X., Wang, Y.L., Chan, T.F., Thompson, T.M., Yau, S.T.: Genus zero surface conformal mapping and its application to brain surface mapping. IEEE Transactions on Medical Imaging 23, 1–10 (2004)
10. Haznedar, M.M., Buchsbaum, M.S., Wei, T.C., Hof, P.R., Cartwright, C., Bienstock, E., Hollander, C.A.: Limbic circuitry in patients with autism spectrum disorders studied with positron emission tomography and magnetic resonance imaging. American Journal of Psychiatry 157, 1994–2001 (2000)
11. Hurdal, M.K., Stephenson, K.: Cortical cartography using the discrete conformal approach of circle packings. NeuroImage 23, S119–S128 (2004)
12. Kelemen, A., Szekely, G., Gerig, G.: Elastic model-based segmentation of 3-d neuroradiological data sets. IEEE Transactions on Medical Imaging 18, 828–839 (1999)
13. Miller, M.I., Banerjee, A., Christensen, G.E., Joshi, S.C., Khaneja, N., Grenander, U., Matejic, L.: Statistical methods in computational anatomy. Statistical Methods in Medical Research 6, 267–299 (1997)
14. Nacewicz, B.M., Dalton, K.M., Johnstone, T., Long, M.T., McAuliff, E.M., Oakes, T.R., Alexander, A.L., Davidson, R.J.: Amygdala volume and nonverbal social impairment in adolescent and adult males with autism. Arch. Gen. Psychiatry. 63, 1417–1428 (2006)
15. Shen, L., Ford, J., Makedon, F., Saykin, A.: surface-based approach for classification of 3d neuroanatomical structures. Intelligent Data Analysis 8, 519–542 (2004)
16. Sparks, B.F., Friedman, S.D., Shaw, D.W., Aylward, E.H., Echelard, D., Artru, A.A., Maravilla, K.R., Giedd, J.N., Munson, J., Dawson, G., Dager, S.R.: Brain structural abnormalities in young children with autism spectrum disorder. Neurology 59, 184–192 (2002)
17. Timsari, B., Leahy, R.: An optimization method for creating semi-isometric flat maps of the cerebral cortex. In: The Proceedings of SPIE, Medical Imaging (2000)
18. Worsley, K.J., Marrett, S., Neelin, P., Vandal, A.C., Friston, K.J., Evans, A.C.: A unified statistical approach for determining significant signals in images of cerebral activation. Human Brain Mapping 4, 58–73 (1996)

Kalman Filtering for Frame-by-Frame CT to Ultrasound Rigid Registration

Haydar Talib[1], Matthias Peterhans[1], Jaime García[1],
Martin Styner[2], and Miguel A. González Ballester[1]

[1] MEM Research Center, Institute for Surgical Technology and Biomechanics
University of Bern, Switzerland
[2] Departments of Computer Science and Psychiatry, Neurodevelopmental Disorders
Research Center, University of North Carolina at Chapel Hill, USA
{Haydar.Talib, Matthias.Peterhans}@MEMcenter.unibe.ch*

Abstract. This paper presents a method for CT-US rigid registration in minimally-invasive computer-assisted orthopaedic surgery, whereby the registration procedure is reformulated to enable effectively real-time registrations. A linear Kalman filter based algorithm is compared to an Unscented Kalman filter based method in simulated and experimental scenarios. The validation schemes demonstrate that the linear Kalman filter is more accurate, more robust, and converges quicker than the UKF, yielding an effectively real-time method for rigid registration applications, circumventing surgeons' waiting times.

1 Introduction

In computer-assisted orthopaedic surgery (CAOS), surgeons often benefit from enhanced visualization by registering a pre-operatively acquired medical image, such as from CT or MRI, to the patient's anatomy during surgery. Registration is usually achieved by digitizing bone surface points from the patient using a navigated pointer, and determining the optimal transformation between the pre-operative data and the points. The use of navigated ultrasound (US) imaging for acquiring bone surface points to be used in registration is an ongoing area of research, and one of the main advantages of using US is that points can be acquired non-invasively [1,2,3].

The use of the Unscented Kalman Filter (UKF) was recently proposed for rigid registration in CAOS, and was shown to have improved performance compared to the Iterative Closest Point method [4]. The advantage of the Kalman filter is that it is a computationally efficient least-squares solver, which is an ideal feature for intra-operative registration applications. Furthermore, the UKF was originally formulated to avoid some of the linearizations that occur in the classic formulation of the Kalman filter.

* The authors thank the NCCR Co-Me and BrainLab AG for funding this project, as well as colleagues Urs Rohrer, Erland Mühlheim, Sebastian Marti, and Ronald Ramseier for the experimental set-up.

T. Dohi, I. Sakuma, and H. Liao (Eds.): MIAR 2008, LNCS 5128, pp. 185–192, 2008.
© Springer-Verlag Berlin Heidelberg 2008

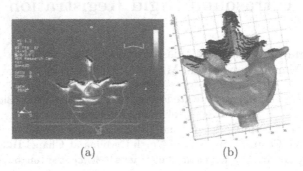

(a)   (b)

Fig. 1. (a) Typical result of US segmentation (dark points) overlaid onto an US image and a contour generated from the ground truth (light grey) (b) segmented US points overlaid onto ground truth

We consider a US-based registration application in this paper, and reformulate the registration procedure such that the registration is effectively real-time. US images are considered as sequential signals, where each frame provides surface points of the anatomy. The registration is updated as frames are acquired, implying that iterations are no longer dependent on the number of points [4]. The registration itself begins during data acquisition, which implies that there is no need to wait until a full set of points is obtained before starting the algorithm.

The linear Kalman filter formulation used in this paper is akin to the perturbation Kalman filter [5]. The Extended Kalman Filter (EKF) could have been an alternative formulation, but the linearizations employed for this study were much simpler than the computation of Jacobian matrices [6]. We will demonstrate that the linear Kalman filter converges more quickly than the UKF, and is more robust with respect to starting positions. To evaluate the performance of these methods, we consider minimally-invasive interventions around the spine as potential target applications. The methods are compared using synthetic data and also in an experimental set-up using navigated 2D US, whereby the accuracy of the proposed registration method shows promise for use in clinical applications.

2   CT to US Rigid Registration

In the usual US-based registration scenario, navigated US images provide a set of bone surface points in the coordinate space of the patient's anatomy, which is referenced by the navigation system. To enhance the limited information provided by US, a surface model representation of the anatomy, as obtained from a CT for instance, is then registered to the US-acquired bone surface points.

The problem at hand is in finding the transformation that would place the CT-generated surface model in the coordinate space of the anatomy. For the Kalman filters, the measurement, z_k, is a set of points in world coordinates acquired by segmenting the US images. At a given time step k, the state x_k

is comprised of the true parameters that represent the transformation between the US points and the corresponding points on the surface model, $\hat{z}_k^-$, which are found by searching for closest points using Euclidean distances. The estimate of this state is denoted $\hat{x}_k$, and is a 6×1 vector $[\alpha, \beta, \gamma, t_x, t_y, t_z]^T$.

2.1   Kalman Filtering for Registration

For the UKF and the EKF, the state x_k represents the transformation from the CT surface model to the set of US-acquired points [4,6], and can be regarded as time-invariant. For the linear Kalman filter used here, however, we consider that x_k is time-variant, meaning that the state represents incremental transformations during the registration procedure [5]. For a given measurement z_k, the corresponding points $\hat{z}_k^-$ are found from the surface at the prior position, S_{k-1}.

To illustrate the registration method, consider the prediction and correction steps of the linear Kalman filter equations [7], with the unused terms omitted:

$$\hat{x}_k^- = \hat{x}_{k-1} \tag{1}$$

$$\hat{x}_k = \hat{x}_k^- + K_k (z_k - H\hat{x}_k^-) \tag{2}$$

At a given time step k, the correspondence is found between the new measurement z_k and S_{k-1}, yielding $\hat{z}_k^-$. The predicted state $\hat{x}_k^-$ is then updated (1) and applied to $\hat{z}_k^-$, yielding the estimated measurement $\hat{z}_k = H\hat{x}_k^-$. The predicted state is then corrected (2) and applied to the surface S_{k-1}, yielding S_k.

No model was used for propagating the state $\hat{x}_k$. z_k and corresponding points $\hat{z}_k^-$ are sets of vertically concatenated points such that they each become $3N \times 1$ column vectors. For instance, $\hat{z}_k^-$ is written as $[\hat{z}_{x1}^-, \hat{z}_{y1}^-, \hat{z}_{z1}^-, \ldots, \hat{z}_{xN}^-, \hat{z}_{yN}^-, \hat{z}_{zN}^-]_k^T$, where N is the number of points segmented from US [4].

The matrix H relates the measurement z_k to the state $\hat{x}_k$, and is used in all the correction steps of the Kalman filter. In the registration scenario, H should relate points in Cartesian coordinates to the parameters of a rigid transformation matrix, which is denoted T, such that:

$$\hat{z}_k = T\hat{z}_k^- = H\hat{x}_k^- \tag{3}$$

In order to determine H, it becomes necessary to employ approximations for the terms in T. We employ a zeroth order truncation of the Taylor Series representations of cosine and sine, such that for a given angle θ, $\cos\theta \approx 1$ and $\sin\theta \approx \theta$, which should be valid for small angles. We denote the approximation of T by T_A (using the $\alpha\beta\gamma$ convention), and (3) for a single point can be written as:

$$T_A\hat{z}_k^- = \begin{pmatrix} 1 & \gamma + \alpha\beta & \alpha\gamma - \beta & t_x \\ -\gamma & 1 - \alpha\beta\gamma & \alpha + \beta\gamma & t_y \\ \beta & -\alpha & 1 & t_z \end{pmatrix} \begin{pmatrix} \hat{z}_{xk}^- \\ \hat{z}_{yk}^- \\ \hat{z}_{zk}^- \\ 1 \end{pmatrix} \tag{4}$$

The residual in the Kalman filter update step (2), $\mathbf{z}_k - \mathbf{H}\hat{\mathbf{x}}_k^-$, can be reinterpreted as $\mathbf{z}_k - \mathbf{T}_A \hat{\mathbf{z}}_k^-$, and $\mathbf{T}_A \hat{\mathbf{z}}_k^-$ can finally be expressed as:

$$\mathbf{T}_A \hat{\mathbf{z}}_k^- = \begin{pmatrix} \hat{z}_{xk}^- \\ \hat{z}_{yk}^- \\ \hat{z}_{zk}^- \end{pmatrix} + \mathbf{H}\hat{\mathbf{x}}_k^- + \begin{pmatrix} \alpha\beta\hat{z}_{yk}^- + \alpha\gamma\hat{z}_{zk}^- \\ \beta\gamma\hat{z}_{zk}^- - \alpha\beta\gamma\hat{z}_{yk}^- \\ 0 \end{pmatrix} \tag{5}$$

Where $\mathbf{H}$, to be used in the Kalman filter equations, becomes:

$$\mathbf{H} = \begin{pmatrix} 0 & -\hat{z}_{zk}^- & \hat{z}_{yk}^- & 1 & 0 & 0 \\ \hat{z}_{zk}^- & 0 & -\hat{z}_{xk}^- & 0 & 1 & 0 \\ -\hat{z}_{yk}^- & \hat{z}_{xk}^- & 0 & 0 & 0 & 1 \end{pmatrix} \tag{6}$$

For a single point, $\mathbf{H}$ is a 3×6 matrix that comprises the cross product matrix on the left side, and $\mathbf{I}_3$ on the right side. For N points, where $\hat{\mathbf{z}}_k^-$ is a $3N \times 1$ vector, $\mathbf{H}$ is a $3N \times 6$ matrix.

Moghari et al. [4] applied the UKF to estimate rigid transformation parameters in US-to-CT registration. By their implementation, the UKF iterates N times, where N is the number of points in their $\mathbf{z}_k$, and for each iteration, the number of points is gradually increasing. While this approach usually provides smooth filter behavior, it does not take advantage of the Kalman filter's sequential real-time nature.

With the UKF, no explicit relationship between the transformation parameters $\hat{\mathbf{x}}_k$ and the points $\mathbf{z}_k$ needs to be defined, but rather the UKF operates on the principle of an implicit linearization of the relationship. At each prediction step, the estimated state $\hat{\mathbf{x}}_k$ is applied to the surface at the initial position, S_1, producing S_k. Correspondence is determined between the measurement and S_k, and when the registration is completed, the resulting state is applied to S_1.

2.2   Frame-by-Frame Registration Procedure

In the usual approach to registration, the registration procedure does not begin until a full set of points is acquired from the anatomy. For the work presented here, we propose using the Kalman filter to update the registration as navigated 2D US images are acquired.

For both Kalman filters, each US frame is treated as one signal, which yields a coplanar cloud of points, $\mathbf{z}_k$. The registration is updated with each newly acquired frame, and so the time step k is now related to the number of US frames, as they are acquired, rather than the number of points. During image acquisition, the surgeon can then receive visual (fig. 1(b)) and numerical feedback in terms of how well the Kalman filter fits the surface to the US-acquired points. The result of this approach is that fewer iterations are needed for the registrations. To stabilize the frame-by-frame processing of the filters, a small subset of points from prior US frames is used to complement the point sets of new frames. In §3, the original UKF registration algorithm is compared to the frame-by-frame UKF and linear Kalman filter registration methods.

3 Results

3.1 Simulated Data

In order to compare their performance on ideal data, the three Kalman filter registration methods were used with synthetic data. For the measurement, consider 100 randomly selected points from a 3D surface model of an L4 vertebra, in the area that would be accessible by US. $\mathcal{N}(0, 1[mm^2])$ noise was added to the coordinates of the points. In the original UKF registration method (point-by-point UKF), each point is treated 99/2 times on average. To achieve a comparison using

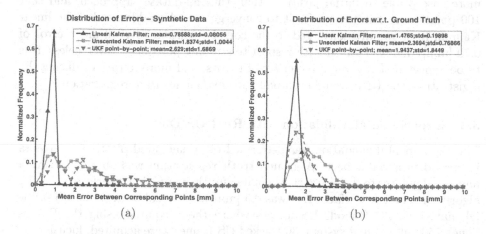

Fig. 2. Distribution of RMS corresponding point-to-point errors, computed between surfaces at estimated positions and the ground truth, for (a) synthetic data and (b) experimental validation, comparing the three Kalman filter-based approaches

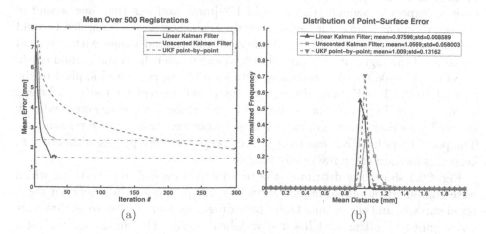

Fig. 3. (a) Mean errors plotted with respect to number of iterations and (b) distribution of RMS point-to-surface errors, computed using nearest points between estimated surfaces and ground truth

the full-dataset approach, the frame-by-frame filters were iterated 50 times over the 100 points. A set of 500 randomly-generated rigid transformations (within a range of ± 5 [deg.] for the three angles, ± 10 [mm] for two translations and 0-20 [mm] in the US scanning direction) was applied to the surface model, and each Kalman filter was used to register the surface to the points for each transformation. Errors were computed by measuring the distances between corresponding points on the registered surface and the surface at the true position.

As can be inferred from the graph in fig. 2(a), the two UKF methods have similarly distributed mean errors, but the point-by-point UKF had much higher errors in several cases. This result indicates that the point-by-point UKF was more susceptible to initial positions than the full-dataset approach, and that 100 points were not enough for it to converge to a desirable result. The linear Kalman filter rapidly converged to the correct solution (overall mean error of 0.79 [mm]) and was robust with respect to starting positions. Nevertheless, it is to be expected that given a larger set of points, and more iterations during the registration, the UKF would eventually achieve an accurate registration.

3.2   Experimental Validation with Real US Data

The experimental validation was performed on a navigated plastic L4 vertebra immersed in a water bath. A ground truth registration was obtained using a navigated pointer to digitize surface points and then applying a surface matching algorithm (point-to-surface error was 0.5 [mm]). After calibrating the US probe [8], navigated 2D B-mode US images where then acquired using the Philips Sonos 7500 ultrasound system. 36 tracked US frames were acquired, focusing on the areas that would be visible in a real patient set-up (fig. 1(b)). Bone contour points were then automatically extracted by combining Otsu thresholding with a morphological opening, and a thinning of the resulting border along the US scan lines. This preliminary segmentation method is suitable for water bath scans, with an expected segmentation error of 1-2 [mm], and less than one second of computation per frame. For each frame, the segmentation was sampled to yield 100 bone contour points. Fig. 1(a) shows an ultrasound image with a typical outcome of the segmentation procedure and the contour from the ground truth.

As in §3.1, 500 transformations were randomly generated and applied to the ground truth. The Kalman filters were then used to register the transformed surface to the US points. For the frame-by-frame filters, 8 points were randomly selected from each prior US image as new frames were used for the registration. The point-by-point UKF was halted once 300 points were processed in order to keep this method computationally feasible.

Fig. 2(b) shows the distribution of mean errors over all registrations, which were computed by measuring distances of corresponding points between registered surfaces and the ground truth, providing a measure in the areas that were not scanned by ultrasound (i.e. the vertebral body). The linear Kalman filter presented in this paper showed superior performance in terms of accuracy (overall mean error of 1.48 [mm]) and robustness with respect to starting positions (standard deviation of 0.20 [mm]). Although the point-by-point UKF achieved a

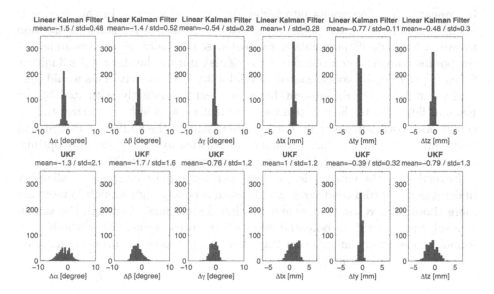

Fig. 4. Distributions of transformation parameter errors

lower mean error than the frame-by-frame UKF, it demonstrated higher sensitivity to starting positions in 6 cases, when it had mean errors higher than 5 [mm]. The point-by-point UKF results may have been improved if it was iterated over more points, but this would have led to an exorbitant amount of computation (e.g. for N points, computing matrix inverses for $3N \times 3N$ matrices).

Fig. 3(a) shows the trend of mean errors with respect to iteration number for each of the three methods. The point-by-point UKF was iterated 300 times, and showed a generally smooth behavior in its estimation. The frame-by-frame methods, which were iterated 36 times, demonstrated much quicker convergence in their estimation, with the linear Kalman filter converging the quickest. Fig. 3(b) shows the distribution of mean distances between the US points and the surface. This result is analogous to the result in [4], and consistent with the the more reliable measure in fig. 2(b).

The histograms in fig. 4 reflect the differences between transformation parameters obtained by the frame-by-frame Kalman filters and those of the 500 randomly-generated transformations, whereby the linear Kalman filter showed a more consistent estimation of the parameters than the UKF.

4 Conclusions

The experimental results suggest that the linear Kalman filter produces more accurate results compared to the Unscented Kalman Filter in the frame-by-frame registration framework presented in this paper. The greatest reason for this unexpected outcome stems from the approach to the design of the filters. Both in this work and in [4], batch processing of points for each iteration was performed by concatenating the points into higher-dimensional vectors. In this way, it is assumed that noise on the points is independent, which is the same assumption as would be made if the points were treated sequentially [6]. In concatenating the points, however, their covariance as calculated from the state, a 3×3 matrix for each point, is also concatenated to yield a $3N \times 3N$ matrix. This would then lead to an ill-conditioned system, but this effect is implicitly mitigated by the Kalman filter due to the additive measurement noise, which regularizes the ill-conditioned covariance matrix. Further discussion on the additive measurement noise can be found in [4], but it would be interesting to investigate more optimal approaches to the sequential batch processing employed here [9].

Nevertheless, the current design demonstrated rapid convergence, reliability under different initial conditions, as well as an accuracy high enough to motivate more thorough investigation, nearer to clinical situations. Although the validation schemes focused on potential applications in the spine, the methods were formulated generally enough that they may be applicable to various minimally-invasive orthopedic procedures.

References

1. Barratt, D., Penney, G., Chan, C., Slomczykowski, M., Carter, T., Edwards, P., Hawkes, D.: Self-calibrating 3d-ultrasound-based bone registration for minimally invasive orthopedic surgery. IEEE Trans. Med. Imaging 25(3), 312–323 (2006)
2. Muratore, D.M., Russ, J.H., Dawant, B.M., Galloway, R.L.: Three-dimensional image registration of phantom vertebrae for image-guided surgery: a preliminary study. Comput. Aided Surg. 7(6), 342–352 (2002)
3. Talib, H., Rajamani, K., Kowal, J., Nolte, L.P., Styner, M., Ballester, M.A.G.: A comparison study assessing the feasibility of ultrasound-initialized deformable bone models. Comput Aided Surg 10(5-6), 293–299 (2005)
4. Moghari, M.H., Abolmaesumi, P.: Point-based rigid-body registration using an unscented kalman filter. IEEE Transactions on Medical Imaging 26(12), 1708–1728 (2007)
5. Grewal, M.S., Andrews, A.P.: Kalman Filtering Theory and Practice. Information and System Sciences Series. Prentice-Hall, Englewood Cliffs (1993)
6. Pennec, X., Thirion, J.: A framework for uncertainty and validation of 3d registration methods based on points and frames. International Journal of Computer Vision 25(3), 203–229 (1997)
7. Welch, G., Bishop, G.: An introduction to the kalman filter. Technical Report TR 95-041, University of North Carolina, Chapel Hill (1995)
8. Kowal, J., Amstutz, C., Nolte, L.P.: On the development and comparative evaluation of an ultrasound b-mode probe calibration unit. Comput. Aided Surg. 8(3), 107–119 (2003)
9. Maybeck, P.S.: Stochastic Models, Estimation, and Control. 1 of Mathematics in Science and Engineering, vol. 141. Academic Press, London (1979)

Cardiac PET Motion Correction Using Materially Constrained Transform Models

Adrian J. Chung[1], Paolo G. Camici[1], and Guang-Zhong Yang[2]

[1] PET Cardiology, MRC Clinical Sciences Centre, Hammersmith Hospital, London, UK
[2] Royal Society/Wolfson MIC Laboratory, Imperial College, London, UK
ajchung@imperial.ac.uk, paolo.camici@csc.mrc.ac.uk,
g.z.yang@imperial.ac.uk

Abstract. Recent improvements in the resolution of Positron Emission Tomography (PET) imaging have not translated into equivalent advances in diagnostic accuracy. Due to long acquisition times involved, the functional imaging modality is hampered by motion artefacts due to respiratory motion. In this paper, two methods for correcting reconstructed PET images through a list-mode re-binning process are investigated. The first method rebins the list-mode data according to a globally defined 3D affine transformation. The second is a novel approach that combines multiple independent 2D affine transforms in order to exploit the specific properties of 2D tomographic reconstruction. Each affine transformation method is applied to the respiratory gated sequence of line-of-response events prior to image reconstruction, thus compensating for any respiratory motion. The deformation models are derived from a non-rigid 3D/3D registration model applied to retrospectively gated MRI acquired during free-breathing. The motion correction schemes are validated using a simulation framework with respiratory gated MRI scans of 10 subjects to generate the required activity maps for estimating emission sinograms. This allows the ground truth solution to be derived so that the motion corrected reconstruction can be compared quantitatively. It is shown that the higher degrees of freedom of the 2D affine motion compensation model is superior to the 3D affine transform provided one incorporates weak material constraints to avoid ill conditioning and can tolerate the lower SNR that 2D reconstruction implies.

Keywords: PET, Lung, Motion, Motion Correction, Gating, MRI, Myocardium, Affine.

1 Introduction

Positron Emission Tomography (PET) imaging has proven to be an invaluable tool in the diagnosis and management of coronary artery disease. The technique has been especially beneficial in the metabolic imaging of viable myocardial tissue, whereby the uptake of a radioactive glucose analogue, fluorine-18 fluorodeoxyglucose (FDG) is quantified [1]. This facilitates high predictive value of positive outcomes for surgical revascularization. The technique, however, is sensitive to patient motion, particularly respiratory induced cardiac motion [2]. Compensating for respiratory deformation in

T. Dohi, I. Sakuma, and H. Liao (Eds.): MIAR 2008, LNCS 5128, pp. 193–201, 2008.
© Springer-Verlag Berlin Heidelberg 2008

the reconstruction of PET images typically entails adopting respiratory gating techniques similar to that applied to Magnetic Resonance Imaging (MRI) [3]. By using motion tracking to the gated images, the deformation of the anatomical structure can be estimated [4], thus allowing each image to be transformed to a common phase of the respiratory cycle [5]. Due to the lowered counts, gated images suffer from a much reduced Signal-to-Noise Ratio (SNR).

Recently, the availability of low cost high-capacity data storage has facilitated the gated acquisition of the PET data in list-mode [6], whereby the line-of-response (LOR) geometry for every positron decay event detected in the scanner is individually recorded. Motion correction can be applied to this intermediate representation of the data prior to final image reconstruction [7]. An alternative approach is to integrate motion compensation in the reconstruction process itself. This allows for elastic transformation with much higher degrees-of-freedom. PET reconstruction can be reformulated over a 4D domain so that motion compensation is incorporated into a unified optimisation process [8]. By extending the expectation maximisation framework over a 4D domain, the parameters of the motion model can also be estimated from the emission data alone [9].

In this paper, two list-mode methods for correcting respiratory induced cardiac deformation are proposed and validated using MRI data. By applying the motion model at the list-mode re-binning stage, it is possible to compensate for respiratory motion in PET independent of the method chosen for volume reconstruction. The motion model parameters are estimated from the gated MRI scans which are also used to derive the activity maps driving the simulator that generates the list-mode data. To simulate the effect of respiratory motion, the reconstructed MRI volume in which the myocardium has been delineated is transformed via deformations recovered from different respiratory phases. There is a significant risk that motion models with many degrees of freedom will be under-constrained and this can result in unrealistic motion. For this reason, two materially-inspired constraints are proposed and have been integrated into the model. Reconstruction errors are quantified relative to uncorrected data so that the benefits of the proposed correction schemes and material constraints can be assessed.

2   Method

2.1   List Mode Transformation Based on Respiratory Motion Modelling

In PET, the list-mode data format allows time-stamp information to be embedded within the file, thus enabling the appropriate correction transformations to be applied to various sections of the list-mode stream. Respiratory phase can be determined by a number of external trackers or via instrumentation mechanically coupled to the patient's torso. Unlike with head-tracking [10], external motion due to respiration will be non-rigid, however optimal placement of trackers [11] will ensure all major modes of respiratory related displacement will be captured.

For motion compensation, each list-mode event recorded is first converted into a pair of 3D Cartesian coordinates $(x_0, y_0, z_0), (x_1, y_1, z_1)$, where the line-of-response (LOR) meets the cylinder of detectors. The basic principle of PET implies that correction transforms applied to LOR events must map straight lines to straight lines, so one is limited to using affine transforms. The 3D affine transform, A_{3D}, in its most general form can be specified by the 12 components of the 3D transformation matrix[7], $\Gamma_{3D} = (a_{00}, ..., a_{23})$. Image reconstruction methods, such as 2D filtered back projection, discard all events where $z_0 \neq z_1$ at the expense of lower signal-to-noise. Hence LOR events associated with any given slice or ring of detectors can be independently transformed by a local 2D affine transformation, A_{2D}. Events can also be re-binned in adjacent slices $z_i' = z_i + \delta z$. Thus, for each slice there are seven correction parameters, six specifying the 2D affine transform $(b_{00}, b_{01}, b_{02}, b_{10}, b_{11}, b_{12})$ plus the parameter, δz, controlling the inter-slice re-binning process. Specifying seven parameters per detector ring yields an excessive number of degrees of freedom. In practice, the dimensionality is reduced by specifying the affine transform for a small subset of slices and then interpolating for the remaining slices:

$$b_{st} = (1 - \lambda)c_{st}^{(k)} + \lambda c_{st}^{(k+1)}, \delta z = (1 - \lambda)\delta z^{(k)} + \lambda \delta z^{(k+1)} \tag{1}$$

where $\lambda = (z_i - z^{(k)})/(z^{(k+1)} - z^{(k)})$, with parameters $(c_{00}^{(k)}, c_{01}^{(k)}, c_{02}^{(k)}, c_{10}^{(k)}, c_{11}^{(k)}, c_{12}^{(k)}, \delta z^{(k)})$ being defined for r slices located at $z^{(k)} < z^{(k+1)}$ for $k = 1...r$.

In general, the transformed coordinates $(x_0', y_0', z_0'), (x_1', y_1', z_1')$ will no longer lie on the ring of detectors. To determine the new detector pair, the intersections of the straight line passing through the two points with the cylinder of detectors must be calculated by solving a quadratic equation [12]. For large deformations, a significant number of LOR events may fail to be mapped to valid detectors, thus causing significant problems in the reconstruction process [13]. Techniques to compensate for this were deemed unnecessary in practice as the number of discarded events was found to be minimal over the ten subjects in the dataset.

Given the set P of all the respiratory gates reconstructed from the MRI data, the correction parameters for either affine correction method can be estimated using the elastic transformation, B_l, $l \in P$, that maps from each respiratory position to the end-inspiration position. To this end, virtual landmarks (which are simply points with position vectors $\mathbf{q}_j$) were distributed evenly throughout the myocardium of the left ventricle on each slice, using random placement constrained by a lower bound on separation distance, followed by rejection of any landmarks positioned outside of the myocardial segmentation boundary. The vectors $\mathbf{p}_j$ are defined such that $\mathbf{q}_j = B_l(\mathbf{p}_j)$, in effect applying the B_l transform in reverse to map the virtual landmarks back to the end-inspiration position. The correction parameters, $\Gamma_{3D} = (a_{00}, ..., a_{23})$, can thus be estimated by minimisation of the following cost function:

$$\Omega_{3D}(\Gamma_{3D}) = \sum_{j}^{m} |A_{3D}(\mathbf{q}_j) - \mathbf{p}_j|^2 \tag{2}$$

Similarly, the correction parameters, $\Gamma_{2D} = (..., c_{st}^{(k)}, \delta z^{(k)}, ...)$, are estimated by minimising the cost function:

$$\Omega_{2D}(\Gamma_{2D}) = \frac{1}{m}\sum_{j}^{m}\left|A_{2D}(\mathbf{q}_j) - \mathbf{p}_j\right|^2 + w_V V(\Gamma_{2D}) + w_S S(\Gamma_{2D}) \tag{3}$$

where V and S are penalty functions for implementing weak material constraints which avoid excessive distortion when there are insufficient landmarks for the degrees of freedom processed by the model. This tends to occur when the end slices intersect the cardiac tissue at a single point or small region, and is further exacerbated by the fact that end slices only have one adjacent slice with which to participate in linear interpolation.

$$V(\Gamma_{2D}) = \frac{1}{r-1}\sum_{k}^{r-1}\left(\left(\nu_k(\Gamma_{2D}) + \nu_{k+1}(\Gamma_{2D})\right)\left(1 + \frac{\delta z^{(k+1)} - \delta z^{(k)}}{z^{(k+1)} - z^{(k)}}\right) - 2\right)^2 \tag{4}$$

where $\nu_k(\Gamma_{2D}) = c_{00}^{(k)}c_{11}^{(k)} - c_{01}^{(k)}c_{10}^{(k)}$ and V is the sum of the squares of the volume change ratio due to the interpolated 2D affine transformation. In this study, its effect on the correction parameter estimation is moderated by non-negative weight w_V and it biases the model toward incompressible deformation. In Eq. (3), S is a measure of shape distortion defined as:

$$S(\Gamma_{2D}) = \sum_{k\in\{1,r\}} w_A\left(\rho_0 - \rho_1\right)^2 + \rho_2^2 \tag{5}$$

where

$$\begin{bmatrix}\rho_0 & \rho_2 \\ \rho_2 & \rho_1\end{bmatrix} = \mathbf{C}^T\mathbf{C} \text{ and } \mathbf{C} = \begin{bmatrix}c_{00}^{(k)} & c_{01}^{(k)} \\ c_{10}^{(k)} & c_{11}^{(k)}\end{bmatrix}$$

and w_A is a non-negative weight governing the relative importance of maintaining a 1:1 aspect ratio. The shape distortion penalty is moderated by non-negative weight w_S. Note that S is zero if $\mathbf{C}$ consists of a rotation and uniform scaling only, and increases according to how far $\mathbf{C}$ deviates from this form. This penalty function has only been applied to the end slices, but can be applied to every slice as needed.

2.2 Photon Emission Simulation and Reconstruction

For photon emission simulation, SimSET is used as a photon history generator (PHG) to estimate a multidimensional LOR-event histogram (*i.e.* sinogram) whose structure mirrors that of the PET scanner being modelled, the Siemens ECAT EXACT3D 962. This scanner has the equivalent of 32 detector rings, with an inter-ring separation of 4.85 mm, an inner radius of 41.2 cm, and a total of 576 detectors per ring for use in coincidence detection. The Software for Tomographic Image Reconstruction (STIR) is used to reconstruct volume data from list-mode data.

One of the input files required by the PHG is a 3D activity map which specifies the uptake region of FDG in the patient. The left ventricular myocardium delineated from MRI was used to specify map, I_o, corresponding to the end-inspiration respiratory phase. The final activity maps, I_o', were produced by remapping the short axis aligned volume to one that is axially aligned with the PET scanner geometry. The MR stack of short axis slices was found to be unsuitable for use as an attenuation map, so instead, a simulated cylinder of water of radius 8-10 cm surrounding the myocardium shaped activity volume was positioned in the centre of, and oriented parallel to, the scanner geometry so that photon scattering effects would be simulated.

A list of 120 million LOR events were randomly generated for each list-mode file L_l. The list-mode data were converted to sinograms and the 3D volumetric data set, V_l, was then reconstructed by applying the standard 2D filtered back projection algorithm to multiple slices. Although an iterative maximum likelihood reconstruction method could have been employed, FBP uses only a fraction of computational power. The higher image quality of the ML method was also found to be unnecessary to illustrate comparative results between the proposed correction methods. The volume, V_0, thus generated from the activity map, I'_0, served as the ground truth for quantitative comparisons. To simulate the effect of respiratory deformation on the PET acquisition, the activity maps for the other respiratory positions were obtained by forward deformation of I'_0 using the freeform transformations B_i. List-mode event files, L_l, for each respiratory position, $l \in P$, were generated and interleaved together to create list-mode file, L_R. To be truly representative of actual respiratory motion, the number of events included from L_l should be proportional to the time the patient spent in the respiratory position, $l \in P$. The corresponding 3D reconstruction, V_R, was compared with reference reconstruction, V_0, to determine the effect of respiratory motion on image quality.

2.3 MRI Acquisition and Respiratory Deformation

Instead of using a PET phantom or a generalised heart model averaged over a patient set, this study used the respiratory induced cardiac deformation specific to individual patients directly. This ensured the correction scheme was evaluated against realistic cardiac motion induced by respiration of real patients as opposed to that of an idealised model. The use of multiple patients also helped to assess how well the proposed method would perform over a wider variety of breathing movements instead of being restricted to that permitted by a given phantom implementation. Ten subjects who consented to be scanned via a Siemens Sonata 1.5T MR scanner were recruited for this study in order to obtain a set of patient specific respiratory-gated cardiac deformation data. The imaging sequence consisted of segmented 3D TrueFISP with an RF flip angle of $65°$, The subjects maintained free breathing in the supine position. The acquisition volume was $256 \times 102 \times 14$ and the voxel size was 1.56 mm $\times 2.70$ mm $\times 8.78$ mm. The FOV spanned from the valve plane to the apex and the sequence was repeated 20 times to ensure adequate sampling over the full range of respiratory movement. The diaphragm position was determined from an interleaved 1D navigator echo. This allowed retrospective respiratory gating to be used to reconstruct the 3D volumes I_p at different respiratory phases p. Furthermore, the respiratory gates are specifically chosen to ensure that each phase has been sufficiently populated with K-space samples that would permit accurate and reliable reconstruction. This has the added benefit that when the MRI gates are used for generating PET data, one simply concatenates equal numbers of line-of-response events for each respiratory position in order to realistically simulate the respiratory artefacts in the PET modality. For each of the ten subjects studied, up to seven image volumes were reconstructed, covering different respiratory positions from end-inspiration to end-expiration. The freeform elastic transformation B_p relating each volume to the end-inspiration volume was estimated by using non-rigid 3D image registration and modelled as a 3D B-spline mapping[14]. Although the 3D and slicewise 2D affine models could have been derived directly at this stage, this intermediate high degree of freedom motion model was used to demonstrate the flexibility of the method, and to decouple the models used for PET correction from the similarity measures used in volume registration.

3   Results

Evaluation of the proposed motion correction scheme required that the segmented myocardium, derived from MRI of the 10 subjects studied, be deformed into each respiratory phase and input into the PET simulation. The PHG executed for 12-18 hours on 3GHz Pentium IV PCs to trace 500 million photons for each subject at each respiratory position. The resulting 3D sinograms were used to randomly generate list-mode files, each containing over 120 million events. Under the assumption of accurate respiratory gating, the list-mode files for all respiratory phases were transformed to the end-inspiration phase using the two methods of affine correction. The corrected

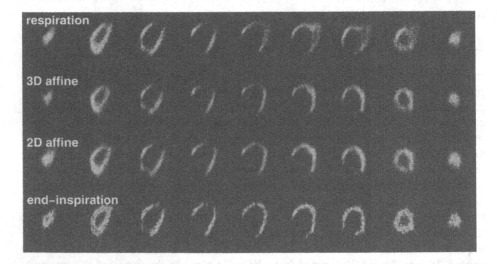

Fig. 1. Visual comparison of 2D and 3D affine list-mode correction methods for one of the subjects studied. The top row represents the slices of the volume data reconstruction without any correction being applied. The bottom row shows the reconstructed volume using data for subjects in full inspiration and is used as the reference. The 2nd and 3rd rows show the results of applying 3D affine and 2D affine correction methods. The results from 2D affine correction appear to be superior owing to the higher degree of freedom however quantitative analysis would yield a more conclusive comparison. 3D affine correction can be applied to 3D reconstruction methods and thus yield less image noise.

volume was reconstructed using the merged results and then compared against reconstructions derived from the end-inspiration list-mode data only, and also from the merged list-mode of all phases without any correction being applied. Figure 1 shows transverse slices for one of the subjects studied for visual comparison. Subjective examination reveals that the uncorrected volumes exhibit motion artefacts and structural flaws that are noticeably reduced using the motion correction algorithm. Initial inspection seems to suggest that interpolated 2D affine, with interpolation over every $r = 4$ rings, is superior to global 3D affine, which is to be expected due to the higher degree of freedom. However visual inspection tends to be subjective, so for a more conclusive assessment a quantitative analysis was performed.

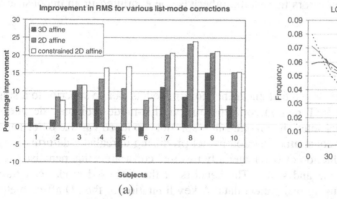 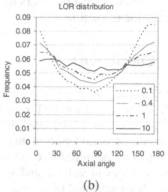

(a)   (b)

Fig. 2. (a) Improvements in RMS error for different list-mode correction method, where 9 out of ten subjects the interpolated 2D affine correction performs better than global 3D affine. Introducing the volume constraint with weight $w_V = 1.0$ shows further improvement in 7 of the subjects however the change is marginal in all but 2 of the subjects where the RMS improvement due to the weak material constraint was clearly significant. (b) The effect of the shape constraint is demonstrated in the distribution of axial angles of the LOR events for different values of w_S, ($w_A = 0.05$, bin width $10°$). A uniform distribution minimises errors introduced by attenuation correction.

The root mean squared error over all voxel values was used as an objective quantitative assessment of the effectiveness of the motion correction algorithm. By using the V_0 reconstruction as ground truth, the RMS error of the interpolated 2D corrected and global 3D corrected data sets were calculated and compared to that of the uncorrected volume V_R. The results are shown in Figure 2, where 8 out of 10 subjects showed improved RMS by using the global 3D affine method, whereas interpolated 2D affine correction yielded improvements in all of the 10 subjects studied. On average, 3D affine yields a mean relative reduction in RMS error of 5.2%, 2D affine yields a 13.1% improvement, rising to 14.2% when the volume constraint is applied.

The simulation as designed only caters for the emission phase of a typical FDG patient study. Another essential data acquisition stage in PET procedures is the transmission scan, which is used to correct for attenuation of the emitted photons according to variations in tissue density and absorption properties. This is typically determined using an external radiation source that is rotated outside the patient, or via a traditional CT scan performed in situ. Since the patient dataset used in this study did not include CT, and MRI is unsuited for deriving attenuation maps, errors due to attenuation correction could not be evaluated in the current framework. Instead, the angular distribution of the LOR events was plotted to judge the effectiveness of the shape constraint penalty $S(\Gamma_{2D})$ for ensuring the risk of artefacts being introduced at the attenuation correction stage was minimal. The distribution of axial angles should remain evenly uniform after correction and this was confirmed for values of weights, $w_S = 10.0, w_A = 0.05$. One can infer from the results shown in Figure 2(b) that the proposed material constraints are necessary for minimising attenuation correction errors that would otherwise be exhibited in an unconstrained 2D affine correction.

4 Conclusions

In this study, we have shown that 2D affine motion models can be superior to a single 3D affine model for PET motion compensation via list-mode rebinning despite the presence of non-trivial inter-slice motion in respiratory induced cardiac deformation. The risk of an under-constrained motion model producing unrealistic deformations is avoided by the introduction of two materially inspired constraints that penalise excessive changes in volume and shape. The benefits of the proposed model constraints have been validated using real patient data. A key limitation of the 2D affine method is its incompatibility with 3D PET reconstruction methods which are desirable for their significantly higher SNR [15]. However, there is also a higher risk of Compton scattering artefacts in 3D PET imaging and existing scatter correction schemes will need to be factored into the motion compensation models in order to assess the relative merits on an application specific basis. Furthermore, the assumption that respiratory phase can be consistently measured in both the MRI and PET context to the accuracy required may be difficult to achieve for a given patient. However, the advent of combined PET/CT and PET/MRI scanners holds promise that these risks can eventually be minimised. Future research will quantify the impact of motion correction schemes on attenuation correction, explore the advantages of using weak material constraints in elastic 3D iterative reconstruction, and assess the impact of respiratory phase errors between the PET and MRI modalities.

References

1. Camici, P.G.: Positron emission tomography and myocardial imaging. Heart 83, 475–480 (2000)
2. Reutter, B.W., Lim, S., Huesman, R.H., Coxson, P.G., Klein, G.J., Budinger, T.F.: Cardiac creep during rest/stress myocardial perfusion studies – patient motion and lung air redistribution. Journal of Nuclear Medicine 37 (suppl. 5), 131 (1996)
3. Runge, V.M., Clanton, J.A., Partain, C.L., James Jr., A.E.: Respiratory gating in magnetic resonance imaging at 0.5 Tesla. Radiology 151, 521–523 (1984)

4. Dawood, M., Lang, N., Jiang, X., Schäfers, K.P.: Lung Motion Correction on Respiratory Gated 3D PET/CT Images. IEEE Transactions on Medical Imaging: Special Issue on Pulmonary Imaging 25(4) (2006)
5. Picard, Y., Thompson, C.J.: Motion correction of PET images using multiple acquisition frames. IEEE Transactions on Medical Imaging 16(2), 137–144 (1997)
6. Livieratos, L., Rajappan, K., Stegger, L., Schafers, K., Bailey, D., Camici, P.: Respiratory gating of cardiac PET data in list-mode acquisition. European Journal of Nuclear Medicine and Molecular Imaging, 1–5 (2006)
7. Lamare, F., Cresson, T., Savean, J., Cheze-Le Rest, C., Turzo, A., Bizais, Y., Reader, A.J., Visvikis, D.: Affine transformation of list mode data for respiratory motion correction in PET. In: Proceedings of Nuclear Science Symposium Conference Record. IEEE Computer Society Press, Los Alamitos (2004)
8. Qiao, F., Pan, T., Clark Jr., J.W., Mawlawi, O.R.: A motion-incorporated reconstruction method for gated PET studies. Physics in Medicine and Biology 51(15), 3769 (2006)
9. Lalush, D.S., Cui, L., Tsui, B.M.W.: A priori motion models for four-dimensional reconstruction in gated cardiac SPECT. In: Proceedings of Nuclear Science Symposium, 1996. Conference Record. IEEE Computer Society Press, Los Alamitos (1996)
10. Goldstein, S.R., Daube-Witherspoon, M.E., Green, M.V., Eidsath, A.: A head motion measurement system suitable for emission computed tomography. IEEE Transactions on Medical Imaging 16(1), 17–27 (1997)
11. Wu, Q., Chung, A.J., Yang, G.-Z.: Optimal Sensor Placement for Predictive Cardiac Motion Modeling. In: Larsen, R., Nielsen, M., Sporring, J. (eds.) MICCAI 2006. LNCS, vol. 4190. Springer, Heidelberg (2006)
12. Livieratos, L., Stegger, L., Bloomfield, P.M., Schafers, K., Bailey, D.L., Camici, P.G.: Rigid-body transformation of list-mode projection data for respiratory motion correction in cardiac PET. Physics in Medicine and Biology 50(14), 3313–3322 (2005)
13. Thielemans, K., Mustafovic, S., Schnorr, L.: Image reconstruction of motion corrected sinograms. In: Proceedings of Nuclear Science Symposium Conference Record. IEEE Computer Society Press, Los Alamitos (2003)
14. Ablitt, N.A., Gao, J., Keegan, J., Stegger, L., Firmin, D.N., Yang, G.-Z.: Predictive Cardiac Motion Modeling and Correction with Partial Least Squares Regression. IEEE Transactions on Medical Imaging 23(10), 1315–1324 (2004)
15. Li, H.H., Votaw, J.R.: Spatial variation of SNR in 2D and 3D neuro PET. In: Proceedings of IEEE Nuclear Science Symposium and Medical Imaging Conference Record (1995)

Image Guidance for Robotic Minimally Invasive Coronary Artery Bypass

Michael Figl[1], Daniel Rueckert[1], David Hawkes[3], Roberto Casula[4],
Mingxing Hu[3], Ose Pedro[1], Dong Ping Zhang[1],
Graeme Penney[5], Fernando Bello[2], and Philip Edwards[2]

[1] Department of Computing, Imperial College London, UK
[2] Department of Biosurgery and Surgical Technology, Imperial College London, UK
[3] Centre of Medical Image Computing, University College London, UK
[4] Cardiothoracic Surgery, St. Mary's Hospital, London, UK
[5] Division of Imaging Sciences, King's College London, UK

Abstract. A novel system for image guidance in totally endoscopic coronary artery bypass (TECAB) is presented. Key requirement is the availability of 2D-3D registration techniques that can deal with non-rigid motion and deformation. Image guidance for TECAB is mainly required before the mechanical stabilization of the heart, thus the most dominant source of non-rigid deformation is the motion of the beating heart.

To augment the images in the endoscope of the da Vinci robot, we have to find the transformation from the coordinate system of the preoperative imaging modality to the system of the endoscopic cameras.

In a first step we build a 4D motion model of the beating heart. Intraoperatively we can use the ECG or video processing to determine the phase of the cardiac cycle. We can then take the heart surface from the motion model and register it to the stereo-endoscopic images of the da Vinci robot using 2D-3D registration methods. We are investigating robust feature tracking and intensity-based methods for this purpose.

Images of the vessels available in the preoperative coordinate system can then be transformed to the camera system and projected into the calibrated endoscope view using two video mixers with chroma keying. It is hoped that the augmented view can improve the efficiency of TECAB surgery and reduce the conversion rate to more conventional procedures.

1   Introduction

1.1   Augmented Reality Applications in Surgery

Augmented reality (AR) systems applied to surgery aim to overlay additional information, most often in form of images or renderings, onto the real view of the surgeon. Using a stereoscopic device has the potential advantage of enabling 3-D perception of both the surgical field and overlays, potentially allowing virtual structures appear beneath the real surface as though the tissue were transparent.

In this paper we describe a system for image-guided robotic surgical treatment of coronary artery disease. We aim to enhance the endoscopic view provided by

T. Dohi, I. Sakuma, and H. Liao (Eds.): MIAR 2008, LNCS 5128, pp. 202–209, 2008.

the da Vinci robot with information from preoperative imaging. This requires construction of a fully 4D model of the patient from coronary CT, both temporal and spatial registration of this model to physical space and visualisation as overlays on the endoscopic view.

1.2 Clinical Need

Totally endoscopic coronary artery bypass (TECAB) has the potential to treat coronary artery disease without the need for invasive sternotomy or heart-lung bypass. However there is still a conversion rate to more invasive methods of 20-30% [1,2,3]. This can occur if there is misidentification of the target vessel or difficulty in locating the artery if it is hidden by fat.

We have identified two critical points in the procedure that might gain from intraoperative guidance. During harvesting of the left internal mammary artery the position of the bifurcation would be useful to know to allow surgery to progress rapidly to this point. After opening of the pericardium overlay of the target vessel will allow accurate location and identification. It is hoped that such guidance will make surgery more efficient and reduce the conversion rate for TECAB.

2 Methods

The layout of the system can be seen in figure 1.

The workstation has two dual output graphics adapters (nVidia Quadro FX 1500) that provide the overlays to each eye and a multiple input frame grabbing device (Active Silicon, Uxbridge, UK) for the purposes of registration.

Overlay on the view through the da Vinci is provided using two video mixers (Panasonic WJ-MX 50) with chroma-keying functionality. This ensures that there is no increased lag introduced by the system. An idea of the quality of chroma keyed overlay can be found in figure 2

To achieve guidance we require a 4D model of the beating heart. This must be both temporally and spatially registered to the patient. Finally the model must be visualised using the calibrated endoscope view.

2.1 4D Model Construction

The preoperative model of the patient comes from coronary CT, which provides a fully 4D representation of the patient. The CT can be reconstructed at up to 20 multiple even phases throughout the cardiac cycle, see figure 3 for an example. The relevant vessels must be segmented along with the surface of the myocardium.

The motion of the heart can potentially be obtained from image registration [4,5]. We are investigating the use of a 4D statistical model to produce a segmentation [6] and also the use of a subdivision surface representation of the

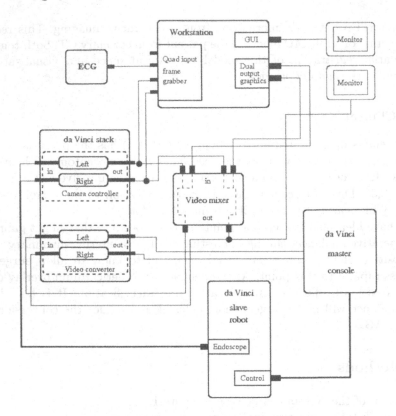

Fig. 1. The layout of the system in theatre. ECG and the stereo video are grabbed by the machine to gain parameters we need for the image overlay, as e.g. the heart and breathing frequencies. The resulting images from the dual graphics output are overlaid to the real video images using video mixers. There is no delay of the real video images in the view of the surgeon as they are just copied to our PC (there direct connection from the camera controller via the video mixer to the converter and the master console).

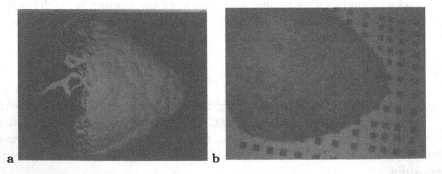

Fig. 2. The surface of a heart phantom and the overlay using chroma keying. **a** shows the rendering of the surface. The surface file is truncated to visualise the difference to the heart phantom underneath as can be seen in **b**.

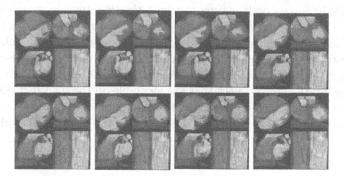

Fig. 3. The phases of a heart displayed using the software rview. Only about half of the 20 phases are shown.

heart with volume preservation to track the motion of the myocardium [7]. We will also apply the registration method in [8] to our volumes.

An example of a patient model can be seen in figure 6(a).

2.2 Model-Based 2D-3D Registration Techniques

Having obtained a preoperative model of the patient we now need to align this model to the video view through the da Vinci endoscope. In this step we will develop suitable non-rigid 2D-3D registration algorithms.

Our strategy in performing registration will be to separate the temporal and spatial alignment of the preoperative model. Temporal alignment may be obtained using the ECG signal, e.g. in figure 1 the video output from the ECG is connected to the frame grabber. However, there may be residual lag between the ECG and the video and we are investigating whether feature tracking in the video images could be used for this purpose. Feature tracking has been proposed as a means of reconstructing the surface viewed through the endoscope and tracking its motion [9].

If corresponding features can be tracked in the left and right views through the da Vinci stereo-endoscope, these can provide 3D tracked points on the viewed surface. We propose this technique to measure the motion of the heart and to separate cardiac and respiratory motion. We are also examining whether geometry constraints can be used as an accurate means of finding the period of the heart cycle, in the present of rigid motion of the camera or near rigid motion due to breathing.

Having established temporal registration, the remaining motion will be rigid apart from possible deformation of the heart due to breathing. Preliminary work has shown that 3D-3D non-rigid registration can be used to build separate models of respiratory motion of the liver [10] and heart [11]. Since both respiratory and cardiac motion are smooth and continuous, we will develop 4D parametric motion models based on 4D B-splines. These motion models will provide compact representations of cardiac motions.

To establish correspondence we are investigating two approaches. We are adopting a similar approach to that of [9] to reconstruct the motion of the viewed surface, which can then be registered to the preoperative 4D model. Secondly we are investigating whether intensity-based similarity metrics can be developed. We are using the concept of photo- consistency [12,13] as a similarity measure using the calibrated stereo views that are available on the da Vinci system. It is hoped that a combination of these techniques will be able to provide alignment of the 4D model from the cardiac CT images with the series of 2D video images grabbed through the endoscope.

2.3   Visualisation

The da Vinci system provides the surgeon with endoscopic stereo video images of the surgical scene during coronary artery bypass. The goal of this step is to provide an augmented reality facility for the da Vinci system during this procedure.

In order to achieve this we need to establish the relationship between camera coordinates and image coordinates (determined by the intrinsic transformation parameters) as well as the relationship between world coordinates and camera coordinates (determined by the extrinsic transformation parameters). Since the intrinsic parameters describe the internal properties of the stereo endoscopic cameras of the da Vinci system, we use an offline camera calibration technique to determine these parameters [14,15].

As the image fusion is done by use of chroma keying with two video mixers, an additional 2D-2D transformation from the graphical output to the input channels of the mixer is needed. This is achieved by point to point registration.

We will then use the model-based 2D-3D registration algorithm described previously to estimate the extrinsic transformation parameters. The resulting visualisation will be able to guide the surgeon during critical parts of the procedure.

3   Results

3.1   4D Model Construction

For preoperative model building we use coronary CT images reconstructed at 20 even phases throughout the cardiac cycle. To produce a 4D model we segment the first phase by hand and propagate this to the other 19 phases by non-rigid registration [8]. This is similar to the method used by Szpala et al [5], but here it is demonstrated on clinical coronary CT scans rather than phantom data. Figure 4 gives an idea of the quality of the registration.

In figure 5 we the heart and breathing frequencies, needed as parameters for the 4D model.

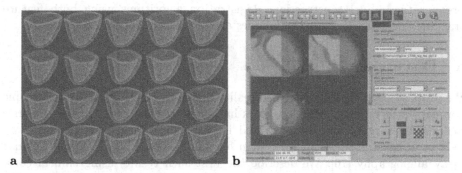

Fig. 4. Non-rigid registration was used to register the first image to the other images. In **a** the deformation of the ventricle is displayed. **b** shows the registered image slices from different phases (0% and 60 %) of the cardiac cycle.

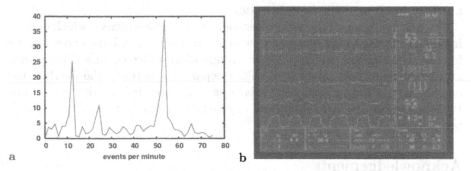

Fig. 5. **a** shows the Fourier transform of the cross-correlation from the image number 12 to the other images of a video sequence of the beating heart like 6 **c**. Two main frequencies can be seen 12 and 54 beats per minute, breathing and the heart beat. **b** shows the corresponding ECG display grabbed with the frame grabber.

Fig. 6. A rendering of the preoperative model showing the myocardial surface, left internal mammary artery, left anterior descending artery and a diagonal branch (a), an aligned rendering (b) and its corresponding endoscope view (c)

3.2   Visualisation

An example of retrospectively aligned images is shown in figure 6. We have a number of clinical coronary CT images that are being used to investigate preoperative model construction. Registration algorithms using both feature tracking and intensity-based techniques are being developed.

4 Discussion

We propose a system for augmented reality image guidance of totally endoscopic coronary artery bypass. Previous work has suggested the use of image guidance in TECAB surgery and demonstrated its feasibility on a heart phantom [5]. Falk et al have demonstrated a system for AR guidance based on multi-planar x-ray angiography [16]. We describe the first such results using clinical coronary CT scans to provide the 4D patient model using non-rigid registration. We also propose two novel strategies for alignment of this model to the endoscopic view. The first uses robust feature tracking to reconstruct the viewed surface, which can then be matched to the preoperative model. The second strategy uses intensity-based methods for registration.

For augmentation of the endoscopic view we use video mixers, which does not introduce any lag to the surgeons view of the real surface. We use chroma-keying for the image fusion, which limits the range of available colours. This is not a significant limitation as we want colour separation between the overlaid view and the largely red surgical view. It is hoped that such information can improve the efficiency of TECAB surgery and reduce the conversion rate to more invasive procedures.

Acknowledgements

We would like to thank the EPSRC for funding this project. We are also grateful to the theatre staff at St Mary's hospital, London and to the radiology staff in St Mary's and the Royal Brompton hospitals for their cooperation.

References

1. Kappert, U., Cichon, R., Schneider, J., Gulielmos, V., Ahmadzade, T., Nicolai, J., Tugtekin, S.M., Schueler, S.: Technique of closed chest coronary artery surgery on the beating heart. Eur. J. Cardio-Thorac. Surg. 20, 765–769 (2001)
2. Dogan, S., Aybek, T., Andressen, E., Byhahn, C., Mierdl, S., Westphal, K., Matheis, G., Moritz, A., Wimmer-Greinecker, G.: Totally endoscopic coronary artery bypass grafting on cardiopulmonary bypass with robotically enhanced telemanipulation: Report of forty-five cases. J. Thorac. Cardiovasc. Surg. 123, 1125–1131 (2002)
3. Falk, V., Diegeler, A., Walther, T., Banusch, J., Brucerius, J., Raumans, J., Autschbach, R., Mohr, F.W.: Total endoscopic computer enhanced coronary artery bypass grafting. Eur. J. Cardio-Thorac. Surg. 17, 38–45 (2000)
4. Wierzbicki, M., Peters, T.M.: Determining Epicardial Surface Motion Using Elastic Registration: Towards Vitual Reality Guidance of Minimal Invasive Cardiac Interventions. In: Ellis, R.E., Peters, T.M. (eds.) MICCAI 2003. LNCS, vol. 2878, pp. 722–729. Springer, Heidelberg (2003)

5. Szpala, S., Wierzbicki, M., Guiraudon, G., Peters, T.M.: Real-time fusion of endoscopic views with dynamic 3-d cardiac images: A phantom study. IEEE Trans. Med. Imaging 24, 1207–1215 (2005)
6. Perperidis, D., Mohiaddin, R., Edwards, P., Hill, R.D.: Segmentation of cardiac MR and CT image sequences using model-based registration of a 4D statistical model. In: Proc. SPIE Medical Imaging 2007, vol. 6512 (2007)
7. Chandrashekara, R., Mohiaddin, R., Razavi, R., Rueckert, R.: Nonrigid image registration with subdivision lattices: Application to cardiac mr image analysis. In: Taylor, C., Colchester, A. (eds.) MICCAI 1999. LNCS, vol. 1679, pp. 335–342. Springer, Heidelberg (1999)
8. Rueckert, D., Sonoda, L.I., Hayes, C., Hill, D.L.G., Leach, M.O., Hawkes, D.J.: Nonrigid registration using free-form deformations: Application to breast MR images. IEEE Trans. Med. Imaging 18(8), 712–721 (1999)
9. Stoyanov, D., Mylonas, G.P., Deligianni, F., Darzi, A., Yang, G.Z.: Soft-tissue motion tracking and structure estimation for robotic assisted mis procedures. In: Duncan, J.S., Gerig, G. (eds.) MICCAI 2005. LNCS, vol. 3749, pp. 139–146. Springer, Heidelberg (2005)
10. Blackall, J.M., Penney, G.P., King, A.P., Hawkes, D.J.: Alignment of sparse freehand 3-d ultrasound with preoperative images of the liver using models of respiratory motion and deformation. IEEE Trans. Med. Imaging 24, 1405–1416 (2005)
11. McLeish, K., Hill, D.L.G., Atkinson, D., Blackall, J.M., Razavi, R.: A study of the motion and deformation of the heart due to respiration. IEEE Trans. Med. Imaging 21, 1142–1150 (2002)
12. Clarkson, M.J., Rueckert, D., Hill, D.L.G., Hawkes, D.J.: A multiple 2D video-3D medical image registration algorithm. In: Proc. SPIE Medical Imaging 2000, vol. 3979, pp. 342–352 (2000)
13. Clarkson, M.J., Rueckert, D., Hill, D.L.G., Hawkes, D.J.: Using photo-consistency to register 2d optical images of the human face to a 3D surface model. IEEE Trans. Pattern Anal. Mach. Intell. 23, 1266–1280 (2001)
14. Bouguet, J.: Camera calibration toolbox for matlab (2007),
    http://www.vision.caltech.edu/bouguetj
15. Tsai, R.Y.: A versatile camera calibration technique for high-accuracy 3D machine vision metrology using off-the-shelf TV cameras and lenses. IEEE J. Robotics and Automation 3(4), 323–344 (1987)
16. Falk, V., Mourgues, F., Adhami, L., Jacobs, S., Thiele, H., Nitzsche, S., Mohr, F.W., Coste-Maniere, T.: Cardio navigation: Planning, simulation, and augmented reality in robotic assisted endoscopic bypass grafting. Ann. Thorac. Surg. 79, 2040–2048 (2005)

MRI-Compatible Rigid and Flexible Outer Sheath Device with Pneumatic Locking Mechanism for Minimally Invasive Surgery

Siyang Zuo[1], Noriaki Yamanaka[1], Ikuma Sato[4], Ken Masamune[1], Hongen Liao[2,3], Kiyoshi Matsumiya[1], and Takeyoshi Dohi[1]

[1] Graduate School of Information Science and Technology, The University of Tokyo
[2] Graduate School of Engineering, The University of Tokyo
[3] Translational Systems Biology and Medicine Initiative, The University of Tokyo
7-3-1, Hongo, Bunkyo-ku, Tokyo 113-8656, Japan
[4] Graduate School of Advanced Science and Technology, Tokyo Denki University
2-2 Kanda-Nishiki-cho, Chiyoda-ku, Tokyo 101-8457, Japan
{sa.siyou, nori-non, ikuma_is, mkiyo}@atre.t.u-tokyo.ac.jp,
{masa, dohi}@i.u-tokyo.ac.jp, liao@bmpe.t.u-tokyo.ac.jp

Abstract. To reduce the invasiveness of surgery, we developed an outer sheath device using a flexible toothed link and pneumatic locking mechanism that works with flexible devices used in minimally invasive surgery. The outer sheath can be switched between flexible and rigid modes, and the angle of its tip can be controlled by a nylon wire. All parts of this device are made of plastic and are MRI-compatible. We manufactured a sheath prototype, 300 mm long, with a 20-mm outer diameter, and an 8-mm inner diameter. Experiment results showed that the outer sheath can protect tissues from high insertion force and secure the path for flexible devices. It can follow a curved path with a reasonable radius.

Keywords: Outer sheath, Pneumatic locking mechanism, Minimally Invasive Surgery, MRI.

1 Introduction

Minimally invasive surgical (MIS) procedures avoid open invasive surgery in favor of closed or local surgery with fewer traumas. These procedures involve use of laparoscopic devices and instruments that enable remote control manipulation with indirect observation of the surgical field through an endoscope or a similar device, and are performed through the skin or through a body cavity or anatomical opening. This can result in shorter hospitalization time or allow outpatient treatment. Many medical procedures, such as endoscopy, laparoscopic surgery, thoracoscopic surgery, and arthroscopic surgery, can be categorized as MIS. We adopt laparoscopic surgery as our focal application. Because of the advantages of minimal invasion, endoscopic surgery has wide use in modern surgery. We consider that endoscopic surgery can effectively use MRI guidance; therefore, an MRI-compatible device is necessary.

T. Dohi, I. Sakuma, and H. Liao (Eds.): MIAR 2008, LNCS 5128, pp. 210–219, 2008.
© Springer-Verlag Berlin Heidelberg 2008

Many instruments have been developed to improve performance and reduce risks and difficulties while performing endoscopic surgery. For instance, a dexterous robotic manipulator added multiple degrees of freedom (DOFs) [1-3] to motion of the instruments and thus improved surgical performance. Master–slave robotic manipulators [4], such as da Vinci, enable surgeons to work with precise movement. However, some problems remain unsolved. First, laparoscopic surgery requires a large space below the abdominal wall. A pneumoperitoneum is commonly used to secure the space, but complications have been reported from this method. Second, laparoscopic surgery is useful when the target can be approached from the anterior of the body. However, it is difficult to approach a target in a deep and narrow area.

Several groups have developed flexible manipulators with a wide curve. Ikuta et al. developed a micromanipulator to approach inaccessible regions [5]. Other flexible manipulators have been developed using shape memory alloys (SMAs) [6] or a wire-driven mechanism [7]. However, flexible instruments cannot be easily inserted in the narrow space between tissues or organs and cannot be completely stabilized when approaching the target.

Systems using lockable sheaths or hybrid gaits involving locking and relaxing have been developed. Robert et al. applied this idea to medical applications [8]. A type of snake robot, called HARP [9], was also developed. Yagi et al. developed a guiding device, which uses flexible manipulators to approach deep regions [10]. However, these manipulators have some limitations. Because the mechanisms of these manipulators are complicated, their diameters must be larger than the space required for the surgery. Moreover, it is difficult to make them MRI-compatible.

On inserting an instrument into an area of interest without causing injury to other tissues requires a surgical instrument with a flexible mode for insertion and a rigid mode for fixing the outer sheath in place. In this study, we developed a rigid flexible outer sheath device using a flexible toothed link and pneumatic locking mechanism for endoscopic surgery. Once in place, the outer sheath provides a path for the surgical instrument inside the human body. The sheath can be twisted to any desired shape and can still retain its shape against external forces. Before inserting a flexible instrument, the surgeon inserts the outer sheath through the narrow gap between the safety areas. When the sheath approaches the target, the surgeon locks the shape and then inserts flexible instruments easily through the path made by the sheath.

This paper reports on the mechanism that enables switching between flexible and rigid modes, a prototype of the outer sheath, and the evaluation experimental results on the stiffness. Moreover, we evaluate the performance of insertion in a phantom experiment in an open MRI environment.

2 Outer Sheath Design

2.1 Design Concept

With the mechanism described below, the outer sheath can be switched between flexible and rigid modes. The outer sheath design consists of flexible toothed links and a bellows tube.

In the flexible mode, because the inside pressure and atmospheric pressure balance out, the sealed cover does not shrink, and the toothed links disengage from the bellows tube. In the rigid mode, the sealed space is evacuated by discharging the internal air, and the atmospheric pressure presses the toothed links into the bellows tube, locking the shape of the outer sheath by pushing the tooth of the link into the chase of the bellows tube (Fig. 1).

The bellows tube and toothed link mechanism can be locked as well as relaxed easily, providing a smooth transition between the flexible and rigid modes.

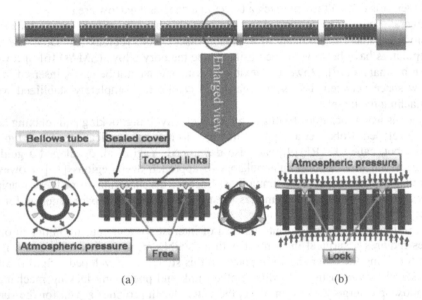

(a)   (b)

Fig. 1. Mechanism of switching between rigid and flexible modes. (a) When there is no vacuum, the links and bellows tube can take any shape. (b) When the pump creates a vacuum, the links move down and mesh with the ditch of the tube, locking the shape of the sheath.

2.2 Prototype

We built a prototype of the outer sheath device and tested it in our laboratory. The prototype has an outer diameter of 20 mm, inner diameter of 8 mm, length of 300 mm, and can achieve a radius of curvature of 8.5 cm. The outer sheath consists of three long flexible toothed links, three nylon wires, a bellows tube, and a polyethylene cover (Fig. 2a). The links and bellows tube are flexible, and the shape is free and changeable. The three toothed links are 120° apart, making it possible to lock the sheath in any direction. The three nylon wires can control the angle of the forward part. The nylon wires are also 120° apart. The outer sheath follows an arbitrary curve in three-dimensional space. The ticks of the bellow tubes are 2 mm apart, and the locking teeth are 17 mm apart. All parts of this device are made of plastic, ensuring excellent MRI compatibility.

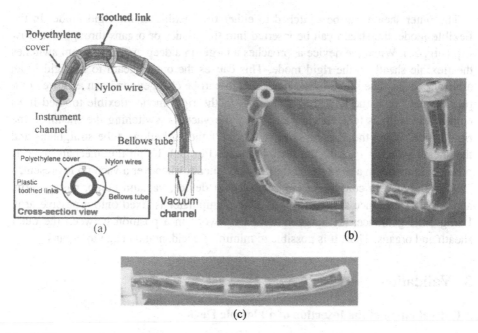

(a)

(b)

(c)

Fig. 2. The outer sheath prototype. (a) The outer sheath mechanism assembly. (b) This image shows that the sheath can curve like a snake and hold its shape. (c) The outer sheath in a flexible mode.

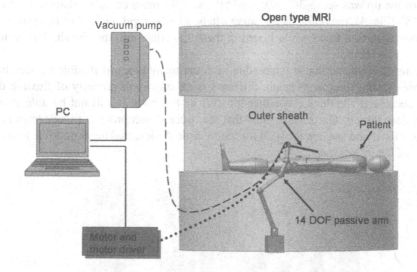

Fig. 3. The system of the outer sheath. The system consists of an outer sheath, a vacuum pump, a passive arm, and an MRI guidance system. Single lines are the electrical connections. The dashed line is the vacuum pump connection and the dotted line represents wires. In future, the wire tension will be controlled by the motor and PC.

The outer sheath can be switched to either the flexible or the rigid mode. In the flexible mode, the sheath can be inserted into the tissues or organs through a narrow gap (Fig. 2c). When the device approaches a target in a deep area, a vacuum switches the flexible sheath to the rigid mode. This causes the outer sheath to be rigid in an arbitrary shape. The shape of the outer sheath can be changed, and can achieve complex shapes, as in the letter "S" (Fig. 2b). In the rigid mode, flexible toothed links engage the bellows tube and are locked by the vacuum, switching the sheath to the rigid mode. When the vacuum is released, the bending bellows tube straightens and the sheath switches back to the flexible mode (Fig. 2c). Using this mechanism, it is possible to maintain a rigid shape for the outer sheath whenever a vacuum is present.

A future system consists of the outer sheath device, vacuum pump, passive arm, and an MRI guidance system (Fig. 3). The manipulator is fixed onto a passive arm. Using MRI guidance, the surgeon can easily work in a position between the outer sheath and organs. Thus, it is possible to minimize accidental damage to organs.

3 Validation

3.1 Evaluation of the Insertion of a Flexible Device

The insertion of flexible devices into the sheath has been tested. Three types of material with properties similar to those of flexible devices were selected-polytetrafluoroethylene (PTFE) rod, soft copper wire, and PTFE tube. The bending angle of the tip was set to 30°, 60°, and 90°, and for more complex shapes, as in the letter "S" (Fig. 4), the outer sheath was switched to the rigid mode. We measured the maximum insertion force while inserting these materials into the sheath. The results are shown in Table 1.

The results indicate that it is possible to insert many types of flexible devices into deep areas using the outer sheath. Stiffness is an important property of flexible devices, because if the device is either too soft or too hard, it will not be able to approach deep targets. Our results show that the outer sheath protects tissues from high insertion force and secures the path for the flexible device, making it possible to use a variety of flexible devices.

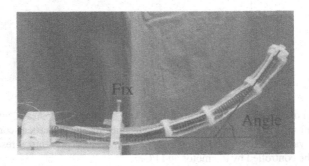

Fig. 4. Experimental device of flexible sheath

Table 1. Maximum insertion force [gf]

		Insertion materials		
		Teflon rod φ2mm	Soft copper wire φ2.5mm	Teflon tube φ3mm
Shape of outer sheath	30° curve	9.25 ± 2.75	26.25 ± 6.13	6.75 ± 0.95
	60° curve	16.75 ± 1.5	24.75 ± 8.77	12.75 ± 2.36
	90° curve	51.75 ± 7.93	27.25 ± 12.63	22.5 ± 4.12
	complex shape	355.75 ± 86.41	99.25 ± 11.44	272.5±33.99

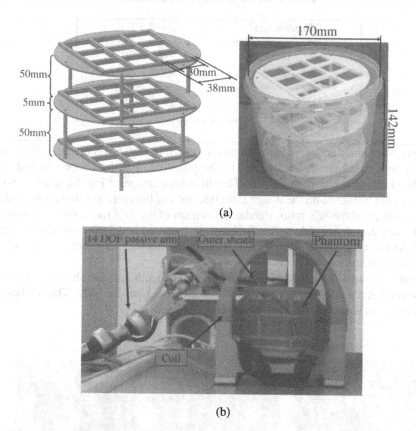

(a)

(b)

Fig. 5. Experiment in an open MRI environment. (a) The MRI phantom and (b) set up for image distortion measurement.

3.2 Evaluation of MR Compliance

The performance of insertion was evaluated in a phantom experiment in an open MRI environment. The materials and drive principle of the device are important in MR compliance. Because the outer sheath manipulator uses vacuum as the locking principle, and all parts of this device are plastic, it should have little influence on MR imaging. We used an open type MRI, with a permanent magnet of 0.2 T. The phantom used for the experiment is showed in Fig. 5a. The phantom consists of three pieces of resin boards, and the boards were superimposed at equal distance. The grids are etched on each resin board. The phantom is kept in a cylindrical container with water. MRI is visible and the positions of grids in the MRI are clear. The size of the circle of the cylindrical container varies in height, but it is about 170 mm at the maximum. The outer sheath is inserted into the grids. The set up of the experiment is shown in Fig. 5b. Table 2 shows the imaging method and conditions.

Table 2. MRI conditions and parameters

Magnetic field	0.2 T
Imaging sequence name	Spin echo (SE)
TR/TE	1000 ms/50 ms
FOV	256 mm × 256 mm
Image resolution	256 × 256 pixels
Pixel resolution	1 mm/pixel
Slice thickness	10 mm

A cross-sectional image of the phantom is shown in Fig. 6. Figure 6a is the image scanned with the outer sheath inserted in the phantom, and the image scanned with only the phantom is shown in Fig. 6b. The difference image of Fig. 6a and b is given in Fig. 6c. No influence on the image from insertion of the outer sheath is observed.

The average of the S/N ratio, standard deviation of the S/N ratio, and S/N decreasing ratio are shown in Table 3. The S/N decreasing ratio is 4.31% from the introduction of the outer sheath into the phantom, indicating that the outer sheath has excellent MRI compatibility.

Figure 7 shows a 3D image of inserting an outer sheath into the phantom. This image shows that the position of outer sheath can be detected by MRI. This makes the sheath useful in surgery with MRI guidance.

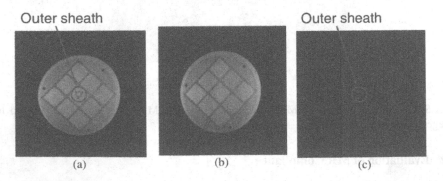

Fig. 6. Measurement results for MR image distortion. (a) The image with the outer sheath, (b) the image with only the phantom, and c) the difference image (a-b).

Table 3. Average and standard deviation of the signal-to-noise ratio and decreasing ratio

		Evaluated value	
		S/N ratio	S/N decreasing ratio (%)
Scan condition	only phantom	73.92 ± 0.17	
	with outer sheath	70.74 ± 0.20	4.31 ± 0.11

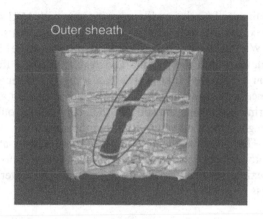

Fig. 7. Measurement result for 3D MR image. This image shows that the outer sheath follows a curved path in the phantom.

4 Discussion

The main advantage of the outer sheath device, besides its simple mechanism, is its ability to achieve curved shapes in three dimensional space (Fig. 2b).

The experiment results showed that our outer sheath mechanism can hold its shape against high insertion force. Laparoscopic manipulators can generate about 500 gf (4.8 N) force perpendicular to the direction of axis to lift heavy organs in the body. Since the outer sheath can be inserted into the required area, avoiding other tissues, it is not necessary for the surgeon to move the organs. Because the outer sheath uses vacuum as the locking mechanism at less than 1 kPa, which is a low pressure, the outer sheath may not damage the tissues around the sheath even if the air leaks and can be used safely. Wire tension is helpful in selecting the direction of route. By transmitting the wire tension to the tip of the outer sheath, it is easier to follow a narrow path. The outer sheath is helpful for manipulators, such as fiber scope and laser knife. We did not consider the situation where flexible manipulators move heavy organs, because the manipulator enters the narrow space between organs and is not necessary for the outer sheath to generate sufficient stiffness to maintain its shape against large forces. Because the outer sheath has excellent MRI compatibility, its position in the human body, especially while inserting the outer sheath, can be detected.

Experiments with our prototype indicate that the design concept is correct. Therefore, we will continue its development, focusing on reducing the diameter, increasing stiffness, and achieving better curvature. Furthermore, by controlling the wire tension with motors and motor drivers will allow controlling the outer sheath with a PC-based program.

5 Conclusion

To perform the minimally invasive endoscopic surgery with MRI guidance, we have developed an MRI-compatible rigid and flexible outer sheath that secures the path for a flexible device. We evaluated the feasibility of the prototype device in terms of inserting flexible devices into the sheath. The results indicate that many types of flexible devices can be inserted into deep areas using the outer sheath. Moreover, insertion performance in a phantom experiment was evaluated in an open MRI environment. The experimental results showed that the outer sheath could follow a curved path with a satisfying radius of curvature, and that the sheath was compatible with an MRI environment. The outer sheath can be inserted into narrow and deep areas that are difficult for conventional laparoscopic tools. Our research to develop an outer sheath, which is flexible yet maintain its shape, is important in terms of minimizing surgical invasiveness.

Acknowledgment

This work was supported in part by Grant-in-aid for Scientific Research (18680042, 1710008) of Ministry of Education, Culture, Sports, Science and Technology (MEXT) in Japan. H. Liao is also supported by the Special Coordination Funds for Promoting Science and Technology commissioned by the MEXT in Japan, Grant-in-Aid for Scientific Research (20650077) of the MEXT in Japan, and Grant for Industrial Technology Research (07C46050), New Energy and Industrial Technology Development Organization, Japan.

References

1. Peirs, J., Reynaerts, D., Van Brussel, H.: A Miniature Manipultor for Integration in a Self-propelling Endoscope. Sensors and Actuators A 92, 343–349 (2001)
2. Nakamura, R., Kobayashi, E., Masamune, K., Sakuma, I., Dohi, T., Yahagi, N., Tsuji, T., Hashimoto, D., Shimada, M., Hashizume, M.: Multi-DOF Forceps Manipulator System for Laparoscopic Surgery. In: Delp, S.L., DiGoia, A.M., Jaramaz, B. (eds.) MICCAI 2000. LNCS, vol. 1935, pp. 653–660. Springer, Heidelberg (2000)
3. Yamashita, H., Hata, N., Kim, D., Hashizume, M., Dohi, T.: Handheld Laparoscopic Forceps Manipulator Using Multi-slider Linkage Mechanisms. In: Barillot, C., Haynor, D.R., Hellier, P. (eds.) MICCAI 2004. LNCS, vol. 3217, pp. 121–128. Springer, Heidelberg (2004)
4. Abbou, C.C., Hoznek, A., Salomon, L., Olsson, L.E., Lobontiu, A., Saint, F., Cicco, A., Antiphon, P., Chopin, D.: Laparoscopic radical prostatectomy with a remote controlled robot. Journal of Urology 165, 1964–1966 (2001)

5. Ikuta, K., Sasaki, K., Yamamoto, K., Shimada, T.: Remote Microsurgery System for Deep and Narrow Space - Development of New Surgical Procedure and Microrobotic Tool. In: Dohi, T., Kikinis, R. (eds.) MICCAI 2002. LNCS, vol. 2488, pp. 163–172. Springer, Heidelberg (2002)
6. Nakamura, Y., Matsui, A., Saito, T.: Shape Memory-Alloy Active Forceps for Laparoscopic Surgery. In: 1995 IEEE International Conference on Robot and Automation, vol. 3, pp. 2320–2327 (1995)
7. Simaan, N., Taylor, R., Flint, P.: High Dexterity Snake-Like Robotic Slaves for Minimally Invasive Telesurgery of the Upper Airway. In: Barillot, C., Haynor, D.R., Hellier, P. (eds.) MICCAI 2004. LNCS, vol. 3217, pp. 17–24. Springer, Heidelberg (2004)
8. Sturges, R.H., Laowattana Jr., S.: A flexible, tendon-controlled device for endoscopy. In: 1991 IEEE International Conference on Robotics and Automation Sacramento, vol. 3, pp. 2582–2591 (1991)
9. Amir, D., Howie, C., Alon, W., Takeyoshi, O., Marco, A.Z.: Percutaneous intrapericardial interventions using a highly articulated robotic probe. In: The First IEEE/RAS-EMBS International Conference on Biomedical Robotics and Biomechatronics, pp. 7–12 (2006)
10. Yagi, A., Matsumiya, K., Masamune, K., Liao, H., Dohi, T.: Rigid-Flexible Outer Sheath Model Using Slider Linkage Locking Mechanism and Air Pressure for Endoscopic Surgery. In: Larsen, R., Nielsen, M., Sporring, J. (eds.) MICCAI 2006. LNCS, vol. 4190, pp. 503–510. Springer, Heidelberg (2006)

MR Compatible Tactile Sensing and Noise Analysis in a 1.5 Tesla MR System

Abbi Hamed[1], Zion Tsz Ho Tse, Ian Young, and Michael Lamperth

[1]Department of Mechanical Engineering, Imperial College London, London SW7 2BX
{a.hamed,t.tse06,m.lamperth}@imperial.ac.uk

Abstract. Medical technologies have undergone significant development to overcome the problems inherent in Minimally Invasive Surgery (MIS) such as inhibited manual dexterity, reduced visual information and lack of direct touch feedback to make it easier for surgeons to operate. An endoscopic tool incorporating haptic feedback is being developed to increase the effectiveness of diagnostic procedures by providing force feedback. Magnetic Resonance Imaging (MRI) guidance is possible to allow tool localisation, however this enforces the requirement of MR compatibility on the device. This paper describes the work done in developing MR compatible sensing devices using piezoelectric sensor elements in two different formats and how each can be used to locate subsurface inclusions in s mined oft substrates. Results show that the position of a hard inclusion can be deterwith both methods.

Keywords: MR Compatible, Force Sensor, Medical robotics.

1 Introduction

In MIS, the main premise is to minimise superfluous trauma to the patient as much as possible, thus ensuring that the patient recovery time is much faster and that the potential for surgery related complications is reduced. To achieve this, the surgical procedure is conducted through the smallest incisions possible using thin handled instruments inserted into the operating area and classically using an instrument with a camera and light source at its distal end (known as an endoscope) for visualisation. The problems associated with this format are that the surgery becomes much more technically demanding, as the surgeon has greatly inhibited visual information, must perform much more complicated and dextrous manipulations and loses touch information almost entirely [1].

As such, MIS is an intuitive direction for the development of surgical robotics, where the accuracy and repeatability of the devices can be made to overcome the limitations of the surgeon by design. It is also possible to incorporate various forms of sensor that can be used to assess forces generated by interaction with tissues or to examine the structure and properties of the tissue itself. Such robots are becoming more common for use in biopsies, MIS tele-surgery and laparoscopic/arthroscopic surgeries [2].

Significant advantages can be achieved when utilising an imaging technology for guidance in conjunction with MIS robotics. This combination provides the advantages

T. Dohi, I. Sakuma, and H. Liao (Eds.): MIAR 2008, LNCS 5128, pp. 220–230, 2008.

of both formats, and allows the possibility of targeting otherwise hidden tissue locations in the body, and by use of trajectory planning; tool entry, operation and extraction can be optimised uniquely for the morphology of each patient. When using image guidance in real time in this way, it is also possible for the system to track both the instruments and the tissues of the body. This is important when operating on mobile pathologies such as the liver. The increased accuracy of the image guided procedures has been shown to statistically improve the outcome of surgery as it is less likely that an operation must be repeated or that complications occur due to surgical inaccuracies [3, 4].

Ultrasound and MRI are most suitable for use in longer duration image guided procedures due to the lack of ionising radiation. However MRI has several advantages, primarily its ability to distinguish clear boundaries between soft tissue structures without the need for contrast agents. Additionally, MRI can also be used to produce tomographic images in several planes without needing to reposition the patient. Also as the scans are programmed sequences, it also has ability to be used in many formats to image brain activity, blood flow and even chemical composition and stiffness of tissues depending on the information required [5]. These advantages have driven the development of mechatronic systems for use with scanners [6-10].

Despite these apparent advantages MRI also poses several challenges when designing mechatronic systems due to its operating principle and physical conformation. The dimensions of the machine restrict the surgeon's access to a patient such that invasive operations are difficult. The presence of a large magnetic field that is required to be highly homogenous within the magnetic isocentre and the use of RF radiation, elicit the necessity of MR Compatibility in all tools and devices that are used close to and within the scanner bore. As such all devices that are designed for use with MRI must have this as one of their primary design specifications.

One of the most active areas of research in the field of MIS robotics has been in the development of force transducers to assess the forces applied by MIS tools and MIS tele-surgical devices used for intervention [11]. Alternatively, it is also beneficial to investigate sensing techniques that can be used in MIS for diagnostic information. Such devices would be used to assess tissue stiffness and textures as well as providing a method of localising sub-surface structures when imaging techniques are insufficient. Such methods require sensors that are placed in contact with the target tissues and therefore need to be transported by a tool or adapted endoscope.

When it comes to force feedback (haptics) in MR compatible medical robotics, there are far fewer examples in literature of developed systems and none that have apparently seen any commercial usage. However, there have been developments of MR compatible haptic devices for various forms of MRI based neuroscience research [12], as well as several new types of sensor specifically for force measurement within the MR environment. [13, 14].

This paper outlines the development to date of a novel tactile sensing device to be used for in vivo tissue stiffness measurements. The perceived benefits of such a device would be to provide the clinician with detailed diagnostic information that could be used to assess the health of tissues and primarily for the detection, localisation and characterisation of suspected tumourous tissue. The device is to be MR compatible for the possibility of application with MRI guidance and combination with other MRI capabilities.

2   Materials and Methods

2.1   Characteristics of the Sensor

The sensing device is to be used as a method for conveying touch information about a target tissue by examination of an area and development of a two dimensional stiffness profile. This force information can be fed back and potentially be represented to the user graphically or mechanically. To complete the haptic feedback loop, the operator can affect the location of assessment by moving the hand or finger in the same way they would if carrying out regular 'palpation' techniques. The requirements of the task depend greatly on the area of application, but for general purpose palpation, the sensitivity, resolution, range and bandwidth are limited only by the operator's capabilities [15].

To define the task more definitely, a study of haptic and medical factors was undertaken. Table 1 has been compiled from a study of literature [16-18]. In addition to these requirements, the general requirements of MR compatibility are also required as discussed above. The specification for compatibility of a device being used within the imaging volume (as the sensing device would need to be), is that the device is MR safe and does not significantly affect imaging quality. The generally accepted quantity here is that the SNR reduction is within 10% [19] and that any image artifact or geometric distortion by the device should be quantified.

Table 1. Values of human touch sense capabilities and tumour characteristics derived from literature. Tumour stiffnesses given are averages for Fibroadenoma and Lobular Carcinoma.

Tissue Elastic Modulus Estimation	90 kPa*	Fingertip Point perception	~1 – 2 mm
Tumour Elastic Modulus Estimation	400 kPa*	Force Resolution	~ 0.1N [17]
Tumour Size	0 -~40cm2. (0-2cm being typical).	Maximum perceivable forces Maximum frequencies for force change perception.	20N @DC 1N @10Hz 5-10 KHz (texture shear force detection) 0-100Hz (static forces) [18]

*Estimations, as tissue stiffness is non-linear [16].

The sensor type selected for this work is piezoelectric. Piezoelectric sensors possess excellent compatibility material-wise and in operation; however the most important aspects that suit this application are the high dimensional scalability and low cost. These are advantages over MR compatible sensors that have been used in other research. Piezoelectric sensors also produce extremely low currents, in the range of nano-Amps, instead outputting charge, meaning that electromagnetic fields generated by them are of much lower magnitude than traditional sensor types thus causing less interference. In terms of performance the sensors can be used over wide frequency and force ranges and due to their high stiffness also have high force resolution [20].

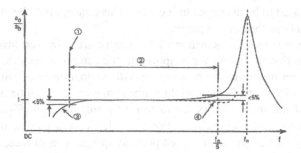

Fig. 1. Frequency dependant characteristics of Piezoelectric Sensors. Vertical scale is shown as output acceleration a$_0$ of the sensor body over the base acceleration a$_b$ applied to the sensor. Natural frequency of vibration f$_n$ is indicated. (1) Low cutoff frequency, (2) Linear operating range, (3) Output amplitude roll-off as 1st Order high-pass filter, (4) Response due to optional filtering. Adapted from [20].

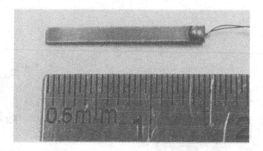

Fig. 2. Piezoelectric bimorph adapted for use in this work

There are several disadvantages associated with using piezoelectric sensors. A major drawback is that they cannot be used to measure static forces; their capacitive nature leading to behaviour analogous to a high-pass filter as shown in Figure 1. Another problem is that their extremely high impedance (>100MΩ) means that it is difficult to use them directly linked to a measuring device as this causes charge to be drawn and hence the reading becomes unreliable [20]. Piezoelectric sensors are normally used by coupling with extremely high impedance MOSFET circuits, or charge amplifiers to ensure much more reliable measurements. Figure 2 depicts a piezoelectric sensor that is adapted for use in this work; the natural frequency f$_n$ of this sensor is determined to be 475 Hz.

2.2 Tactile Sensor Array and MR Compatible Shaker

In the context of this project, it is foreseen that piezoelectric sensors can be scaled down and incorporated onto an array that can be positioned on an endoscopic tool. The tool can be inserted into the body to assess tissue stiffnesses at an area of interest. The sensor array would then be actuated over the target area and a surface stiffness contour is generated to be displayed to the user. This concept is to be demonstrated in two experiments described in this paper.

Two possible schemes for actuation of the sensor are proposed involving the design and construction of mounts for adaption on the actuating devices. Actuating devices are based on piezoceramic motors, the MR compatibility of which have been demonstrated in [9]. These devices produce linear motion, and can be used to provide lateral motion of the sensor across the surface of a soft material (Figure 3 (a)). It is also possible to produce sinusoidal motion in which case a particular frequency of excitation is imparted on the sensor when pressed up against a surface, the magnitude of which is dependant on the force thus applied (Figure 3(b)). In the vibrational scheme of actuation, there is no translation across the material surface, therefore to produce spatial stiffness information, an array of 18 sensors was constructed so that each sensor formed a single sensory 'pixel' in a two dimensional force profile with a resolution equal to the sensor spacing of 1.8 mm.

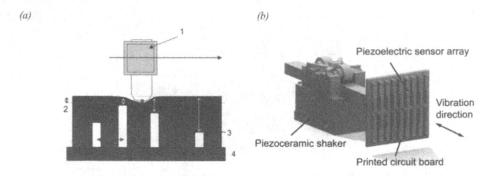

Fig. 3. (a) Concept of sliding actuation scheme. Single sensor is incorporated in a mount (1), and actuated linearly across a material surface at a constant indentation depth (2). Harder inclusions (3) are mounted on a hard base (4), and give different depths below the surface. (b) Vibrational actuation scheme. CAD rendering of a sensor array mounted on an MR compatible shaker.

2.3 Data Transmission Scheme for Noise Elimination

As piezoelectric materials have intrinsically very high impedance but weak output signal, a charge amplifier system coupled with a filtering circuit has been utilised especially for signal processing. For this type of high impedance system, MRI presents a highly noisy environment, therefore a scheme for data transmission and noise elimination shown in Figure 4 is proposed. As long cables connected from the control room to the scanner room constitute potential antennae inducing and amplifying noise, optical fibre is used for data transmission and all electrical pulses are encoded to be optical pulses by optical converters. The sensor array is connected to the charge amplifier system and through to the data acquisition device via twisted cables with good shielding well connected to the ground of the scanner. All electronics in the scanner room are put inside a faraday cage.

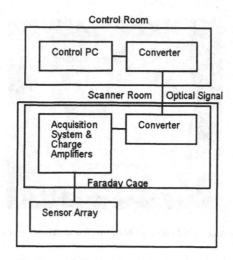

Fig. 4. Proposed data transmission scheme for noise elimination

3 Results and Discussion

3.1 MR Compatibility Tests

Experiments were carried out to determine MR compatibility of the sensor in a 1.5T Siemens Magnetom system. The size of the image artifacts were quantified using the ASTM standard F2119 protocol. The piezoelectric sensor was disconnected and placed in a container of $CuSO_4$ solution. Scans were taken using Gradient Echo (GE) and Turbo Spin Echo (TSE) image sequences as shown in Table 2. The sizes of the artifacts were measured from the device boundary to the artefact edge, the maximum distance is taken.

Table 2. Detail of image sequences selected

	TR (ms)	TE (ms)	FA (degree)	No. of slice	Thickness of slice (mm)	Spacing (mm)	Resolution	FOV (mm)	BW (Hz/px)
TSE	500	20	180°	15	3	3	256✕256	300	130
Gradient Echo	200	15	30°	15	3	3	256✕256	300	130

The maximum artefact size was observed to be 2.2mm × 20 mm in Gradient Echo, which is slightly larger than the sensor body at 1.5mm × 15mm. This artefact size means that the sensor can be placed within the imaging volume without significantly distorting the image of interest. The artefact produced under gradient echo is shown in Figure 5.

MR Safety was shown, as no appreciable force was measured with the sensor placed inside the scanner bore; from literature PZT (Lead Zirconium Titanate), has been determined to have a magnetic susceptibility of -30×10^{-6} or less. The test concludes that the sensor is non-magnetic [21].

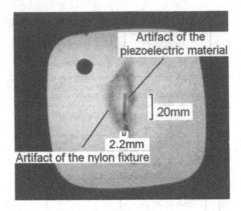

Fig. 5. Sensor is indicated in solution for measurement of artifact

3.2 Application and Noise Analysis in the MR Scanner Room

Experiments were carried out within the MRI scanner bore using models representative of soft tissue with hard inclusions to determine functionality. The model is formed of a hydrogel (Spenco® 'Dermal Pads') substrate with 6mm wide Delrin® inclusions, which being made from polyethylene and plastic are also MR compatible. The MRI scanner was programmed to conduct continuous scanning in both TSE and GE sequences as described above.

The sensor was tested using the sliding actuation scheme. The sensor was actuated over the model to locate the position of a single inclusion at a depth of 3mm. Operation of the system using any scanning sequence revealed an issue of induced noise on the system due to scanning. Figure 6(a) shows the output result of the experiment during a Gradient Echo scan where the indentation is fixed at 1mm. Output values on this chart are scaled to the performance of the charge amplifier the characteristics of which are as follows:

$$GAIN = 0.4 \times 10^9 \, V/C, \, RANGE = +/- \, 10V.$$

The position could be seen as the peak in the waveform between approximately 12 and 16mm; however the signal was clearly corrupted by noise.

Subsequent experiments were conducted to determine the nature of the induced noise.

Sensor output was analysed without actuation at different points in the scanner room to determine noise. This was done during scan sequences (as above) and without. Table 3 gives the results of these experiments where position refers to a sensor position relative to the scanner.

It was found that significant noise only occurred during a scan sequence when the sensor was physically attached to the bore, from which it was concluded that induced noise on the sensor was not electromagnetic but mechanical interference due to the vibration of the scanner body.

Spectrum analysis was carried out on both of the signals using Fourier Transform to further define the characteristics. It was found that the raw signal data acquired

Table 3. Results of MRI induced sensor noise

Position*	Scan	Signal max p-p (mV)	Ave Error (μV)	Ave error – percentage of signal.
A	None	1.22	n/a	
A	GE	1.22	0	0
A	TSE	1.22	12.94	9.4%
B	None	1.22	1.61	1.3%
B	GE	1.22	31.91	20.4%
B	TSE	1.22	32.15	20.5%
C	None	1.22	0	0
C	GE	4.56	369.78	74.8%
C	TSE	4.88	369.62	74.8%

*(A) is 4m from the iscocentre unrestrained, (B) is within scanner bore but unrestrained and (C) is affixed to the inner surface of the bore at the isocentre.

roughly approximated white noise of very low amplitude (Figure 7(a)) in all cases of A and B. However, sensor signals in the case of position C became noisy during either GE or TSE scanning. Fourier Transform of the noisy signals showed definite peaks at 10Hz, 40Hz and most greatly at 100Hz (Figure 7(b)). A 5th order low-pass Finite Impulse Response (FIR) digital filter was applied to the acquired data and it was found that a cut-off frequency of 5Hz was sufficient to greatly improve the output waveform. Figure 6(b) illustrates the effect of filtering on the signal in Figure 6(a).

To further assess the performance of the sensing format, experiments were carried out to determine the relationship between inclusion depth and the minimum sensor indentation. The minimum sensor indentation was taken to be the point at which the signal amplitude was 10% of the maximum output. It was found that the ratio of minimum sensor indentation to inclusion depth increased as inclusion depth increased, and at shallow levels the ratio was as small as 0.125 (Figure 8).

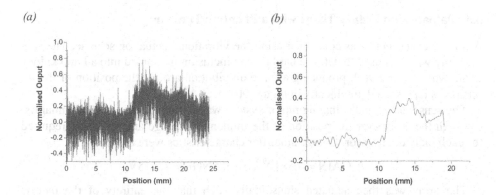

Fig. 6. (a) Output of the sensor within the scanner during a Gradient Echo scan, showing induced noise. Inclusion depth: 3mm, indentation depth 1mm. (b) Sensor output from (a) after application of a 5th order FIR low pass filter with cut-off frequency 5Hz, showing inclusion position between 11 and 17mm.

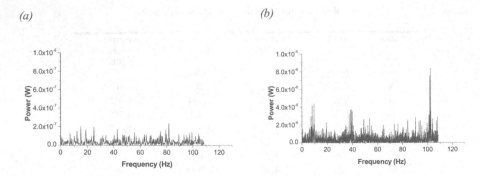

Fig. 7. (a) Fourier Transform of sensor signals in position A, B or C (without scan), show the similar frequency patterns, with low magnitudes. (b) Fourier transform of signal from sensor attached to the scanner bore during any scan. Note the scale in (b) is 10 times larger than (a).

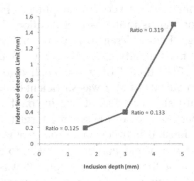

Fig. 8. Minimum indentation at which inclusion is detected increases with deeper inclusions. Also the ratio of that indentation to the inclusion depth increases.

3.3 Palpation on Kidney Tissue with a Phantom Tumour

A further experiment was conducted using the vibrational actuation scheme. The sensor array was then used to detect a hard plastic inclusion implanted into a lamb kidney as shown in Figure 9(a), producing a force distribution around the position of the insertion as represented graphically in Figure 9(b).

The sensor array and actuating motor system was set up adjacent to the animal tissue with the array over the position of the implant. A charge amplifier was required for each individual sensor. Charge amplifier characteristics were as follows:

$$GAIN = 0.8 \times 10^9 \text{ V/C}, RANGE = +/- 15V.$$

The array was then actuated sinusoidally such that the entirety of the motion caused the sensors to be impinged on the tissue. The frequency of vibration and peak to peak amplitude of motion was maintained constant at 5Hz and 1mm respectively within the capabilities of the motor. A sinusoidal force was thus produced on the sensors, the amplitude of which was taken as a direct measure of the force applied on each. A 5th order FIR bandpass filter is also applied to allow 5Hz signals.

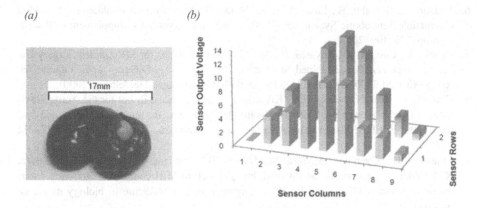

Fig. 9. (a) Measurement setup of a phantom tumour implanted in a normal lamb kidney and (b) its force distribution

4 Conclusions

It has been shown that the principle of force sensing within the MR scanner isocentre is achievable using piezoelectric force transducers although challenges arise from the presence of scanner induced noise. It is conceivable that this noise can be removed by using just digital filtering alone, as the frequencies of the noise were well above the frequencies of useful information. However as the noise has been shown to be almost entirely mechanical, it may also be possible to remove the noise by using a mechanical low pass filter (damper) to decouple the scanner vibration from the sensor. It has been shown that it is possible to generate a force profile of a soft material using two different actuation schemes and locate the position of a harder subsurface inclusion by a mechanical action approximating palpation. It is also possible to use this output to generate quantitative measurements of force to allow more accurate determination of feature characteristics.

Future work involves the incorporation of this technology with positioning devices such that sensor position may be mapped to the output. It is also necessary to miniaturize the components further to allow adaption on endoscopes.

References

1. Mack, M.J.: Minimally invasive and robotic surgery. Jama 285, 568–572 (2001)
2. Eltaib, M.E., Hewit, J.R.: Tactile sensing technology for minimal access surgery–a review. Mechatronics 13, 1163–1177 (2003)
3. Howe, R.D., Matsuoka, Y.: Robotics for surgery. Annu. Rev. Biomed. Eng. 1, 211–240 (1999)
4. Virtanen, J.: Enhancing the Compatibility of Surgical Robots with Magnetic Resonance Imaging. In: Faculty of Technology. University of Oulu, Oulu (2006)
5. McRobbie, D.W.: MRI from picture to proton. Cambridge University Press, Cambridge (2003)

6. Melzer, A., Gutnabb, B., Lukoschek, A., Mark, M.: Experimental Evaluation of an MRI Compatible Telerobotic System for CT MRI Guided Interventions. Supplement to Radiology, pp. 226–409 (2003)
7. Koseki, Y., Chinzei, K., Koyachi, N., Arai, T.: Robotic Assist for MR-Guided Surgery Using Leverage and Parallelepiped Mechanism. In: Delp, S.L., DiGoia, A.M., Jaramaz, B. (eds.) MICCAI 2000. LNCS, vol. 1935, pp. 940–948. Springer, Heidelberg (2000)
8. Chinzei, K., Hata, N., Jolesz, F.A., Kikinis, R.: Surgical Assist Robot for the Active Navigation in the Intraoperative MRI: Hardware Design Issues. In: Intelligent robots and systems; 2000 IEEE/RSJ International Conference, Takamatsu, Japan, vol. 1, pp. 727–732 (2000)
9. Elhawary, H., Zivanovic, A., Rea, M., Davies, B.L., Besant, C., McRobbie, D., Souza, N.D., Young, I., Lamperth, M.: A modular approach to MRI compatible Robotics: Interconnectable one DOF stages. In: IEEE Engineering and Medicine in biology magazine (in press, 2007)
10. Stoianovici, D., Patriciu, A., Mazilu, D., Petrisor, D.: Multi imager compatible robot for transperineal percutaneous prostate access. IEEE Transactions on Information Robotics (2005)
11. Madhani, A.J., Niemeyer, G., Salisbury, J.K.: The Black Falcon: a Teleoperated Surgical Instrument for Minimally Invasive Surgery. In: Intelligent robots and systems, Victoria, Canada, vol. 2, pp. 936–944 (1998)
12. Burdet, E., Gassert, R., Gowrishankar, G., Chapuis, D., Bleuler, H.: fMRI Compatible Haptic Interfaces to Investigate Human Motor Control. In: International symposium on experimental robotics, Singapore, vol. 2, pp. 25–34 (2004)
13. Tada, M., Kanade, T.: Design of an MR-compatible three-axis force sensor. In: 2005 IEEE/RSJ International Conference on Intelligent Robots and Systems (IROS 2005), pp. 3505–3510 (2005)
14. Moser, R.G., Burdet, E., Sache, L., Woodtli, H.R., Erni, J., Maeder, W., Bleuler, H.: An MR compatible robot technology. In: Robotics and Automation. Proceedings of IEEE International Conference on ICRA 2003, vol. 1, p. 15 (2003)
15. Field, D.: Anatomy: Palpation and Surface Markings, 2nd edn. Butterworth-Heinemann, Oxford (1997)
16. Wellman, P.H., Dalton, R., Kern, E.: Breast Tissue Stiffness in Compression is Correlated to Histological Diagnosis, Technical Report Harvard BioRobotics Laboratory, Division of Engineering and Applied Sciences, Harvard University
17. Burdea, G.: Force and touch feedback for virtual reality. John Wiley, Chichester (1996)
18. Dargahi, J.S.N.: Human tactile perception as a standard for artificial tactile sensing - a review. The International Journal of Medical Robotics and Computer Assisted Surgery 1, 23–35 (2004)
19. Chinzei, K., Kikinis, R., Jolesz, F.A.: MR Compatibility of Mechatronic Devices: Design Criteria. In: Taylor, C., Colchester, A. (eds.) MICCAI 1999. LNCS, vol. 1679, pp. 1020–1030. Springer, Heidelberg (1999)
20. Kistler, I.C.: The Piezoelectric Effect, Theory, Design and Usage (2007),
   http://www.GlobalSpec.com,
   http://www.designinfo.com/kistler/ref/tech_theory_text.htm
21. Grimes, C.A.: High-frequency, transient magnetic susceptibility of ferroelectrics. Journal of applied physics 80, 4548–4552 (1996)

A Framework of the Non-invasive Ultrasound Theragnostic System

Norihiro Koizumi[1,2], Deukhee Lee[1], Kohei Ota[1], Shin Yoshizawa[1], Kiyoshi Yoshinaka[1], Yoichiro Matsumoto[1], and Mamoru Mitsuishi[1]

[1] School of Engineering, The Univ. of Tokyo
7-3-1, Hongo, Bunkyo-ku, Tokyo 113-8656, Japan
nkoizumi@nml.t.u-tokyo.ac.jp
[2] Translational Systems Biology and Medicine Initiative (TSBMI)

Abstract. The authors have developed an Non-Invasive Ultrasound Theragnostic System to decrease the strain of patients and medical doctors. The system we propose tracks and follows movement in an affected area –kidney stones here– while High-Intensity Focused Ultrasound (HIFU) is irradiated onto the area. In this paper, a framework of the non-invasive ultrasound theragnostic system is proposed and illustrated. Specifically, the concept of the system is proposed at first. Secondly, decomposing and reconstructing (structuring) of the functional requirements are discussed. Third, the constructed system, which is based on those structured functional requirements, is illustrated. Fourth, the result of the servoing experiments of the model stone is reported to confirm the effectiveness of the proposed construction methodology and constructed system.

Keywords: High-Intensity Focused Ultrasound (HIFU), Non-Invasive Diagnosis and Therapy, Theragnostics, Motion Tracking.

1 Introduction

Areas can be selectively diagnosed and treated non-invasively by using high-intensity focused ultrasound (HIFU), based on the same principle as conventional ultrasound. It propagates harmlessly through living tissue. If the ultrasound beam is focused too tightly, however, energy in the focal volume may raise temperature locally [1].

It is thus possible to treat affected area in focal volume without damaging surrounding or overlying tissues, which is a promising alternative to current abdominal and endoscopic surgeries thanks to its noninvasiveness (Fig.1 (a)).

A number of reports have been made since Lynn, et al. demonstrated the potential medical application of HIFU [1][2]. e.g., the noninvasive destruction of kidney stones (Fig.1 (b)) by energy generated by cavitation. One advantage is that debris from such stones is small enough to avoid problems with adjacent organs [3].

JC HIFU is widely used in clinical practice [4][5]. Some 19 devices in clinical use were used to treat 1050 patients with a variety of tumors [6][7].Compensation was not made, however, for movement in the affected area, mainly due to respiration. The

T. Dohi, I. Sakuma, and H. Liao (Eds.): MIAR 2008, LNCS 5128, pp. 231–240, 2008.
© Springer-Verlag Berlin Heidelberg 2008

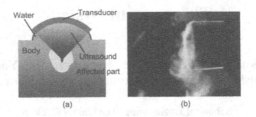

Fig. 1. (a) High Intensity Focused Ultrasound (HIFU), (b) Destruction of kidney stone by HIFU

need to prevent such movement when irradiating focused ultrasound on the affected area thus conventionally places a large burden on the physician and patient.

In the integrated system we propose for noninvasive ultrasound diagnosis and treatment. Movement is compensated for by tracking and following the affected area through stereo ultrasound imaging while simultaneously irradiating the affected area. The concept behind our proposal focuses on destroying tumors and stones. Using focused ultrasound directly without damaging healthy tissue while tracking and following the affected area - kidney stones in this case - during movement due, for example to the patient's respiration.

Pernot et al.[8], Nakamura et al., Thankral et al., and Ginhoux et al. have studied how to compensate for organ movement[9-12]. Pernot et al. proposed 3-dimensional (3D) motion canceling using multiple ultrasound transducers on a spherical surface but servoing performance is insufficient. Nakamura proposed synchronization between organ movement and slave manipulator operation using a 955 fps high-speed CCD camera and robot controlled based on control theory. Thankral et al. proposed modeling physiological movement based on a Fourier linear combiner (FLC) algorithm [10]. But did not shown how to apply the algorithm to actual robotic servoing.

Ginhoux et al. proposed model predictive control (MPC) with an adaptive observer [11]. as applied to a living pig, and verified the proposal's effectiveness. Their system is based on a 500 fps high-speed CCD camera.

Such a camera cannot be used for noninvasive diagnosis and treatment, however, due to the need to avoid damaging healthy tissue. Tracking and following organ movement - kidney stones here - while simultaneously irradiating the affected area raises a problem with servoing error mainly due to ultrasound imaging and its dead time, which differs from the case when a high-speed camera is used. To solve this problem, we propose feed-forward control using semi-regular kidney movement, focusing on enhancing servoing performance.

We proceed by presenting the concepts, required functions and the system configuration of integrated noninvasive ultrasound diagnosis and treatment, then discuss factors of dead time. We then analyze kidney movement mainly due to respiration, and propose feed-forward control using regular movement in the affected area to enhance servoing performance. We then review experimental results demonstrating the effectiveness of our proposed feed-forward control.

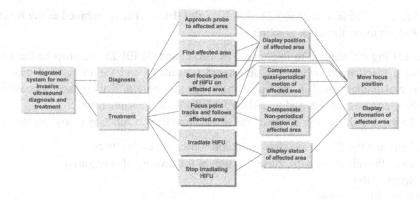

Fig. 2. Decomposing and Reconstructing (Structuring) functions to implement in the system

2 Construction Methodology

2.1 Decomposition and Reconstruction of Required Functions

It is required to be made clear the required functions for the system to realize the efficient system. An overview of the decomposing and reconstructing (Structuring) functions is shown in Fig.2. First, the required function of the integrated system for Non-Invasive Ultrasound Diagnosis and Treatment system is decomposed into these 2 functions as mentioned below.

(FR-1) Function to diagnose
(FR-2) Function to treat
Among those, (FR-1) is decomposed into these 2 sub functional requirements.
(FR-1.1) Function to approach the probe to the affected area.
(FR-1.2) Function to find the affected area.
(FR-2) is decomposed into these 4 sub functional requirements.
(FR-2.1) Function to set the focus of HIFU on the affected area.
(FR-2.2) Function for the focus of HIFU to track and follow the affected area
(FR-2.3) Function to irradiate HIFU to the affected area.
(FR-2.4) Function to stop irradiating HIFU..

Next, functional requirements are reconstructed, considering the implementation of the system. Among those, the functional requirements (FR-1.1), (FR-1.2), (FR-2.1), and (FR-2.2) are combined as the function (R-FR-1.1) to display position of the affected area to the medical doctor. Same as this, (FR-2.3) and (FR-2.4) are combined as the function (R-FR-1.4) to display the states of the affected area to the medical doctor. (R-FR-1.1) and (R-FR-1.4) are combined as the function (R-FR-2) to display information of the affected area.

For (FR-2.2), these 2 functions below should be realized.
(R-FR-1.2): Compensate the quasi-periodic motion of the affected area.
(R-FR-1.3): Compensate the non-periodic motion of the affected area.

(R-FR-1.2), (R-FR-1.3), (FR-1.1), (FR-1.2), and (FR-2.1) are combined as the function (R-FR-1) to move the focus position.

Considering the method to implement (R-FR-1) and (R-FR-2), we propose the united hardware mechanism, where the ultrasound transducer and the ultrasound probe are united and implemented in the tip of the hardware system. This makes it possible to acquire diagnostic images and treat the affected area at the same time.

To diagnose and treat the affected area at the same time, a function below is required.

(i) HIFU and the diagnostic ultrasound don't interfere each other.

To adopt the robotic system, these function as follows are also required.

(ii) Secure safety.

(iii) Lessen uneasiness.

(iv) Secure ultrasound paths to the affected area.

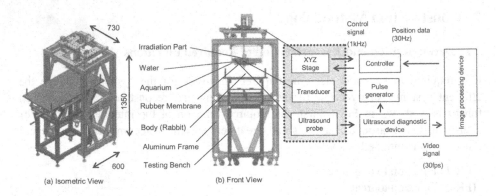

Fig. 3. Overview and system configuration of the constructed non-invasive ultrasoundtheragnostic system

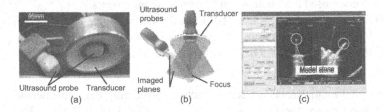

Fig. 4. (a) Overview of the configuration of the probes and transducer, (b) Image planes and the focus of HIFU, (c) Ultrasound images and the visual tracking of the renal stone by image processing

2.2 Implementation of Reconstructed Required Functions

The constructed non-invasive ultrasound theragnostic system is shown in Fig.3. Stereo diagnostic images are acquired using two ultrasound diagnostic probes.

Based on stereo images, 3D positioning data of the affected area, the relative value to the focused position of the HIFU, is obtained. In control, the focus tracks and follows the kidney stone using 3D positioning data.

Focused ultrasound is irradiated onto the kidney stone using the pulse generator and transducer. The specification of irradiation of focused ultrasound is detailed in reference [13].

The robot has a spherical piezoelectric transducer and two ultrasound probes (Fig.4 (a) and (b)) --one in the center of the piezoelectric transducer and the other one is located in the lateral side of the piezoelectric transducer. These two probes meet two conditions:

(i) Image planes, acquired by probes, are mutually perpendicular.

(ii) The focus of HIFU, irradiated by piezoelectric transducers, is on both image planes acquired by probes.

The two ultrasound image planes are shown in Fig.4 (c). The stone is shown as bright regions in yellow circles in left and right ultrasound images.

The left ultrasound image is acquired by the probe in the center of the piezoelectric transducer and that at right by the probe on the lateral side of the piezoelectric transducer.

The kidney stone is tracked by imaging left and right ultrasound images based on the Matrox Imaging Library (MIL8.0) processing cycle (Fig.6), which involves 5 steps:

1: Grabbing ultrasound images. 2: Processing grabbed images to enhance image quality for tracking the kidney stone. 3: Pattern matching to detect the 3D location of the stone. 4: Finding and updating the target by blob analysis if the kidney stone is lost during tracking.

The 3D relative positioning data between the stone and the focus of high-intensity focused ultrasound is thus acquired. Positioning data is transmitted to the controller of the XYZ stage. The focused position tracks and follows the stone by activating the the XYZ stage based on transmitted positioning data. In Fig.4 (c), the left ultrasound image is acquired by the probe, which is located in the centre of the piezo transducer. The right ultrasound image is acquired by the probe, which is located in the lateral side of the piezo transducer (Fig.4 (a) and (b)).

The position of the renal stone is tracked by image processing on both left and right ultrasound images. The image tracking system for the stone motion is constructed based on the Matrox Imaging Library (MIL8.0). There are mainly 5 steps in a processing cycle.

[Step 1] A step to grab ultrasound images as shown in Fig.4 (c). [Step 2] A step to process the grabbed images to enhance the image quality for the image tracking of the model stone. [Step 3] A step to execute the image processing to detect the 3 dimensional position of the renal stone. [Step 4] A step to find and update the target model by the blob analysis when the system fails to track the renal stone. [Step 5] A step to report the result of the image processing.

Thus, 3 dimensional relative position data between the model stone and the focus of the high intensity focused ultrasound is acquired. Then, the position data is transmitted to the controller of the XYZ stage. The focused position tracks and follows the model stone by actuating the XYZ stage based on the transmitted position data.

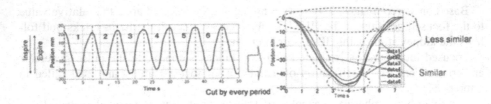

Fig. 5. Quasi-periodical kidney motion

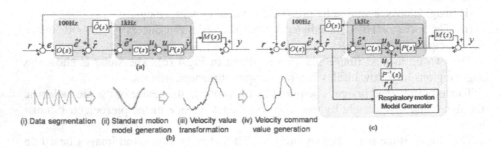

Fig. 6. (a) Block diagram of the fundamental controller, (b) An algorithm to generate feed-forward term, (c) Block diagram of the proposed feed-forward controller

3 Controller by Utilizing the Semi-periodical Motion of the Organ by Respiration

3.1 Semi-periodical Organ Motion by Respiration

Fig.5 show a quasi-periodical kidney motion in a body, which is acquired by an ultra-sound probe. It is confirmed that [Feature 1] the motion path of the kidney in a period is similar to the one in another period, as shown in Fig.5. It is also confirmed that [Feature 2] Similar during in the high speed motion area, [Feature 3] Less similar during in the low speed motion area.

3.2 Control Methodology

The block diagram of the fundamental controller is shown in Fig 6 (a). Here, r : Target position, e : Servoing error, $\hat{e}'$: Referred servoing error (100Hz), $\hat{r}$: Presumed target position, $\hat{e}''$: Presumed servoing error (1kHz), u : velocity command value, y :Focus position of HIFU, $\hat{y}$: Presumed focus position of HIFU. Our system is composed of position acquisition part $O(s)$, Controller part $C(s)$, motor driving part of XYZ stage $P(s)$, Oscillation part of the hardware mechanism $M(s)$, The presumed value $\hat{O}(s)$ of $O(s)$. Those mathematical model are expressed below.

$$O(s) = \hat{O}(s) + d_o \tag{1}$$

$$M(s) = -\frac{s^2}{s^2 + 24s + 3.1\times10^3} + d_m \tag{2}$$

$$P(s) = \frac{s + 7.5\times10^{-4}}{s(s + 2.2\times10^{-3})} \exp(-0.003s) \tag{3}$$

Here, d_o is the disturbance, which is mainly caused by the noize of the ultrasound image, tracking error, etc. d_m is the mechanical disturbance, which cannot be expressed in $M(s)$. Target position is acquired by the ultrasound machine at the limited sampling rate of 100Hz. While, the XYZ stage is controlled at the rate of 1kHz in the presented system. PID Feedback control is applied, at first, by error between the target and the focus position. The integral part is implemented in $P(s)$.

PD part is expressed as $C'(s) = K_P(1 + T_D s)$. Here, we applied Ziegler-Nichols ultimate sensitivity method to determine proportional gain $K_P = 19.4$ and derivative time $T_D = 0.014$. The controller is designed $C(s) = (19.4 + 0.26)F(s)$.

In the kidney motion tracking by utilizing ultrasound image, there exist some problems and difficulties. First, due to the effect of dead time, servoing error increases with feedback control alone. The shape changes when the servoing error becomes large and the quality of the ultrasound image becomes worse for visual tracking. Second, the visual tracking error occurs promptly during the HIFU irradiation. This is mainly caused by the bubbles generated by HIFU around the crushed pieces of the kidney stone.

To solve this problem, we propose feed-forward control method by utilizing the quasi-periodical motion of the organ due to respiration. The procedures for the feed-forward term generation is shown in Fig.6 (b). The block diagram of the feed-forward control is shown in Fig.6 (c).

The period and the amplitude fluctuates, while the kidney motion is quasi-periodical. Then, (i) the kidney motion is segmented into each period at first. Second, (ii) the standard motion model r_f is generated based on the last several segments. Third, (iii) the standard motion model is transformed into the velocity data and (iv) the velocity command value u_f is generated by $P^{-1}(s)$. Then, the u_f is input to $P(s)$ with the feedback term u_b.

4   Experiments

Servoing experiments of the model stone are conducted to confirm the effectiveness of the proposed feed-forward controller by utilizing the quasi-periodical motion of the kidney. The tracking and following target is the artificial model stone[13]. Overview of

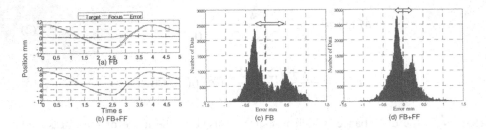

Fig. 7. (a) Servoing performance only by feedback control, (b) Servoing performance by the proposed feed-forward control with feedback control, (c) Tracking error only by feedback control, (d) Tracking error by the proposed feed-forward control with feedback control

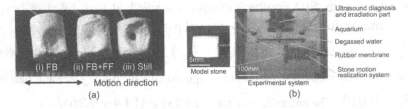

Fig. 8. (a) Stone destruction by HIFU, (i) With only the feedback, (ii) With the proposed control, (iii) The stone is still, (b) Overview of the experimental setup

the model stone and its motion mechanism is shown in Fig.8 (b). Here, these parameters as follows are set by considering the position and motion of the human kidney.

$d_1 = 55$ [mm]: Distance from the water surface

$d_2 = 10 \sim 50$ [mm]: Motion range

The moving direction of the stone model is the translational axis that corresponds to the axis of the human body. The real kidney motion is input to the stone model. Specifically, we compared the tracking and following performance of the model stone under these 2 conditions.

[FB] Servoing only by the feedback control.

[FB+FF] Servoing not only by the feedback control but also by the proposed feed-forward control by utilizing the quasi-periodical motion of the kidney.

CCL (Cavitation Cloud Lithotripsy [3]) is applied to crush the model stone. Irradiation time is set 30 minutes.

The experimental result is shown in Figs.7 (a)-(d) and 8 (a). The transition of the position of the model stone, the focus, the motion tracking error between the stone and the focus in each condition, is shown in Figs.7(a) and (b). The maximum tracking error is 1.5mm, the average tracking error is 0.38mm, only by the feedback control. On the other hand, the maximum tracking error is 1.2mm, the average tracking error is 0.24mm, with the feed-forward control.

The distribution of the motion tracking error during 120 s with the sampling rate 1kHz (Total amount 120,000 points) is shown in Figs.7(c)(d). The standard deviation of the tracking error is 0.44mm (FB), 0.29mm (FB+FF) in the experiment. The crushed model stone after the 30 minutes is shown in Figs 8(a). In the figure, (i) is under the condition [FB], (ii) is under the condition [FB+FF], and (iii) is under the condition where the kidney stone is still.

It is confirmed that the servoing performance could be enhanced by the proposed the proposed feed-forward control by utilizing the quasi-periodical motion of the kidney. I think the improvement of the phase delay, which is mainly caused by dead times, is effective. Phase delay between the target position and the focus position of HIFU is calculated as (a) 56ms, (b) 26ms. Concerning the destruction of the model stone, the crushed shape is almost circle within the 5mm diameter model stone among in the condition (a)-(c). This is the sufficient results for the purpose to crush the stone. Usual stones in the human body is about 20-30mm in diameter. Stones within the diameter 4mm could be emitted out of the body with the unine.

5 Conclusion

In this paper, a non-invasive ultrasound theragnostic system is proposed. The concept of the proposed system is to destroy tumors or stones non-invasively. The proposed system tracks and follows the motion of the affected area (renal stones in the presented system). High Intensity Focused Ultrasound (HIFU) is irradiated to the affected area at the same time.

Specifically, the functional requirements for the system are made clear at first. Second, those extracted functional requirements are decomposed and reconstructed (structured). Third, the non-invasive ultrasound theragnostic system is constructed based on the introduced requirements. Fourth, the dead time and the required servoing precision are discussed. Fifth, the controller by utilizing the periodical motion of the affected area, which is mainly caused by respiration, is proposed and implemented to enhance the servoing performance. Fifth, the result of the servoing experiment for the model stone is reported and the effectiveness of the proposed control method and the constructed system was confirmed.

Acknowledgements

This work was supported by the "Translational Systems Biology and Medicine Initiative (TSBMI)", "Mechanical Systems Innovation," supported by JSPS Program, Ministry of Education, Culture, Sports, Science, and Technology.

References

1. Kennedy, J.E., Ter Harr, G.R., Cranston, D.: High-intensity focused ultrasound: surgery of the future? The British Journal of Radiology 76, 590–599 (2003)
2. Lynn, J.G., Zwemer, R.L., Chick, A.J., Miller, A.E.: A new method for the generation and use of focused ultrasound in experimental biology. J. Gen. Physiol. 26, 179–193 (1942)

3. Ikeda, T., Yoshizawa, S., Tosaki, M., Allen, J.S., Takagi, S., Ohta, N., Kitamura, T., Matsumoto, Y.: Cloud Cavitation Control for Lithotripsy Using High Intensity Focused Ultrasound. Ultrasound Med. Biol. 32(9), 1383–1397 (2006)
4. Wu, F., Wang, Z.L., Zhang, Z., et al.: Acute biological effects of high-intensity focused ultrasound on H22 liver tumours in vivo. Chin. Ultrasound Med. J. 13(3), 1–4 (1997)
5. Tu, G., Qiao, T.Y., He, S.: An experimental study on highintensity focused ultrasound in the treatment of VX-2 rabbit kidney tumours. Chin. Ultrasound Med. J. 20(8), 456–458 (1999)
6. Wu, F., Chen, W.Z., Bai, J., Zou, J.Z., Wang, Z.L., Zhu, H., Wang, Z.B.: Pathological changes in malignant carcinoma treated with high-intensity focused ultrasound. Ultrasound Med. Biol. 27(8), 1099–1106 (2001)
7. Kennedy, J.E., Wub, F., ter Haarc, G.R., Gleesond, F.V., Phillipsd, R.R., Middletone, M.R., Cranstona, D.: Highintensity focused ultrasound for the treatment of liver tumours. Ultrasonics 41, 931–935 (2004)
8. Pernot, M., et al.: 3-D Real-Time Motion Correction in High-Intensity Focused Ultrasound Therapy. Ultrasound Med. & Biol. 30(9), 1239–1249 (2004)
9. Nakamura, Y., Kishi, H., Kawakami, H.: Robotic Stabilization that Assists Cardiac Surgery on Beating Hearts. In: Proc. of Medicine Meets Virtual Reality 2001, pp. 355–361 (2001)
10. Nakamura, Y., Kishi, H., Kawakami, H.: Heartbeat Synchronization for Robotic Cardiac Surgery. In: Proc. 2001 Int. Conf. Robotics and Automation, pp. 2014–2019 (2001)
11. Thankral, A., Wallace, J., Tomlin, D., Seth, N., Thakor, N.V.: Beating heart tracking in robotic surgery using 500 Hz visual servoing, model predictive control and an adaptice observer. In: Proc. 2004 Int. Conf. Robotics and Automation, vol. 1, pp. 274–279 (2004)
12. Ginhoux, R., Gangloff, J.A., Mathelin, M.F., Soler, L., Sanchez, M.A., Marescaux, J.: Beating heart tracking in robotic surgery using 500 Hz visual servoing, model predictive control and an adaptice observer. In: Proc. 2004 Int. Conf. Robotics and Automation, vol. 1, pp. 274–279 (2004)
13. McAteer, J.A., Williams, J.C., Evan, A.P., Cleveland, R.O., Cauwelaert, J.V., Bailey, M.R., Lifshitz, D.A.: The impact of the geometry of the lithotripter aperture on fragmentation effect at extracorporeal shock wave lithotripsy treatment. In: Urol. Res., vol. 33, pp. 429–434 (2004)

In Vivo Evaluation of a Guidance System for Computer Assisted Robotized Needle Insertion Devoted to Small Animals

S.A. Nicolau, L. Mendoza-Burgos, L. Soler, D. Mutter, and J. Marescaux

IRCAD-Hopital Civil, Virtual-Surg, 1 Place de l'Hopital, 67091 Strasbourg Cedex
Phone number: +33 388119095
{stephane.nicolau, luc.soler}@ircad.u-strasbg.fr
http://www.virtual-surg.com

Abstract. To improve therapy research against cancer, we propose a robotized computer assisted system for needle insertion devoted to the small animal. The system is composed of a robotic arm on which the needle is attached and two cameras rigidly linked. It needs a preoperative CT acquisition in which the biologist defines an entry point and the target he wants to reach. The needle guidance is ensured by a visual servoing and the needle is registered in the CT frame using radio-opaque markers stuck beforehand on the small animal.

Biologists estimate that such a system can be beneficial if the time preparation per animal remains below 15 minutes and if the insertion accuracy is within 1 mm. Several error sources can be identified : the error due to the system only, the organ repositioning error (due to breathing motions) and the error induced by the needle insertion.

In this paper, we report an evaluation on living rats of the system error and of the organ repositioning error. Encouraging results show that a global accuracy of 0.9 mm may be reached with an acceptable preparation time.

1   Introduction

In order to develop new medical therapies, we often begin to evaluate their feasibility and effectiveness on small animals like mice or rats. This helps the biologist to develop specific parameters for safe and effective therapies on human beings, especially for the research of new therapies against cancer. A standard protocol consists in performing a first dissection of the skin to inject artificial tumors inside the animal via a needle. Tumor evolution is then observed and therapeutic agents are injected after a second dissection. The effectiveness of this protocol depends mainly on the gesture accuracy during needle insertion. There are many problems arising when doing a manual needle insertion. During the therapeutic agent injection, the accuracy can be very coarse mainly due to the difficulty to visually locate tumors when they are deep inside the organ. Our biologist evaluations show that in half the cases the therapeutic agents are not injected inside the tumor. Hand tremor can also decrease the accuracy and

T. Dohi, I. Sakuma, and H. Liao (Eds.): MIAR 2008, LNCS 5128, pp. 241–250, 2008.

damage tissues. Moreover, the overall task can be very time consuming and thus can be an issue when dealing with many animals.

Since a reliable biopsy is not possible when the tumor is deep inside the organ, the observation of tumor evolution is commonly based on two tests. The first test is based on medical imagery like a CT or PET-scan. The second test is based on an *ex vivo* statistical analysis which involves that some animals need to be killed at each step of observation. Obviously, the evaluation effectiveness of the therapeutic agent would be much better if the biologist could perform an accurate biopsy to analyse tumor cells. Indeed, the evolution of the same tumor could be observed in all animals.

To perform a percutaneous puncture with high accuracy, minimal preparation time, less animal trauma and that allows a reliable biopsy, a robotized computer assisted system can be used in order to improve the needle insertion task.

Previous works. In [10,7], Kazanzides et. al. developed a robotic system to perform an automatic needle insertion inside a tumor. However, the angle insertion is limited and can only be done along a vertical direction. This can be a limitation when targets are located under the ribs or near fragile structures that need to be avoided with an oblique orientation. Other robotic systems have been proposed in [13,5,2] for humans. Nevertheless, they are not adapted to our application for small animals, since the needle calibration is done manually and is very time consuming. Waspe et. al. proposed a system which is based on a remote center of motion (RCM) design to perform a needle insertion in small animals guided by a micro-imaging system [14,15]. It provides a high kinematics accuracy needle positioning. However, needle calibration is time consuming (1h) and requires a specific needle-tip positioning.

Our aim is to design a robotized computer assisted system for needle insertion devoted to the small animal. We propose an alternative method based on a visual servoing of the needle position by a stereoscopic system. This approach avoids the calibration step between the robot and the CT frame.

For such a system to be useful for biologists, it has firstly to avoid a too long manual preparation step. Secondly this system needs to be able to insert a needle without orientation constraints and to manipulate it independently of its model (length, thickness and shape). Thirdly the targeting accuracy on the small animal has to remain below 1 mm. This accuracy threshold has been discussed with several biologists that consider that they rarely need to puncture targets of a diameter below 2 mm.

There are different sources of errors that can corrupt needle insertion. The first one depends on the system only and comprises the needle calibration error, the needle tracking error and the CT model registration error. The second one is the breathing motion: although we plan the needle insertion during expiratory phases only to reduce its influence, there is still an organ repositioning error since the breathing is not perfectly cyclical. The third one is the deformation of the surrounding tissues induced by the needle when it is inserted. In this paper, we report in-vivo experiments to assess the first two kinds of error (i.e. the error due to the system only and the organ repositioning error) and the time needed to prepare the small animal. The last error will be evaluated in a future paper.

Firstly we describe the different components of our system. Secondly we detail the protocol we designed to evaluate the accuracy of the system. Finally we present the encouraging results that highlight that an average accuracy of 0.9 mm may be reached.

2   System Description

Our system consists of a robotic manipulator that can orientate and move its end-effector with six degrees of freedom (Mitsubishi RV1A ©) and of a stereo-scopic system to register in a same frame the small animal position and the needle (cf. Fig. 1 for a general view of the system). In our protocol, the biologist firstly shaves the animal skin and sticks several radio-opaque markers on its abdomen. These markers will be used to register the needle and the CT model in a common frame. Then it is strapped on its bed and scanned in order to acquire its CT-model. From this 3D image, the biologist selects two points : the skin-entry point and the target (tumor) to be reached. Afterwards, the bed in which the animal lies is moved out of the scanner and placed in front of the robot and the stereoscopic system. To reduce the influence of the breathing motion the CT acquisition is performed during expiratory phases as well as the needle positioning. The respiratory phases are tracked using a pressure transducer which is attached onto the abdomen with a belt. To guide the needle insertion according to the planned path, several registrations are needed.

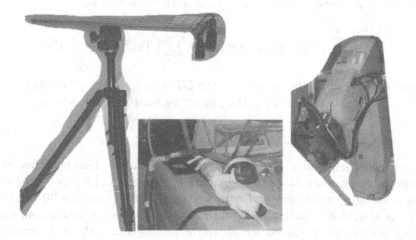

Fig. 1. Illustration of the relative position of each system component. The rat is lying on a table between the camera tripod and the robotic arm. The stereoscopic system is located above the rat and the robotic arm is positioned so that both rat skin and needle can be seen by the cameras.

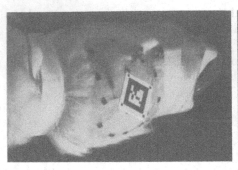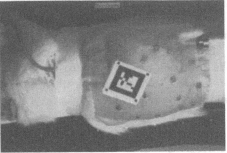

Fig. 2. Left : left camera view of the rat attached on the CT bed. One can see the black radio-opaque markers that are previously stuck on its abdomen and the square pattern attached to the needle. This pattern is tracked in real-time with the ARTag library [4]. Right : superimposition of the CT model on the right camera view. One can see that the radio-opaque markers segmented from the CT model are correctly registered on the markers visible in the video image.

2.1   3D Model Registration

To register the CT model we use radio-opaque markers stuck on the small animal abdomen (cf. Fig 2). These markers provide a high response in the CT image (cf. left Fig. 5) and can easily be thresholded and extracted automatically. Marker extraction in the video images is performed using a color and size thresholding. Then, the markers are automatically matched using the epipolar geometry followed by a prediction/verification algorithm (cf. [11] for further details on the method and accuracy analysis). Finally, the registration is performed by minimizing the reprojection error C in both video views :

$$C = \sum_{i=1}^{N} \| P_1(T \star M_i) - m_i^1 \|^2 + \sum_{i=1}^{N} \| P_2(T \star M_i) - m_i^2 \|^2$$

where M_i is the ith marker position in the CT image, m_i^j the ith marker position in the jth video image and P_j is the projective matrix of jth camera.

2.2   Needle Servoing

The needle is attached to the end-effector of the robot. This end-effector is a pneumatic device that allows to insert with a high speed ($1.8\ m.s^{-1}$) the needle along a straight orientation and with a known depth (typically 30 mm). This device is mandatory since mouse and rat skins are highly elastic and do not allow a needle that is moved too slowly to be inserted without deforming the surrounding tissues. Therefore, the needle has to be firstly positioned at 30 mm of the target and oriented along the lines defined by the skin entry point and the target center.

To guide the robotic arm so that the needle reaches this initial position, we choose to perform an image based visual servoing using the stereoscopic system. This servoing requires features that we are able to extract in real time and that are rigid w. r. t. the needle. We choose to attach a known square pattern to the needle, its four corners are tracked automatically in both video images (cf. Fig 2). The needle position w. r. t. the pattern is determined using the method described in the next subsection.

The robotic movements that have to be done to lead the needle to the correct position and orientation are computed from the four corners' movements in the video images using the interaction matrix theory proposed in [3,6,8].

Note that the guiding accuracy highly depends on the jitter due to the camera sensor intrinsic noise. The impact of this jitter is usually important with planar target when only one camera is used. However, we use two calibrated cameras to locate the square pattern: this reduces considerably the jitter impact. Quantitatively, we observe a jitter on the corner extraction of less than 0.03 pixel which corresponds to a needle tip jitter below 0.2 mm.

2.3   Needle to Square Pattern Calibration

The needle tip is calibrated with respect to the pattern using the pivot method [9]. The needle is moved whilst its tip remains at a fixed point. Therefore, the pattern center of gravity moves along a sphere, its center being the needle tip. Needle orientation is computed by rotating it along its axis. In that case, the pattern center moves on a plane, the normal vector of which corresponds to the needle orientation. Please refer to [12] for an accuracy evaluation of the calibration method.

Image processing techniques could also be used to calibrate the needle position with respect to the pattern [1,15]. There are still no comparison experiments showing the superiority of one of the approaches. The main advantage of image processing techniques is that they can be performed automatically using the robot. However, the light conditions have to be perfectly controlled. That is why we prefered to perform a manual calibration.

3   Evaluation Protocol

In this section, we propose a protocol that allows us to evaluate the error due to the system, the organ repositioning error and the duration of the mandatory manual steps.

- 1) The small animal is shaved and about fifteen radio-opaque markers are stuck on its abdomen.
- 2) The pattern is attached to the needle and it is calibrated.
- 3) The needle is inserted through the skin into the kidney.
- 4) The animal is scanned with the needle in expiratory phases
- 5) Radio-opaque markers are automatically extracted from the CT image
- 6) Needle position is semi-interactively segmented in the CT image

- 7) The cameras are placed so as to view the animal with the markers and the needle
- 8) Radio-opaque markers are automatically extracted in both video images and the CT model of the animal and of the needle are registered in the stereoscopic frame
- 9) The needle position is tracked using the pattern
- 10) The distance D between the estimated position of the needle by the stereoscopic system and its registered 3D model is measured at expiratory phases

The observed distance D corresponds in fact to an evaluation of the cumulated error induced by the CT model registration error, the needle calibration error and the needle tracking error.

To evaluate the preparation time of one animal, we kept time of steps 1) and 2). The other steps are either performed in real-time or not included in the robotic insertion process we described in Sec. 2.

Since the needle is inserted in the animal and that we can locate its tip using the pattern, this means we can also measure the repositioning error of the needle tip, which should correspond to the repositioning error of a point in the animal kidney. We assume here that the rigid needle in the animal body has no influence on internal movements. To assess this error, we follow the needle tip position along the animal's breathing during 1 minute and record the positions of the tip during each expiration phase. We measure two kinds of repositioning errors. The first one corresponds to the tip movements inside each expiration phase (we call it the intra-expiration standard deviation) and the second one is the position difference of the needle tip between each expiration (so called inter-expiration standard deviation).

4   Results on 5 Rats

We have followed the described protocols on 5 rats. Their average weight was 220 g and they were under isoflurane during the whole procedure. Both cameras had a resolution of 640x480 (F046C from Allied Vision Tech ©) and were calibrated together with the method of Zhang [16]. The CT-scan device is a MicroCat II from Imtek ©. It incorporates a respiratory gating system using a pressure transducer that has to be belted on the animal abdomen. This system ensures that the CT acquisition is performed during expiratory phases only.

Preparation duration. The average time needed to shave a rat and to stick markers is of 6 minutes $\pm$ 1 min. The main part of this duration is waiting for the effect of the depilatory cream we use to shave the rat. This duration is not negligible, however we can shave several rats simultaneously. This seems acceptable for our biologists.

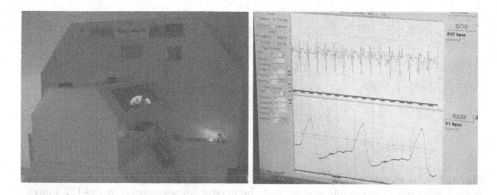

Fig. 3. Left: the MicroCat II from Imtek ©. Right: illustration of the respiratory gating software that monitors the breathing cycle from the pressure transducer information (bottom curve).

Table 1. Repositioning errors of the needle tip after the needle insertion. Two kinds of errors are reported : the intra-expiration repositioning error and the inter-expiration repositioning error.

Rat number	1	2	3	4	5
Intra expiration repositioning error (mm)	0.06 ± 0.02	0.08 ± 0.02	0.04 ± 0.03	0.05 ± 0.03	0.07 ± 0.04
Inter expiration repositioning error (mm)	0.16 ± 0.04	0.21 ± 0.05	0.18 ± 0.04	0.17 ± 0.05	0.15 ± 0.03

Attaching the pattern to the needle and calibrating it took on average 4 minutes $\pm$ 40 sec. Since this step can be performed during the CT acquisition (which lasts on average 30 minutes), this is not a problem for biologists.

Evaluation of the needle tip repositioning error. For each rat, the needle was inserted in the kidney. This organ was chosen because its size and shape are very similar to usual targeted tumors. We report in Tab. 1 the two kinds of repositioning errors we measured.

Evaluation of the system error. We report for two rats on Fig. 4 the distance along the breathing between the needle tip located with our stereoscopic system and the needle tip extracted in the CT image. Obviously, it evolves cyclically with the rat breathing and is minimal during the expiratory phases (around 0.7 mm). Tab. 2 shows that the average error due to the system only remains below 0.9 mm for the 5 rats. We show in Fig. 5 left an example of a rat CT scan with the inserted needle. In Fig. 5 right, the CT model is registered in the camera frame during an expiratory phase and the tracked needle is then displayed with respect to the CT frame. One can see the slight discrepancy between the two needle tips.

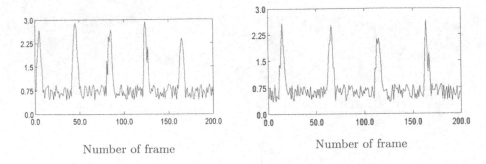

Number of frame   Number of frame

Fig. 4. Evolution on two rats during 20 sec. of the distance D between the needle tip located with our stereoscopic system and the needle tip segmented in the CT image. The abscissa corresponds to the number of the video frame (there are roughly 10 frames per second) and the ordinate to the distance D in mm. This distance is minimal during expiratory phases with a magnitude about 0.7 mm.

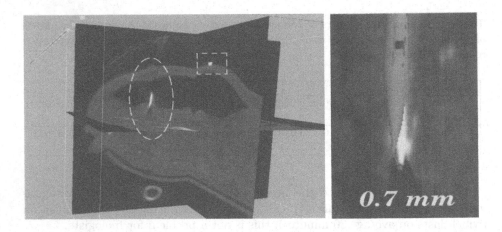

0.7 mm

Fig. 5. Left: example of a rat CT image after needle insertion. One can see in the axial slice the needle inside the animal body (highlighted in the ellipse) and in the sagittal slice one of the marker used for the registration (highlighted in the square). Right: 3D visualisation of the needle localized by the stereoscopic system after the CT model registration at an expiratory phase. One can see the slight discrepancy between the two tips.

Table 2. Average error due to the system only. This error comprises the needle calibration error, the needle tracking error and the CT model registration error.

Rat number	1	2	3	4	5
System error (mm)	0.76 ± 0.06	0.85 ± 0.05	0.63 ± 0.04	0.82 ± 0.04	0.68 ± 0.05

5   Conclusions

In this paper, we have proposed a robotized computer assisted system for needle insertion devoted to small animals. The insertion procedure is guided by a stereoscopic system that realises an image based servoing of the needle. To register the CT model of the animal in the camera frame, we use radio-opaque markers that are visible in both CT and video images.

In this paper we have evaluated on 5 living rats the influence of the main part of the error sources i.e. the needle calibration error, the needle tracking error, the CT registration error and the organ repositioning error. Results show that the error due to the system only is on average within 0.7 mm and that the average organ repositioning error is below 0.2 mm. We point out that this latter error is incompressible since we cannot prevent the animal from breathing during the whole procedure without killing it. This shows that targeting a tumor with a diameter below 0.4 mm requires another approach that includes the tumor position monitoring in real time.

Obviously, we have evaluated here the repositioning error of the kidney only. The results we obtained may not be generalized. However, parallel experiments we recently performed on the liver seem to confirm the uncompressible error of 0.2 mm. More studies will be carried on to assess the repositioning error on other organs.

In the next step we will evaluate the deformation induced to the surrounding organs with respect to the needle insertion speed. Our latest tests (not reported here) seem to show that the slower the needle during insertion, the higher the induced deformation. After this step, we will assess the accuracy of the entire computer assisted robotized process.

References

1. Ayadi, A., Nicolau, S., Bayle, B., Graebling, P., Gangloff, J.: Fully automatic needle calibration for robotic-assisted puncture on small animals. In: IEEE Workshop Life Science Systems and Applications Workshop, LISSA 2007, pp. 85–88 (2007)
2. Boctor, E.M., Taylor, R., Fichtinger, G., Choti, M.: Robotically assisted intraoperative ultrasound with application to ablative therapy of liver cancer. In: SPIE Annual Conference on Medical Imaging 2003, vol. 5029, pp. 281–291 (2003)
3. Espiau, B., Chaumette, F., Rives, P.: A new approach to visual servoing in robotics. IEEE Transactions on Robotics and Automation 8, 313–326 (1992)
4. Fiala, M.: Artag, a fiducial marker system using digital techniques. In: IEEE Computer Society Conference on Computer Vision and Pattern Recognition (CVPR 2005), pp. 590–596 (2005)
5. Fichtinger, G., DeWeese, T., Patriciu, A., Tanacs, A., Mazilu, D., Anderson, J., Masamune, K., Taylor, R., Stoianovici, D.: System for robotically assisted prostate biopsy and therapy with intraoperative CT guidance. Journal of Academic Radiology 9(1), 60–74 (2002)
6. Hutchinson, S., Hager, G.D., Corke, P.I.: A tutorial on visual servo control. Robotics and Automation 12(5), 651–670 (1996)

7. Kazanzides, P., Chang, J., Iordachita, I., Li, J., Ling, C., Fichtinger, G.: Design and validation of an image-guided robot for small animal research. In: Larsen, R., Nielsen, M., Sporring, J. (eds.) MICCAI 2006. LNCS, vol. 4190, pp. 50–57. Springer, Heidelberg (2006)

8. Lapreste, J.T., Jurie, F., Dhome, M., Chaumette, F.: An efficient method to compute the inverse jacobian matrix in visual servoing. In: ICRA, Avril, vol. 1, pp. 727–732 (2004)

9. Lavalle, S., Cinquin, P., Troccaz, J.: Computer Integrated Surgery and Therapy: State of the Art. ch. 10, Roux and J.L. Coatrieux edn., pp. 239–310. IS Press, Amsterdam (1997)

10. Li, J.C., Iordachita, I., Balogh, E., Fichtinger, G., Kazanzides, P.: Validation of an image-guided robot system for measurement, biopsy and injection in rodents. In: Proceedings of the IEEE 31st Annual Northeast Bioengineering Conference, pp. 131–133 (2005)

11. Nicolau, S., Garcia, A., Pennec, X., Soler, L., Ayache, N.: An augmented reality system to guide radio-frequency tumor ablation. In the Journal of Computer Animation and Virtual World 16(1), 1–10 (2005)

12. Nicolau, S., Goffin, L., Soler, L.: A low cost and accurate guidance system for laparoscopic surgery: Validation on an abdominal phantom. In: Proceedings of ACM Symposium on Virtual Reality Software and Technology (VRST 2005), Monterey, pp. 124–133 (2005)

13. Patriciu, A., Solomon, S., Kavoussi, L.R., Stoianovici, D.: Robotic kidney and spine percutaneous procedures using a new laser-based ct registration method. In: Niessen, W.J., Viergever, M.A. (eds.) MICCAI 2001. LNCS, vol. 2208, pp. 249–257. Springer, Heidelberg (2001)

14. Waspe, A., Cakiroglu, H., Lacefield, J., Fenster, A.: Design and validation of a robotic needle positioning system for small animal imaging applications. In: Engineering in Medicine and Biology Society, pp. 412–415 (2006)

15. Waspe, A., Cakiroglu, H., Lacefield, J., Fenster, A.: Design, calibration and evaluation of a robotic needle-positioning system for small animal imaging applications. Physics in Medicine and Biology 52, 1863–1878 (2007)

16. Zhang, Z.: Flexible camera calibration by viewing a plane from unknown orientations. In: Proceedings of the Nineth International Conference on Computer Vision (ICCV 1999), pp. 666–673 (1999)

Composite-Type Optical Fiberscope for Laser Surgery for Twin-to-Twin Transfusion Syndrome

Kiyoshi Oka[1], Akihiro Naganawa[2], Hiromasa Yamashita[3], Tetsuya Nakamura[4], and Toshio Chiba[3]

[1] Japan Atomic Energy Agency, Tokai-mura, Naka-gun, Ibaraki, Japan
oka.kiyoshi@jaea.go.jp
[2] Akita University, 1-1 Tegata Gakuen-machi, Akita-shi, Akita, Japan
naganawa@control.mech.akita-u.ac.jp
[3] National Center for Child Health and Development, Setagaya-ku, Tokyo, Japan
{yamashita-h, chiba-t}@ncchd.go.jp
[4] PENTAX Corporation, 1-9-30 Shirako, Wako-shi, Saitama, Japan
t.nakamura@aoc.pentax.co.jp

Abstract. We present our new laser device for prospective human fetoplacental surgery including that of twin-twin transfusion syndrome. We developed a composite-type optical fiberscope (2.2-mm in diameter) that enables transmission of 40-W Yb fiber laser light alongside of coaxial fetoscopic images. Using a laser condensing lens on the fiberscope tip, Yb fiber laser light can be focused 10-mm off. Using porcine liver tissue, despite changes in delivered laser energy, the diameter and depth of cauterized areas remained constant when the liver position agreed with the laser focal point, although the laser output altered the extent of tissue ablation. In conclusion, the performance of the fiberscope can be well controlled with accurate and efficient ablation of the target tissue. This Yb fiber laser fiberscope is expected to work much better if mounted on a miniature bending manipulator and if provided with additional functions (real-time distance and blood flow measurements).

Keywords: Fetoscopic surgery, Yb fiber laser ablation, Composite-type optical fiberscope.

1 Introduction

Prenatal treatment of fetoplacental abnormalities such as twin-twin transfusion syndrome (TTTS) and fetal myelomeningocele is still technically demanding and has limited postnatal outcome. Accordingly, substantial technological advancements are required to functionally enhance current endoscopic surgical devices. For this purpose, following issues must be settled: (1) collimation of the laser light is inadequate to precisely operate on the target because the scanning axis of fetoscope is different from that of optical fiber for laser irradiation, (2) sighting the laser focus on the target is occasionally difficult because the distance between the laser fiber tip and the target is unknown, (3) excessive tissue cauterization occasionally occurs because the laser

T. Dohi, I. Sakuma, and H. Liao (Eds.): MIAR 2008, LNCS 5128, pp. 251–259, 2008.

energy required for sufficient cauterization can not be estimated accurately before-hand, and (4) perpendicular access to the placental surface is occasionally difficult because the straight rigid fetoscope in current use cannot be mechanically bent.

In this regard, technological advancement has been achieved at the Japan Atomic Energy Agency (JAEA) for remote manipulation of the thermonuclear experimental reactor (ITER) [1]-[3]. Based on this technology, we developed the composite-type optical fiberscope which enables transmission of the laser energy alongside the endo-scopic images coaxially. In this article, we report a new endoscopic device, the com-posite-type optical fiberscope, which is flexible, small in diameter and capable of transmitting laser energy. The design and specifications are presented along with the outcome of feasibility study of tissue ablation performance.

2 Materials and Methods

We developed a flexible and ultra-fine endoscopic device equipped with a laser irra-diating function, a composite-type optical fiberscope (Fig. 1). To develop the device, following issues had to be resolved; (1) the device must be fine in diameter so as to be available for fetoscopic surgery, (2) the device can transmit laser beam with a narrow focal point, (3) the device must be equipped with a coupled function of transmitting both laser light and object images coaxially.

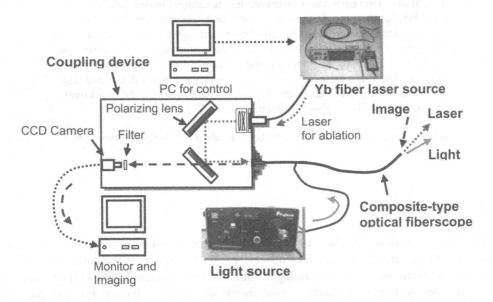

Fig. 1. System configuration of the composite-type optical fiberscope

2.1 Composite-Type Optical Fiberscope

Based on our experiences of welding / cutting by the Yb fiber laser light, the diame-ter of an optical fiber core needs to be around 0.7 mm in diameter to transmit high output (several kW) and collected laser light from a laser oscillator. In addition, the optical fibers for fetoscopic image transmission should have 2,000 - 20,000 pixels to ensure an acceptable resolution and field of vision. Furthermore, the optical fiber for laser transmission is designed as thin as 0.1 mm in diameter because the minimum laser output of around 40 W is required for fetoscopic surgery. A small collecting lens attached onto the tip of the optical fiberscope was designed for focusing laser beam and obtaining object images concurrently. The illuminating optical fibers were arranged to encircle the entire optical fibers for both laser and image transmissions. The whole outer diameter was designed for an intrauterine fetoscopic use.

Specifications of the composite-type optical fiberscope are shown in Table 1 and Fig. 2.

Table 1. Specifications of the composite-type optical fiberscope

Item	Specification
Core diameter for laser	About 100 μm
Cladding surface diameter for laser	About 120 μm
Core materials	A quartz glass
Cladding materials	A quartz glass
The number of the picture element	About 9,000
An angle of view	About 54 degrees
Materials of an object lens	A quartz glass
A total external diameter of a scope (a flexible part)	φ2.2 mm
Full length of a scope	3 m
Flexibility of a scope (a flexible part)	Smallest bending radius of 45 mm
Waterproofing	A tip is a waterproofing structure
Disinfection processing	EOG sterilization is capable

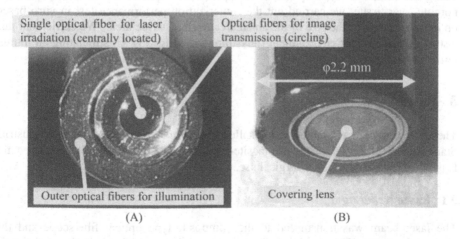

Single optical fiber for laser irradiation (centrally located)

Optical fibers for image transmission (circling)

φ2.2 mm

Outer optical fibers for illumination

Covering lens

(A)   (B)

Fig. 2. The tip of the composite-type optical fiberscope. (A) Front view, (B) Oblique view.

2.2 Laser Source

A laser source with an adequate condensing performance is required because the laser beam emitted by an oscillator could potentially spread over a given distance of its path and the laser light cannot be condensed into a smaller spot. In designing the composite-type optical fiberscope, it is required to condense the laser beam so as to make the spot diameter smaller than that of the optical fiber for laser transmission.

For this purpose, we selected a Yb fiber laser having a wavelength of 1,075 nm, not the conventional Nd:YAG laser oscillator with a wavelength of 1,064 nm. This selected fiber-laser can condense the laser beam into the diameter of a minimum of φ0.05 mm. In addition, with the use of this system, a power of 100V-20A can be provided with a laser output of 50W.

2.3 Coupling Device

A coupling device was developed in order to transmit the laser light to the composite-type optical fiberscope after collection of the emitted laser beam. This coupling device is composed of a beam splitter which can transmit a visible light of wavelength 400 - 780nm and reflect the fiber-laser of wavelength 1,075 nm. Fine adjustment mechanisms were installed in each optical system to secure an accurate link with its interface. The imaging system was integrated with a condenser system consisting of dielectric multi-layer coated mirror and an imaging lens. Each optical component has an anti-reflection (AR) coating. A CCD camera for imaging was 1/4 -inch digital color camera. The image signal is NTSC signal output with a BNC connector.

2.4 In Vitro Laser Ablation of Porcine Liver

Using the composite-type optical fiberscope (with a quartz lens at the tip) and the porcine liver tissue, we carried out the cauterization performance test in vitro based on measurements of the size of the ablated/cauterized tissue area. We carried out this test in the underwater environment (physiological saline, 37°C) simulating an intrauterine environment.

3 Results

These devices were assembled and installed in a 19 inches rack of Japanese Industrial Standards. A prototype of the composite-type optical fiberscope was developed for feasibility tests of fetoscopic surgical use.

3.1 Laser Irradiation

The laser beam was transmitted to the composite-type optical fiberscope and the phases of cauterization of colored chart paper are shown in Fig. 3. In this test, the tip of the scope was kept 10 mm above the chart paper in the atmospheric environment

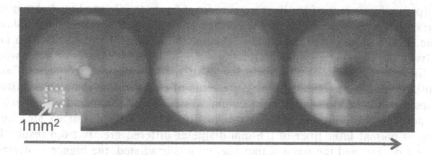

Fig. 3. Laser irradiation test using a color chart paper

and the laser beam (3 W at the tip) was irradiated for two seconds. Based on the test results, it was demonstrated that the device can well achieve both observation and cauterization of the chart paper concurrently.

3.2 Laser Transmission Efficiency (Table 2)

The efficiency of laser power transmission between the laser source (output; 10 - 90%) and the composite-type optical fiberscope was measured. A power sensor (LM-100HTD, COHERENT JAPAN Inc.) and an energy meter (Field Master-GS, COHERENT JAPAN Inc.) were used for measuring laser output. When the laser source output was set at 55 W (setting point of 90%) and the laser was transmitted to the composite-type optical fiberscope through the coupling device, the laser output was 46 W at the tip of the fiberscope (the transmission efficiency; 83.6%). When the output at the laser source was ranging between 10% and 90%, the transmission efficiency was 84.7% in average.

Table 2. Laser transmission efficiency of the composite-type optical fiberscope

Output from laser source		Output from the composite-type optical fiberscope tip	
Set-point (%)	Power (W)	Power (W)	Efficiency (%)
10	0.72	0.60	83.3
20	7.07	6.0	85.3
30	13.7	11.8	86.1
40	20.6	17.6	85.4
50	27.4	23.4	85.4
60	34.2	29.1	85.1
70	41.2	34.9	84.7
80	48.0	40.1	83.5
90	55.0	46.0	83.6

3.3 In Vitro Laser Ablation of Porcine Liver

During the in vitro laser ablation of porcine liver in 37°C normal saline, the laser power at the tip of the fiber ranged from 10W to 40W with the distance between the tip and the surface of the liver ranging from 5 mm to 20 mm. Fig. 4 shows the matrix of macroscopic views of (A) surface and (B) cross section of the ablated tissue. Fig. 5 shows the relationship between the distance between fiber tip and the liver and the size of ablated area by our new device. Worthy of note, when the distance was kept 10 mm (focal length of the new device's condensed laser beam), both diameter and depth measurements of cauterization remained constant irrespective of the changes in laser output which altered the extent of cauterization accordingly. In contrast as shown in Fig. 6, the size of ablated area by a previous normal laser fiber of 0.6-mm diameter differed greatly from results by the new device, and the more output energy was irradiated, the bigger cauterized sizes became accordingly. In addition, the cauterization performance substantially decreased with even a minimal change of the distance from 10mm. This probably happened because the laser beam is likely to spread when the distance does not agree with the focal length of the lens mounted on the fiber tip. Then, it is suggested that steady balanced cauterization can be accomplished with the use of our laser treatment system.

4 Discussion

We developed a 2.2-mm composite-type optical fiberscope with a core-fiber for Yb fiber laser irradiation encircled by around 9000 fibers for fetoscopic imaging. The laser irradiation can be focused by a quartz condensing lens 10-mm away from the fiber tip. Based on the results of feasibility tests, the new fiberscope worked well with high transfer efficiency of Yb fiber laser and an efficient laser ablation/cauterization of in vitro porcine liver tissue was accomplished especially when the distance between the fiber tip and the tissue surface was set at the focal length (10-mm) without causing inadvertent spread of coagulation. And the range of laser focus can be expected to cancel small positioning error without major clinical problem. Accordingly, the new fiberscope can cauterize the underwater porcine liver tissue in vitro with specified diameter and depth based on the predetermined planning.

During the use of our device, however, the distance between the fiberscope tip and the irradiated tissue becomes significant because it occasionally seems essential to prevent the fiberscope tip from an inadvertent contact to the targeted tissues. Our fiberscope is capable of detecting reflected light with different wavelength through the same optic fiber. Then, we might be able to measure the distance between fiberscope tip and the targeted tissue surface in real time securing safety issue associated with an inadequate positioning of the fiberscope. Furthermore in ablation of blood vessels, we should catch in real time whether the targeted vessel is definitely occluded or not. To resolve this issue, it might be useful to apply Doppler blood flow measurement through the same laser fibers in our fiberscope (composite-type). Moreover, to manipulate the direction of laser beam within a narrow restricted space (e.g. in utero) freely and accurately, the fiberscope might have to be mounted on a kind of miniature bending robotic manipulators [4][5].

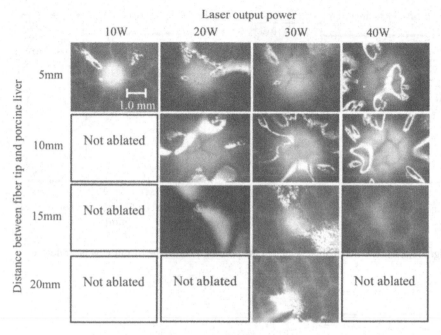

(A) Appearance of ablated porcine liver tissues

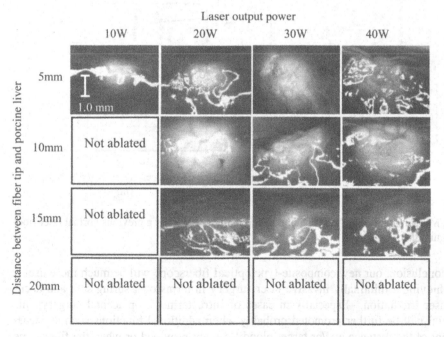

(B) Cross section of ablated porcine liver tissues

Fig. 4. Results of laser ablation to the porcine liver tissue by our new device

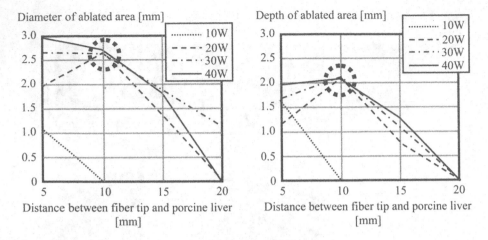

Fig. 5. Measurements of ablated area in the porcine liver tissue by our new laser device

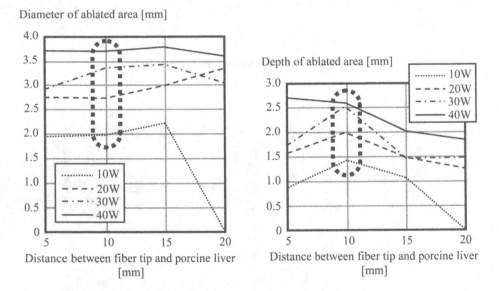

Fig. 6. Measurements of ablated area in the porcine liver tissue by a previous normal laser fiber of 0.6-mm diameter

In conclusion, our new composite-type optical fiberscope will be much more useful for achieving a minimally invasive laser surgery in terms of assuring safe and accurate laser irradiation. Especially in cases of intrauterine fetoplacental surgery, this potential will be further promoted probably when additional functions such as measurement of the distance and/or target blood flow are provided or when the fiberscope is mounted on a miniature bending manipulator.

Acknowledgments. This study was carried out as a part of physicofunctional device development research enterprise of the Ministry of Health, Labour and Welfare.

References

1. Shibanuma, K., Honda, T.: ITER R&D: Remote handling systems: Blanket remote handling systems. Fusion Engineering and Design 55(2-3), 249–257 (2001)
2. Oka, K.: A new optical fiber system with hybrid functions of power delivery and real-time remote observation for YAG laser welding. The Review of Laser Engineering 31(9), 612–617 (2003)
3. Oka, K., Itou, A., Takiguchi, Y.: Development of bore tools for pipe welding and cutting. Journal of Robotics and Mechatronics 10(2), 104–109 (1999)
4. Harada, K., Nakamura, T., Chiba, T., Fujie, M.: Bending Laser Manipulator for Intrauterine Surgery. In: The first IEEE / RAS-EMBS International Conference on Biomedical Robotics and Biomechatronics, pp. 238–242 (2006)
5. Yamashita, H., Matsumiya, K., Masamune, K., Liao, H., Chiba, T., Dohi, T.: Miniature bending manipulator for fetoscopic intrauterine laser therapy in twin-to-twin transfusion syndrome. Surgical Endoscopy 22(2), 430–435 (2007)

Surgical Manipulator with Balloon for Stabilizing Fetus in Utero under Ultrasound Guidance

Noriaki Yamanaka[1], Hiromasa Yamashita[1], Kiyoshi Matsumiya[1], Hongen Liao[2,3],
Ken Masamune[1], Toshio Chiba[4], and Takeyoshi Dohi[1]

[1] Graduate School of Information Science and Technology, The University of Tokyo, Japan
[2] Graduate School of Engineering, The University of Tokyo, Japan
[3] Translational Systems Biology and Medicine Initiative, The University of Tokyo, Japan
[4] Department of Strategic Medicine, National Center for Child Health and Development, Japan

Abstract. This paper describes a surgical manipulator to stabilize intrauterine
fetus with ultrasound image guidance. The manipulator includes an outline of 4
mm in diameter, a mechanism with 7 joints, and a set of balloons. The manipulator is arranged as straight form and the balloon is fold to be a minimum size
before the insertion. Accuracy evaluation of bending performance showed that
the standard deviations were ±3.6 degrees on wired-driven mechanism and ±1.6
degrees on linkage-driven mechanism. Experimental results also demonstrated
high repeatability of the mechanisms. In feasibility experiments, ultrasound images in 2D and 3D modes were examined for guiding the manipulator. The 2D
images provided wide view and easily viewable display of the balloon inflation.
The 3D images provided easily viewable display of bending motion of the arm
and the relative position of a phantom. It is possible to operate the manipulator
in utero under the ultrasound guidance in 2D and 3D by switching them in each
procedural stage.

Keywords: Stabilizer, Intrauterine fetal surgery, Myelomeningocele, Balloon,
Ultrasound guidance.

1   Introduction

Myelomeningocele (MMC) is one of the most common in spina bifida, which is a
devastating congenital defect of the central neural system. The patient suffers from
orthopedic disabilities, bowel and bladder dysfunctions and mental retardation after
birth. This disease occurs 1 case per 2000 births [1].

The process is not completely performed and the tube is left opened when neural
cord is constructed in early gestation suffered MMC. Additionally vertebral arches
and skin on it are also not closed. Although these primary defects occur, the neural
tissue itself is normal in early gestation. Since the spinal cord is exposed in uterus, the
spinal cord in whole period of gestation suffered secondary injuries such as direct
trauma, hydrodynamic pressure and chemical stimulus by the amniotic fluid. Furthermore, leak of cerebrospinal fluid through the opened spinal cord may cause Ar-
nold-Chiari malformation (hindbrain hernia) leading to hydrocephalus.

T. Dohi, I. Sakuma, and H. Liao (Eds.): MIAR 2008, LNCS 5128, pp. 260–269, 2008.
© Springer-Verlag Berlin Heidelberg 2008

The treatment for MMC after birth aims to prevent spinal tissues from infections by neurosurgical approach, but it's not an effective method. To prevent dysfunctions, the treatment should be performed before the destruction of the spinal tissue since the functions become irreversible after the birth. Surgical treatments like covering, suture and patch the spinal cord in fetal surgery, could prevent it from secondary damages and maintain the neural functions [2]. The damage on the spinal cord will be small when the earlier repair is performed. However, the treatment before 18 weeks gestation is technically difficult because the skin of the fetus is fragile like gelatin. Most of the treatments on the fetus are performed at 19-25 weeks gestation [1].

Conventionally, fetal treatment for MMC is open surgery. Endoscopic approach is preferable [3,4] because of minimally invasive to the mother and the fetus, which can decrease the risk of complications like prematurely delivery [5,6]. However, endoscopic surgery requires more skill of surgical treatment. Furthermore, it is difficult to perform a precision treatment to the floating fetus in amniotic fluid. To solve these issues, a device is required to stabilize the fetus in endoscopic intrauterine surgery [7].

Previous study included development of a suction type stabilizer with silicone tube in small diameter [8]. However, the area of the fetal skin sucked by negative pressure may be congested with blood. We developed a manipulator with flexible balloon-based stabilizer [9]. The inflated balloon was used to stabilize the fetus with large area contacted to the fetus after insertion into the uterus. However, the umbilical cord might be pressed when the fetus is supported beneath since the balloon was inflated into a circular shape. Furthermore, we developed a prototype manipulator with multiple joints and a covering balloon to support the fetal chest and abdominal sides without pressing the umbilical cord [10]. We report a miniaturized manipulator and ultrasound guidance for it in this study.

2 Methods and Materials

A balloon-type manipulator system is developed to stabilize the fetus around chest and abdominal sides ventrally and keep the fetus from translation movement and rotation. We developed a miniaturized manipulator to support fetus in utero. It has a balloon to make large area touched to the fetus, contrary to small diameter for small incision. And it has bending mechanisms to hold the fetus.

2.1 Procedure to Support Fetus

In fetus stabilizing, it is preferable to support the trunk of the body without charging any load to limb and joints of the fetus because the fetus is still fragile at the target period. If the devices press the umbilical cord, it may disturb blood flow. We hold the fetus especially from abdominal sides to chest ventrally with large space around umbilicus. Small incision should be made especially for intrauterine fetal surgery to reduce the risk of premature delivery.

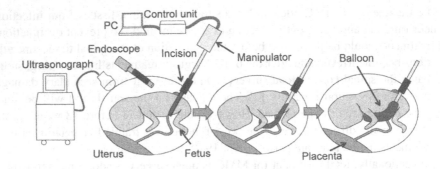

Fig. 1. Procedure of stabilizing fetus. Left: inserting manipulator into uterus. Center: bending manipulator under fetus with balloon being inflated. Right: holding fetus.

The procedure of the manipulator is as below (Fig.1). To ensure the surgical space of intrauterine treatment, the uterus can be inflated with saline or Ringer's solution. The manipulator is arranged as straight form and the balloon is fold to be in minimum size before the insertion. The manipulator is inserted through a trocar fixed on a small incision in the back side of the fetus. The arm of the manipulator is bent to fit the fetal body and the balloon is inflated with saline under a guidance of ultrasound and endoscope.

2.2 Manipulator

The diameter of the developed manipulator is 4mm. It has 3 bending mechanisms to hold fetus (Fig.2). Hook-like mechanism is used for making a balloon on the arm fit fetal body and supporting around chest. It consists of 4 joints and bends 180 degrees in both left and right directions, driven by 2 wire ropes tied to a pulley. It bends from tip-side joint when inserted into uterus to reduce the risk of contact to placenta by making the path of the arm's bending small. Linkage mechanism is for adjusting posture of the arm corresponding to insertion angle and incision placement which is far away from placenta. It consists of 2 joints and bends 90 degrees. Finger-like mechanism is for holding fetal abdominal sides between the tip frame and frames of linkage mechanism. It is bent 45 degrees by a wire and straightened by a super elastic wire. A pulley for wires driving hook-like mechanism, and the rod of linkage mechanism are powered by motors on driving unit which is controlled by PC (Fig.3). The commands are given from a user interface or a dialog on PC.

A balloon is made from plastic sheet which is 0.03 mm in thickness to make incision minimum. It covers the arm and it is sealed up with a heat shrinkable tube. Nodes of the balloon expand in all direction around the frames of the arm and keeps fetus from contact with the frames. The balloon is inflated with saline so that ultrasound passes through it to get information under the manipulator. However, mixture of air is accepted if it is as little as not to prevent imaging.

The manipulator can be easily handled since it is as light as within 350 g. The driven unit meets autoclave sterilization, the driving unit meets EOG sterilization, and the balloon is disposable.

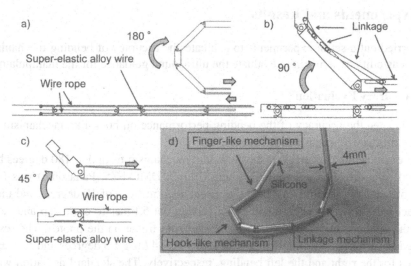

Fig. 2. Bending mechanisms of manipulator. a) hook-like mechanism which bends from tip-side joint by difference of the strength of a super-elastic alloy wire. b) linkage mechanism. c) finger-like mechanism. d) configuration of bent arm of manipulator.

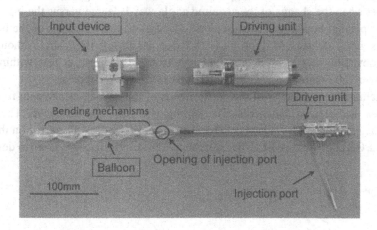

Fig. 3. Units of manipulator. Driven unit is connected to driving unit and bending mechanisms driven by motors on driving unit which are controlled by PC. Signals for driving are given from an input device. Balloon is inflated with saline through an injection port.

2.3 System Configuration

In intrauterine fetal surgery, surgeons handle devices like forceps to treat an affected area, a manipulator to stabilize a fetus, endoscope and ultrasound to guide the treatment. Endoscope has a main role to acquire the detail on the affected area. Ultrasound has a main role to acquire the whole intrauterine condition, including the manipulator and relative position and state of a balloon on it.

3 Experiments and Results

We carried out a set of experiments to evaluate the accuracy of bending mechanisms and a feasibility experiment to evaluate the ultrasound guidance for the manipulator.

3.1 Accuracy Evaluation

We evaluated the accuracy of the bending performance on hook-like mechanism and linkage mechanism controlled by motors.

We examined the accuracy of the hook-like mechanism from 0 to 180 degrees both left and right directions. A digital camera (Lumix DMC-FZ5, Panasonic) was fixed about 50 cm from the arm. We bent the mechanism in steps of 10 degrees and measure each pose from the taken photos. We carried out 5 times to each step and calculated the bending angle between tip frame and root frame on the photos. The results showed the error at target angle of 180 degrees were 47.6 ± 1.3 degrees and 50.0 ± 0.8 degrees for the right and the left bending, respectively. The standard deviation was ± 3.6 degrees maximum around 0 degrees (Fig.4-a).

We extended the acquired bending angle to about 180 degrees and evaluate the repeatability of the mechanism on required range of bending angle. The maximum angle was set when the change of the acquired angle was 1 degree versus the input of 10 degrees to prevent breaking of wire. The results showed that the range of the bending angle was 177.1 degrees in right and 178.2 degrees in left (Fig.4-b). Although the standard deviation was ± 3.6 degrees at most around 0 degrees, it was within ± 2.0 degrees over 150 degrees and within ± 1.0 degrees over 170 degrees.

We examined the accuracy of the performance of the linkage mechanism from 0 to 90 degrees in a step of 5 degrees. The setting was the same as above. The result showed the error on 90 degrees was 2.5 ± 0.1 degrees (Fig.4-c). The error on the path was 17.4 ± 0.2 degrees at most. The maximum standard deviation was ± 1.6 degrees.

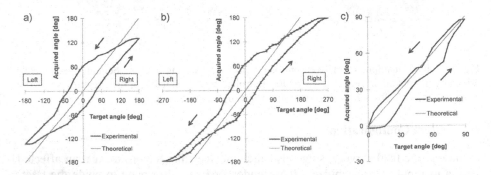

Fig. 4. Result of bending performance. (N=5) a) bending performance of hook-like mechanism. b) bending performance of hook-like mechanism when acquired angle was set about 180 degrees. c) bending performance of linkage mechanism.

3.2 Feasibility Experiment of Ultrasound Guidance

We examined the feasibility of ultrasound for the manipulator guidance under water that is similar to amniotic fluid. We used an ultrasonic imaging (ProSound α10, ALOKA) and a probe (1010) for both 2D and 3D imaging. The imaging mode was OBST on which parameters are adjusted for obstetrics, and frequency of ultrasound was 5 MHz. The arm of the manipulator was located about 150 mm under water surface and the distance between the arm and a probe was about 100 mm. We observed the arm and it's bending performance. Furthermore, we put a phantom in the water and took images of the arm holding it.

(A)Ultrasound image of manipulator

First, we took ultrasound images of the arm (Fig.5-a). The whole arm in straight form was observed on 2D ultrasound image easily at gain 60-70 dB. On the other hand, the arm was clearly shown on 3D ultrasound images at the gain 30 dB. We moved the probe and changed imaging area to recognize the shape of the arm on 3D ultrasound image since the image was narrow. The performance of linkage mechanism was realized on 2D ultrasound image. However, the performance of hook-like mechanism and the configuration of the bent arm were not easily recognized on the image. On the other hand, the performance and the configuration of the arm were easily recognized on 3D ultrasound image (Fig.6-a,b). We observed the hook-like mechanism's bending from tip side joint by handling the probe to follow up the tip of the arm.

Second, we took ultrasound images of the status of balloon's inflating and deflating. Nodes of the balloon inflated from the near side of the opening of the water injection port (Fig.5-b). On 2D ultrasound image, the status of the balloon was easily recognized at the gain 60 dB. The water flow was represented by bubbles in it. The space between the surface of the balloon and the frames of the arm got large and the swelling node went ahead (Fig.6-c). By following up the swelling point, we confirmed that the all nodes were inflated. On 3D ultrasound image, it was difficult to observe the detail of the balloon because it showed only the surface of the balloon and change of the balloon was subtle in a few second. However, finally the appearance of the inflated balloon was bigger than deflated nodes. After that, the inflated balloon was reversely deflated. Although bubbles and water flow were not shown, we observed that the balloon got smaller from the opening of the injection port on 2D ultrasound images. And the balloon got small on 3D ultrasound images.

(B)Ultrasound image of manipulator holding fetal phantom model

We evaluated the feasibility of ultrasound guidance for holding fetus by the arm of the manipulator with the balloon inflated (Fig.7).

A phantom was made of agar so that ultrasound passed through to get information under the phantom. In real case, ultrasound passes through fetus and surgeons acquire the view of inside of the body and condition under the fetus. Mixture ratio of agar was 1.5 % of water. It was visible at the gain about 70 dB on 2D ultrasound image and 60 dB on 3D ultrasound image.

On 2D ultrasound image, the phantom and the arm with inflated balloon under the phantom were both depicted. Although the arm holding the phantom was represented, its configuration and relative position were not easily recognized. On 3D ultrasound image, the model was not represented because the reflective ultrasound was too weak when the configuration of the arm was shown at the gain 30 dB. After turning up the gain to about 55dB, the model was appeared with some noise and we recognized the arm holding it (Fig.8). When the gain was higher than that, the image was too noisy to recognize them.

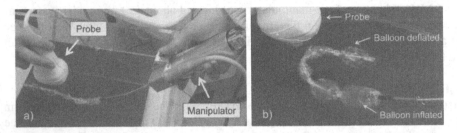

Fig. 5. View of ultrasound imaging arm and balloon on it. a) arm with deflated balloon. b) balloon being inflated with water. A node of the balloon near the opening of the injection port expands first and the next one follows it.

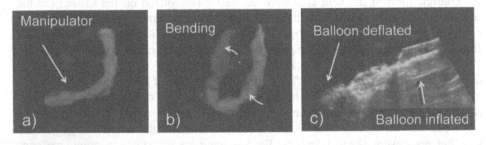

Fig. 6. Ultrasound images of manipulator in insertion procedure. a) performance of hook-like mechanism on 3D ultrasound image. b) the configuration of arm are clearly depicted on 3D ultrasound image. c) balloon being inflated on 2D ultrasound image. The surface of the balloon and frames of arm is shown and space between them enlarges.

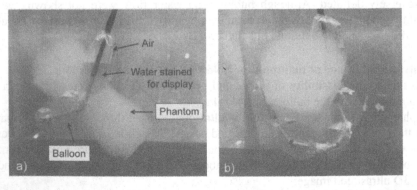

Fig. 7. Manipulator holding a fetal model made of agar. Balloon on the arm is inflated with water and keeps the model from contact to the frame of the arm. Water is stained blue for display. a) long axis of fetal model. b) short axis of fetal model.

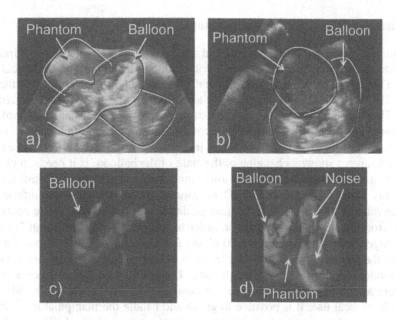

Fig. 8. Ultrasound images of manipulator holding fetal model. a) long axis of fetal model on 2D ultrasound image. b) short axis of fetal model on 2D ultrasound image. c) only balloon is shown at low gain on 3D ultrasound image. d) fetal model held by balloon appears at high gain on 3D ultrasound image.

4 Discussion

4.1 Accuracy of Bending Performance

We carried out the accuracy evaluation of bending performance of hook-like mechanism and linkage mechanism. On hook-like mechanism, the error was large since the wire ropes are loose around 0 degrees for balance of the wire tension with the strength of the super elastic wire. The rate of changing angle follows theoretical one at middle area. And the rate gets smaller because the wire tension became large with bending and the wire ropes elongated. The standard deviation was as small as about ±1.0 degrees around large bending area for holding fetus. The range from 177.1 degrees in right to 178.2 degrees in left is acceptable because a balloon on the arm adjust the space between the tip frame and the root frame in some degree and can fit the fetal abdominal sides. On linkage mechanism, the main cause of the error is the looseness on the joints. The pins on joints slant because the pins are cantilever type. The cause also applies to the cone cave area around 50 degrees in straightening path. The standard deviation was small as ±1.6 degrees for adjusting the pose of the arm. The repeatability of both mechanisms was sufficiently high to operate under ultrasound guidance. The issues on operation can be solved by calibration.

4.2 Ultrasound Guidance for Manipulator

We evaluated the feasibility of ultrasound guidance for the manipulator. First, the arm of the manipulator is inserted into uterus with a deflated balloon in clinical procedure. The results showed that both 2D and 3D ultrasound images indicated the arm clearly. 2D ultrasound image was superior to show whole sight of the arm in straight shape. 3D ultrasound image was superior to represent the performance of hook-like mechanism and the configuration of the arm. 3D image will be often used when the balloon is deflated. Second, the balloon is inflated when the arm is bent. 2D and 3D ultrasound images showed changing of the state of the balloon. If it needs to observe the detail of the inflating balloon, 2D ultrasound image is preferable. Third, the arm holds fetus with inflated balloon. 2D ultrasound image gave a little information about the relative position. 3D ultrasound guidance will be necessary. We controlled the gain from 30 dB to about 55 dB in order to represent the phantom on 3D ultrasound image. The gain is usually set 50-60 dB for real fetus on 3D ultrasound image. Although the phantom has a little smaller ratio of reflection than real fetus, it played a good model for ultrasound to pass through. Images may be clearer in case of real fetus. And as the experiment, the relative position will be recognized by adjusting the gain in clinical use. It is possible to guide and handle the manipulator in clinical use by ultrasound images with switching the imaging procedure of 2D and 3D and adjusting the gain.

5 Conclusion

We have developed a prototype of manipulator with a balloon to stabilize fetus in intrauterine surgery. The arm of the manipulator is 4 mm in diameter and the balloon covers the arm. The arm has bending mechanisms, hook-like mechanism, linkage mechanism and finger-like mechanism, to hold the fetal chest and abdominal sides.

We evaluated accuracy of the mechanical performances and feasibility of ultrasound guidance. The result of bending performance showed that the standard deviation of hook-like mechanism and linkage mechanism were ±3.6 degrees and ±1.6 degrees, respectively. The repeatability is sufficiently high to operate the manipulator under image guidance. Both 2D and 3D ultrasound imaging gave clear appearance of the arm and balloon. The performance and the configuration of the arm were clearly shown on 3D ultrasound image. And we succeeded to control the configuration of the arm under the images. The status of the balloon's being inflated and deflated was well represented on 2D ultrasound images. The relative position between an agar phantom and the arm was shown on 3D ultrasound images. These results showed that it is possible to operate the manipulator in utero under an ultrasound guidance in 2D and 3D by switching them in each procedural stage.

Acknowledgements. This work was supported in part by the the Grant-in-Aid for Scientific Research (17100008, 20650077) of the Ministry of Education, Culture, Sports, Science and Technology (MEXT) in Japan, and Special Coordination Funds for Promoting Science and Technology in Japan.

References

1. Walsh, D.S., Adzick, N.S., Sutton, L.N., Johnson, M.P.: The Rationale for in utero Repair of Myelomeningocele. Fetal. Diagn. Ther. 16, 312–322 (2001)
2. Farmer, D.L., Koch, C.S., Peacock, W.J., Danielpour, M., Gupta, N., Lee, H., Harrison, M.R.: In Utero Repair of Myelomeningocele. Arch. Surg. 138, 872–878 (2003)
3. Bruner, J.P., Richards, W.O., Tulipan, N.B., Arney, T.L.: Endoscopic coverage of fetal myelomeningocele in utero. Am. J. Obstet. Gynccol. 180, 153–158 (1999)
4. Kohl, T., Hering, R., Heep, A., Schaller, C., Meyer, B., Greive, C., et al.: Percutaneous Fetoscopic Patch Coverage of Spina Bifida Aperta in the Human - Early Clinical Experience and Potential. Fetal Diagn Ther. 21, 185–193 (2006)
5. Hamada, A.H., Walsh, W., Heddings, A., Bruner, J.P., Tulipan, N.: Intrauterine myelomeningocele Repair: effect on Short-Term Complications of Prematurity. Fetal Diagn Ther. 19, 83–86 (2004)
6. Barini, R., Weber, M., Barreto, G., Cursino, K., Zambelli, H., Parando, A., Sbragia, L.: Abruptio Placentae during Fetal Myelomeningocele Repair. Fetal Diagn Ther. 2, 115–117 (2006)
7. Oberg, K.C., Robles, A.E., Ducsay, C.A., Rasi, C.R., Rouse, G.A., Childers, B.J., Evans, M.L., Kirsch, W.M., Hardesty, R.A.: Endoscopic intrauterine surgery in primates. Surg. Endosc. 13, 420–426 (1999)
8. Tsubouchi, K., Harada, K., Chiba, T., Enosawa, S., Fujie, M.G.: Development of the drawn-in type stabilizer for a fetus operation. In: The 14th conference of Japan computer-aided-surgery society, pp. 45–46 (2005)
9. Liao, H., Suzuki, H., Matsumiya, K., Masamune, K., Dohi, T., Chiba, T.: Fetus Support Manipulator with Flexible Balloon-Based Stabilizer for Endoscopic Intrauterine Surgery. In: Larsen, R., Nielsen, M., Sporring, J. (eds.) MICCAI 2006. LNCS, vol. 4190, pp. 412–419. Springer, Heidelberg (2006)
10. Yamanaka, N., Yamashita, H., Matsumiya, K., Liao, H., Masamune, K., Chiba, T., Dohi, T.: Balloon-Based Manipulator with Multiple Linkages for Intrauterine Surgery. In: Proceedings of the 2007 IEEE/RSJ International Conference on Intelligent Robots and Systems, pp. 1278–1283 (2007)

Investigation of Partial Directed Coherence for Hand-Eye Coordination in Laparoscopic Training

Julian J.H. Leong, Louis Atallah, George P. Mylonas, Daniel R. Leff,
Roger J. Emery, Ara W. Darzi, and Guang-Zhong Yang

Royal Society/Wolfson Medical Image Computing Laboratory & Department of Biosurgery
and Surgical Technology, Imperial College London, London, United Kingdom
{j.leong,l.atallah,george.mylonas,d.leff,
r.emery,a.darzi,g.z.yang}@imperial.ac.uk

Abstract. Effective hand-eye coordination is an important aspect of training in laparoscopic surgery. This paper investigates the interdependency of the hand and eye movement along with the variability of their temporal relationships based on Granger-causality. Partial directed coherence is used to reveal the subtle effects of improvement in hand-eye coordination, where the causal relationship between instrument and eye movement gradually reverse during simple laparoscopic tasks. For assessing the practical value of the proposed technique for minimally invasive surgery, two laparoscopic experiments have been conducted to examine the ability of the trainees in handling mental rotation tasks, as well as dissection and manipulation skills in laparoscopic surgery. Detailed experimental results highlight the value of the technique in investigating hand-eye coordination in laparoscopic training, particularly during early motor learning for complex bimanual procedures.

1 Introduction

Hand-eye coordination is a complex combinatory problem, involving many sensorimotor coupling including the visual, proprioceptive, tactile, attention, and motor systems. However, the study of hand-eye coordination can be simplified to a model describing the use of the visual system to guide/validate the movements of the hand. This fundamental fact implies a black box approach in the understanding of the function of the whole system [1].

In laparoscopic surgery, two dimensional images are projected on a screen away from the actual operating site, this is coupled with the 'fulcrum' effect intrinsic to the arrangement of the instruments. This disturbance of the visuo-motor axis require prior mental spatial transformation to coordinate the actions of the hands with the images perceived by the eyes, which can explain the steeper learning curve of laparoscopic surgery. The assessment of the intrinsic hand-eye coordination ability could help monitor progression of laparoscopic skills level.

Predictive, rather than reactive, eye movements have been implicated in the feedforward paradigm of visual assistance in well rehearsed movement generation. In learning a new visuospatial task, the spatiotemporal relationship of the eye and

T. Dohi, I. Sakuma, and H. Liao (Eds.): MIAR 2008, LNCS 5128, pp. 270–278, 2008.

effector has been used to provide a framework to divide learning into distinct phases; where vision is first used as a feed-back mechanism until the new coordinate transformation becomes automated [2]. Multiple studies have confirmed that the prediction of the sensory consequences of actions defines early stages of motor learning [3].

Thus far, several techniques have been investigated to describe the interdependency between multivariate series. For example, Graphical interaction models describe the interrelationships among the components of a time series as undirected graphs, where vertices depict the components and edges indicate possible dependencies between the components [4]. Parametric models have also been used to illustrate the dependence structure of a process as a model selection problem [5]. In the frequency domain, cross spectrum analysis and coherence have been used to describe the interdependency between two time series.

However, when causality between time series is of relevance, or when more than two multivariate time series are being observed, the distinction of indirect and direct relationships between them becomes important. While ordinary coherence measures the linear dependence between two signals, directed coherence [6],[7],[8] focuses on the feed-forward and feed-back aspects of relationships between signals.

Causality in general has three essential criteria. First, the cause must precede the effect in time; second, the two variables must be associated; third, the correlation cannot be explained by a third variable. It was also defined that if the prior knowledge of a series predicts another, the former Granger-causes the latter. The purpose of this paper is to evaluate the hypothesis of interdependency of the hand eye movement along with the variability of their temporal relationships. Partial Directed Coherence (PDC) is used as a frequency domain description of Granger-causality for measuring the predictability of hand and eye motions.

2 Measuring Partial Directed Coherence

2.1 Partial Directed Coherence

PDC was introduced for the inference of Granger-causality in the frequency domain [6],[7],[8]. Granger-causality by definition states that an observed time series $x_c(n)$ Granger-causes another series $x_i(n)$ if the knowledge of $x_c(n)$'s past significantly improves the prediction of $x_i(n)$. This type of predictability is not reciprocal. Assessing Granger-causality provides a measure of the strength of interaction between time series, under the rational that predictable variations in a series take place if their mechanisms of generation are intrinsically linked. In a linear framework, Granger-causality is related to multivariate autoregressive models (MVAR).

If $(x_1(t),....x_n(t))'$ is a stationary n-dimensional time series with mean zero, a vector autoregressive model of order p VAR[p] can be abbreviated by:

$$\begin{pmatrix} x_1(t) \\ \vdots \\ x_n(t) \end{pmatrix} = \sum_{r=1}^{p} a_r \begin{pmatrix} x_1(t-r) \\ \vdots \\ x_n(t-r) \end{pmatrix} + \begin{pmatrix} \varepsilon_1(t) \\ \vdots \\ \varepsilon_n(t) \end{pmatrix} \tag{1}$$

The vector $(\varepsilon_1,...,\varepsilon_n)'$ denotes independent Gaussian white noise, and $\mathbf{a}_r$ is the coefficient matrix of the VAR. To guarantee stationarity of the model, the assumption was made that $\det(I - \mathbf{a}(1)z - \cdots - \mathbf{a}(p)z^p) \neq 0$, for all $z \in C$ such that $|z| \leq 1$. In the Eq. (1), the coefficients $a_{ic}(r)$ describe how the present values of x_i depend linearly on the past values of the components x_c. Thus, if all entries $a_{ic}(r)$ are zero for $r = 1....p$, then x_c does not Granger-cause x_i.

In this paper, p_{opt}, the optimal order of an Autoregressive (AR) model was chosen as the optimizer of Schwarz's Bayesian Criterion, this was investigated by Lütkepohl who found that this selection criterion leads, on average, to the smallest mean squared prediction error of the fitted model. Baccala and Sameshima [6] introduced the concept of PDC, where the difference between the n-dimensional identity matrix and the Fourier transform of the coefficient series is:

$$\mathbf{A}(w) = \mathbf{I} - \sum_{r=1}^{p} \mathbf{a}(r)e^{-iwr} \tag{2}$$

and the PDC is defined as [8]:

$$\pi_{i \leftarrow c}(w) = \frac{|\mathbf{A}_{ic}(w)|}{\sqrt{\sum_k |\mathbf{A}_{kc}(w)|^2}} \tag{3}$$

PDC takes a value between 0 and 1 due to the normalization in Eq. (3). This provides a measure of the influence of previous samples of x_c on the present samples of x_i with the effect of x_c on other variables. Thus, it can measure the strengths of interactions between two signals in a directed manner. ARfit was used in this study for the estimation of the parameters of the AR model [9].

2.2 Experiment Setup

For assessing basic hand-eye coordination involved in minimally invasive surgery, two laparoscopic experiments were conducted. The first experiment involved a task of locating two standardized points on a simulated plastic small bowel model using laparoscopic instruments, each point was attached to a circuit switch to mark the beginning and end of the trajectories. The subjects were asked to touch alternatively the two points with the left instrument 10 times, and then the right instrument (Task 1.1). View rotation tasks were introduced in order to increase the complexity of hand-eye coordination, as the ability to handle mental rotation tasks has been suggested to be indicative of the innate capacity in mastering laparoscopy [10]. The subjects were required to repeat the task with the laparoscopic camera rotated 90 degrees counter clockwise for three training sessions (Tasks 1.2-1.4), and clockwise for three further sessions (Tasks 1.5-1.7). Finally, a post training assessment (Task 1.8) using normal camera orientation was completed. Data from nine complete novices was used for this experiment.

For the second experiment, eight complete novices were recruited to perform a more complex laparoscopic procedure. A cadaveric avian model was used to simulate dissection and manipulation skills in laparoscopic surgery. The procedure was broken down into tasks: (2.1) dissecting the subcutaneous connective tissue over the pectoralis muscle, (2.2) dissecting the muscle to reveal a simulated tumor tissue, (2.3) removal of the simulated tissue, (2.4) repositioning the dissected skin layers, and (2.5) returning the instruments to the start position. Each subject completed the procedure ten times in 3 separate sessions. Fig. 1 illustrates the experimental setup and screenshots of the key tasks.

For both experiments, instrument tip positions were obtained by bespoke designed Infrared (IR) tracking devices that were attached rigidly to the handles of the laparoscopic instruments. They were tracked by the Polaris (Experiment 1) and Optotrak Certus (Experiment 2) systems (Northern Digital Inc, Ontario, Canada). The offsets of the instrument tips from the IR markers were calculated using the Pivot function of the NDI software. Data interfacing was achieved through RS-232 and the provided tracking accuracy was 0.35 mm RMS at a sampling rate of 60Hz for Polaris, and 0.15 mm RMS at a sampling rate of 50Hz for Optotrak Certus. A Tobii 1750 eye tracker (Tobii Technology, Stockholm, Sweden) was used to display the laparoscopic scene. It is a remote eye tracking device using the standard binocular video-oculography technique integrated with a 17 inch TFT display, with a sampling rate of 50Hz and an accuracy of 0.5 degrees. It can tolerate moderate head movement thus providing a relatively natural environment for laparoscopic tasks [11],[12].

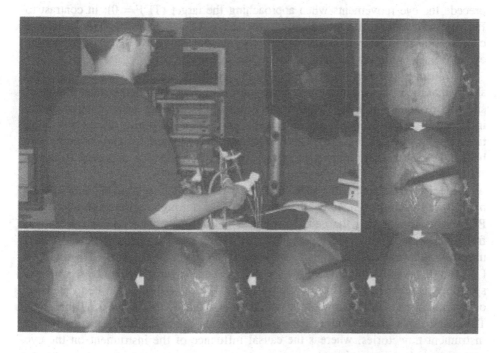

Fig. 1. Experiment setup with screen shots showing the key manipulation steps involved in the laparoscopic workflow of Experiment 2

In order to calculate the two dimensional screen projection of the instrument tips for Experiment 1, the laparoscopic camera with endoscope was calibrated using the camera calibration toolbox. The extrinsic and intrinsic parameters were then obtained after the camera setup was rigidly fixed. The three dimensional instrument tip data was then projected onto two dimensional data corresponding to its position on the laparoscopic monitor screen. For the analysis described above, the Target Distance Function (TDF) was used, where the instrument and eye positions were expressed as the normalized Euclidean distance from the target, this reduces the 2D position data into 1D distance data. For Experiment 2, key steps of the workflow were marked manually. The time to complete each trial was compared across the trials by using repeated Friedman Test for non-parametric related samples. When the trials are no longer significantly different from each other, a performance improvement plateau is reached. The significance level of $p < 0.05$ was used throughout the study

3 Results

3.1 Target Distance Function and PDC

In Fig. 2(a), the TDF of the first camera rotation task (1.2) is illustrated. This is the most difficult task in terms of coordination, as the dissociation of the eye-hand axis was introduced the first time to the subject. The instrument movement was shown to precede the eye movements when approaching the target (TDF = 0); in contrast to Fig. 2(c), illustrating the post training task (1.8), the subject's improved hand-eye coordination after the training was reflected by the predictive eye behavior, where the eye movement approaches the target before the instrument tip.

To illustrate the performance of PDC in detecting causal influences, Fig. 2(b) shows that the influence of the instrument on eye movement is larger than the opposite (off diagonal) in Task 1.2. However, higher PDC values when comparing the influence of eye movements on instrument were observed during the post-training task (1.8) as shown in Fig. 2(d). This corresponds to the hypothesis that predictive eye behavior develops after training in laparoscopic skills, reflecting improved hand-eye coordination.

Table 1(a) summarizes the PDC analysis for all the subjects of the first experiment. In an attempt to quantify the change in PDC throughout the experiment, the PDC values examining the causal influence of the instrument on the eye for all frequencies are summarized for all the tasks. Using non-parametric repeated measure tests, there is a significant decrease in PDC between Task 1.1 and 1.8 ($p < 0.001$) when compared within the subjects at the same frequencies. A corresponding increase in PDC from Task 1.1 to 1.8 was also observed, when the effect of eye on instrument motion was examined ($p < 0.001$) as shown in Table 1(a). This shows that after training, the eye movements are more likely to predict the instrument trajectories, whereas the causal influence of the instrument on the eye was stronger before training.

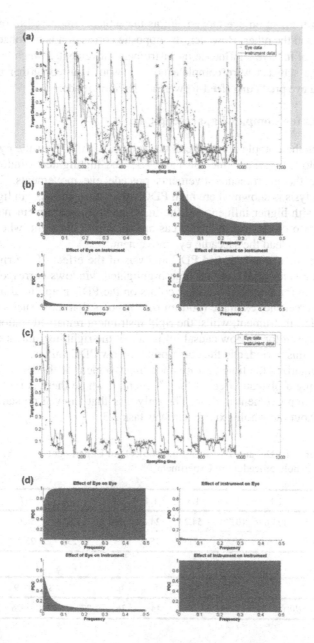

Fig. 2. (a, c) TDF of the instrument and eye data in an example where instrument movement precedes eye movement and vice versa (red dots – eye data, blue line – instrument data). (b, d) the PDC of the instrument and eye data showing the independence of the eye and instrument data.

Moreover, there is a significant negative correlation between PDC and Tasks 1.2 to 1.4 ($r = -0.48$ $p < 0.001$) and Tasks 1.5 to 1.7 ($r = -0.15$ $p < 0.001$) using Spearman's rank correlation, which represent the three successive training sessions with the first and second camera rotations respectively. This describes the decreasing causal influence of the instrument on eye movement, as the subjects improved in one camera rotation condition and the other. However, the opposite correlation is not observed with the PDC measures of the eye's influence on instrument movements, which is explained by the fact that the subjects were complete novices who required further training to reveal an increased eye predicting (feed-forward) behavioral model.

3.2 PDC Analysis for Complex Laparoscopic Task

Fig. 3(a) illustrates the complexity of the data streams, with TDF of the eye and left instrument data plotted against time for Task 2.1. The highlighted windows in red show areas where the instrument movements precede eye movements. The corresponding PDC analysis is shown where high PDC values are expressed in light colors, this is consistent with higher influence of the instrument on eye movements. Screenshot examples of two of the highlighted areas are shown on the right, where the left instrument is shown to lead the saccadic eye movement.

Fig. 3(b) shows the same TDF and PDC analysis of the effect of the right instrument on the eye movements. Here, the blue highlighted windows correspond to low PDC values, and are represented by darker colors on the PDC graph in almost all the frequencies. The screenshot example (bottom right) shows that the visual system was used to guide the left instrument, whilst the right instrument remained stationary. This substantiates the reason for the low causal influence of the right instrument on the eye movements during this period, and the corresponding low PDC values.

Table 1(b) summarizes the time performance improvement of the whole procedure (2.1 to 2.5), showing a plateau effect at the 5th attempt, where there is no further statistical significant improvement in time. The only task that showed no statistical improvement throughout the whole experiment was task 2.3.

Table 1. (a) Summary of PDC analysis for all the subjects in Experiment 1. (b) Median times of completion of the whole procedure in Experiment 2.

Task	1.1	1.2	1.3	1.4	1.5	1.6	1.7	1.8
Instrument on Eye *	123.6	107.7	54.7	24.6	70.5	122.4	58.6	26.5
Eye on Instrument *	37.6	29.8	71	35.4	33.8	23.7	23.7	46.5
Median PDC × 10³								

Attempt	1	2	3	4	5	6	7	8	9	10
Median time (s)	70	52	39	32	44	36	27	23	26	28

The PDC analysis of the latter attempts did not show a causal influence of the eye on the instrument movements. As the subjects improve, visual analysis of the video data showed a significant improvement of predictive eye behavior in the 10th attempt when compared to the 1st attempt. However, this type of predictive behavior is non-sequential: as the subjects improve in this complex laparoscopic procedure, the visual system is used to for target selection, instead of simple feed-forward guidance of the instruments.

Fixations often landed on three to four potential targets, before the instrument was utilized on the selected target. This type of non-sequential causality cannot be measured by PDC due to the cognitive influence of the maneuver.

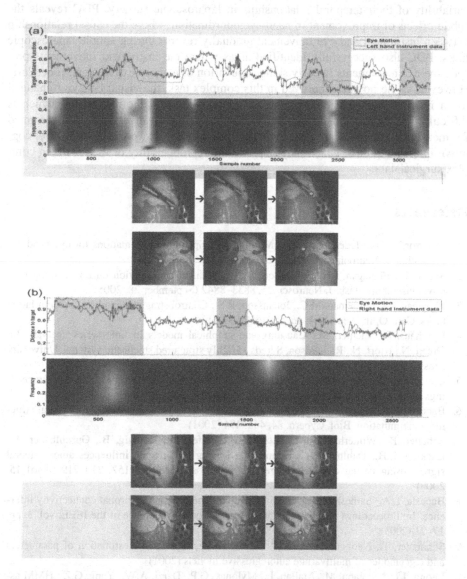

Fig. 3. (a) TDF of eye and instrument data against time (expressed as sample number) for a subject performing Task 2.1, and moving window PDC analysis (300 time samples with 50% overlap) of the causal influence of the *left* instrument on eye movement, the high PDC values of the specific frequencies are expressed in light colors, these areas are highlighted in red. Screen shots of two high PDC windows are illustrated on the right (red/yellow dot = gaze position). (b) TDF and moving window PDC of the causal influence of the *right* instrument on eye movement. Blue highlighted areas represent low PDC levels. Screen shots of one high and one low (bottom) PDC windows are illustrated on the right.

4 Discussion and Conclusions

This paper investigates the interdependency of the hand eye movement along with the variability of their temporal relationships in laparoscopic surgery. PDC reveals the subtle effects of improvement in hand-eye coordination, where the causal relationship between instrument and eye movement gradually reverse during simple laparoscopic tasks. PDC also successfully identified areas where the instrument movements precede the eye movements in early skills acquisition of a complex bimanual procedure. However, as the novices improved in this complex task, the visual behavior changed to an intricate non-sequential predictive relationship with the instrument, which is difficult to be measured using simple PDC analysis. Further investigation is warranted for measuring complex combinatory behavioral data by incorporating high-level cognitive inferencing data, which may improve the reproducibility of the results in complex surgical data.

References

1. Crawford, J.D., Medendorp, W.P., Marotta, J.J.: Spatial transformations for eye-hand coordination. J. Neurophysiol. 92, 10–19 (2004)
2. Sailer, U., Flanagan, J.R., Johansson, R.S.: Eye-hand coordination during learning of a novel visuomotor task. J. Neurosci. 25, 8833–8842 (September 28, 2005)
3. Flanagan, J.R., Bowman, M.C., Johansson, R.S.: Control strategies in object manipu-lation tasks. Curr. Opin. Neurobiol. 16, 650–659 (2006)
4. Dahlhaus, R., Eichler, M.: Causality and graphical models in time series analysis. In: Green, N., Hjort, N., Richardson, S. (eds.) Highly structured stochastic systems, University Press, Oxford (2003)
5. Eichler, M.: Fitting graphical interaction models to multivariate time series. In: Proceedings of the 22nd Conference on Uncertainty in Artificial Intelligence (2006)
6. Baccala, L.A., Sameshima, K.: Partial directed coherence: a new concept in neural structure determination. Biol. Cybern. 84, 463–474 (2001)
7. Schelter, B., Winterhalder, M., Eichler, M., Peifer, M., Hellwig, B., Guschlbauer, B., Lucking, C.H., Dahlhaus, R., Timmer, J.: Testing for directed influences among neural signals using partial directed coherence. J. Neurosci. Methods 152, 210–219 (April 15, 2006)
8. Baccala, L.A., Sameshima, K.: Partial directed coherence and neuronal connectivity inference. In: Proceedings of the 25th Annual International Conference of the IEEE, vol. 3, pp. 17–21 (2003)
9. Schneider, T., Neumaier, A.: ARfit: A Matlab package for the estimation of parameters and eigenmodes of multivariate autoregressive models (2001)
10. Leong, J.J., Nicolaou, M., Atallah, L., Mylonas, G.P., Darzi, A.W., Yang, G.Z.: HMM assessment of quality of movement trajectory in laparoscopic surgery. Comput. Aided Surg. 12, 335–346 (2007)
11. Nicolaou, M., James, A., Darzi, A., Yang, G.Z.: A Study of Saccade Transition for Attention Segregation and Task Strategy in Laparoscopic Surgery. In: Barillot, C., Haynor, D.R., Hellier, P. (eds.) MICCAI 2004. LNCS, vol. 3217, p. 97. Springer, Heidelberg (2004)
12. Yang, G.Z., Dempere-Marco, L., Hu, X.P., Rowe, A.: Visual search: Psychophysical models and practical applications. Image and Vision Computing, pp. 291–305 (2002)

A Virtual Reality Patient and Environments for Image Guided Diagnosis

Barnabas Takacs[1], David Hanak[1], and Kirby G. Voshburg[2]

[1] MTA SZTAKI / VHI Group,
1111 Kende u 13-17, Budapest. HUNGARY
[2] Harvard CIMIT
165 Cambridge St. Suite 702, Boston, MA, USA

Abstract. We describe a real-time virtual reality platform and a novel visualization technique designed to deliver constant rendering speed of highly detailed anatomical structures at interactive rates using portable, and low-cost computers. Our solution represents the torso section of the human body as a volumetric data set and employs label maps as the prime data format of storing anatomical structures. Multi-channel 3D textures are uploaded to the GPU and a simple pixel shader algorithm allows operators to select structures of interest in real-time. The visualization module described herein was successfully integrated into a virtual-reality 3D Anatomical Guidance System for Ultrasound Operators and its rendering performance tested on a "backpack" system.

Keywords: Anatomical Guidance, FAST Exam, Augmented Reality, Virtual Human Interface.

1 Introduction

Anatomical Guidance (AG) combines generic 3D models of the human body with medical real-time imaging devices, such as laparascopic or hand-held ultrasound [1]. The purpose of image-guided interventions is to visually aid medics and operators in correctly identifying anatomical structures for the purposes of examination and planning of subsequent surgical interventions. It has been shown, that such tools doubled the performance of novice users, during the in vivo examination of anesthetized pigs, effectively boosting their skills to reach the accuracy of experts without the AG support. Furthermore experts also performed nearly 150% better when using the AG system in comparison to performing diagnostics without it. These studies indicate that a portable, anatomically guided ultrasound system would find many applications in the field of patient care.

For many decades researchers and medics has been seeking for safe and effective casualty care technologies to address situations where initial emergency life-saving surgery. In such circumstances prompt, aggressive resuscitation may have to be performed within a limited time in which medical care can be effective in saving life and to render a patient transportable. *A leading cause of death in these situations is hemorrhage.* To address these difficulties Ultrasound offers a fast method to detect internal

T. Dohi, I. Sakuma, and H. Liao (Eds.): MIAR 2008, LNCS 5128, pp. 279–288, 2008.

bleedings and help save the life of people in the field. It is currently the imaging solution available in a portable, low power consumption form and therefore it has very high potential for being the first such technology successfully deployed to help *Medical Aid Stations (MAS)*.

This paper describes the architecture and applications of a compact anatomically guided 3D ultrasound solution that employs virtual- and augmented reality to successfully increase the diagnostic capabilities of novice users and experts alike.

2   Internal Bleeding and the FAST Exam

When a medic first reaches a casualty, his or her priorities are to determine signs of life, then to ensure breathing. Among the possible, and necessary, treatments are the insertion of a chest dart or tube to relieve tension pneumothorax. Following these initial steps, the medic's next priorities are to search for bleeding. If there is bleeding from an extremity wound, compresses, active compresses, or, if necessary, a tourniquet are applied. Then, he may attempt to determine whether there is a treatable site of internal hemorrhage. It is unfortunately the case that vital signs, as currently defined and measured, are of minimal use in determining, in the early phase, whether there is excessive internal bleeding. It is well accepted, most notably in recent studies at the Army's Institute of Surgical Research, that conventional vital signs such as arterial blood pressure, body temperature, or blood oxygen saturation, that is, the parameters that are easy to measure in a field setting, are not good prognostic indicators.   On the other hand, it is not possible or even desirable to immediately begin resuscitation with intravenous fluids, for both tactical and medical reasons.

The medic is then faced with a significant diagnostic challenge.   He or she must determine if there is *internal bleeding*, quantify the rate of such bleeding, identify the sources of bleeding, and guide appropriate treatment to the site. If the source is visible and accessible, as it is for the extremity injuries mentioned above, the obvious first choice is the use of hemostatic agents. If this therapy fails, the direct application of coagulative thermal therapies, such as focused ultrasound or, more directly, thermal cautery, might be attempted.

To address *internal hemorrhage*, whether from penetrating or concussive insults, the *diagnostic instrument* of choice that may be deployed in *Medical Aid Stations (MAS)* for the present as well as for the foreseeable near future is transcutaneous lultrasound imaging. This contrasts with the situation in major medical center emergency departments, where Computer Tomography (CT) is the easiest and most definitive choice for detecting pooled blood. Several high quality, low cost, portable (battery powered or low power) instruments are now commercially available, creating the opportunity to design such a system for portable casualty care. However, since ultrasound imaging requires a level of care and sophistication that makes it unlikely that a minimally trained, unsupported operator could perform a diagnostic examination under field conditions, tools for 3D visualization, guidance and telemedicine using the toolset of Image Guided Surgery become a necessity [2].

The *Focused Assessment with Sonography for Trauma (FAST)* [3] examination was originally developed for the assessment of blunt abdominal trauma, but has been shown to be effective for assessing penetrating trauma as well. *FAST* examinations have shown a sensitivity near 85% and a specificity of better than 95% (op. cit.). The primary indicator for a positive reading is the observation of a *pool of intraperitoneal blood* in regions around the liver, spleen or the pelvic organs. The standard treatment after a positive *FAST* examination is an exploratory laparotomy to identify and treat the injury. Before reaching the second echelon of care, however, this is not possible. Rather, the non-incisional approach using focused ultrasound therapy (*High Intensity Focused Ultrasound*, or *HIFU* [4]) is a promising, practical alternative. The effective use of *HIFU* depends on identifying the site to be coagulated and then establishing an acoustic path to the bleeding site. The most challenging problem is site identification in which a minimally trained medic requires the assistance of doctors from remote sites. For *HIFU* (or any coagulative therapy) to be effective, it must be applied to the site of injury.   While it is sometimes very difficult to use the ultrasound imager to detect a region of diffuse bleeding, it is possible to identify a ruptured artery or vein, particularly if Doppler capability is available. In general, these lesions are the most serious and desirable to treat, since they lead to the most rapid exsanguination.

In order to be effective in a mobile environment, the emergency instruments carried on the field must be portable, self contained, easy to operate, and provide clear guidance to personnel who had only limited training. Using ultrasound for imaging the body of an injured person, has many advantages. First, it is the only imaging solution that is available in a portable, low power consumption form that has the potential of successfully being deployed in *MAS* or with paramedics in civilian sector. Second, it offers a low-cost, yet powerful method to detect internal bleedings; and third, it can be used virtually without any restrictions on exposure, i.e. as many times without any risk to the patients' health (unlike X-rays, CT, etc.). However, a critical difficulty when using US is that images are noisy and features are often rather difficult to recognize even for trained personnel. In fact, without knowing the context where the US probe is located, it is almost impossible even for doctors to recognize whet they are looking at. On the other hand several studies have shown that 3D guidance can be of significant help both for novice users and expert users in laparascopic surgical procedures. Based on this premise, in a previous study we have successfully built and demonstrated the power of 3D anatomical guidance and validated its usability. Specifically, using a clinical setup at Harvard we assessed the effectiveness and efficiency of *anatomically guided ultrasound vs. traditional ultrasound* for a standard EUS exam in a porcine model. Novices carrying out EUS reached only 30% in correctly identifying anatomical structures, however their performance increased to 59% when using the *AGU* setup. Note that this is almost the same (only 2% lower) then the performance of experts using traditional EUS (61%), which is a significant result in alone itself from the perspective of the major goals of this project. Furthermore, expert users also benefit from using *AGU*, as their performance too increased above 90%.

3   The CyberCare Portable Virtual Reality System

The power of virtual- and augmented reality (*CyberCare*), systems stems from is its ability to offer *flexibility*, *repeatability* and a *controlled environment* that aids medical personnel to carry out certain tasks. The *CyberCare* VR system we developed is comprised of multiple configurable hardware software components, each addressing key aspects of the goals of specific rehabilitative needs. The doctor may wear a head-mounted display system (HMD) that delivers visual and auditory input directly to his or her eyes and ears. Attached to the HMD is a motion tracker that measures the rotation parameters (yaw, pitch and roll) of the head. Translation (i.e. x,y,z motion in 3D space) is controlled via a joystick device so that patient, if needed, can move freely and navigate in 3D virtual space. The head motion and joystick information are relayed to a computer, which in turn generates the appropriate visual representation of the patient model and the 3D augmented environment. This virtual reality computer is responsible for rendering the high-resolution scene in photo-realistic quality based on the patient's movement information as received from the sensors. Along with the visual stimulus sent directly back to the HMD, the VR computer is also responsible for recording *live video* data, physiological measurements and *biological feedback* from the patient, all displayed in readily accessible form. The video input is used to support real-time interaction with the virtual environment. This virtual environment itself is comprised of a high fidelity digital human model, 3D environments combined with photo-realistic elements, such as a 360° virtual panorama as background, and overlaid animated synthetic objects.

The *CyberCare* system we describe here was built upon our core technology, called the *Virtual Human Interface* or *VHI* [5,6] shown in Figure 1. Each of these modules play a vital part in the process of rehabilitation. As shown in the figure we devised a general architecture that can be freely and easily configured to address the various needs of a large variety of virtual-reality-based applications. Its main features are as follows: *Portable Virtual-Reality Platform, High Fidelity Digital Humans, Real-Time Panoramic Video, Compositing and Augmented Reality, Physical Simulation, Low-Cost Input/Output Devices, Motion Capture (MOCAP) Support.*

One of the key focuses of the *CyberCare* system is the ability to produce virtual scenarios that are not only highly realistic, but also run on portable platforms that may be deployed in the field. Therefore the CyberCare system combines the benefits of *high quality 3D virtual models* with *panoramic spherical video*, both demonstrated in Figure 2. These environments maybe used to show our virtual patient during operation or as lying on the table.

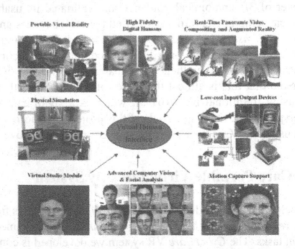

Fig. 1. Core modules of the Virtual Human Interface (VHI) System

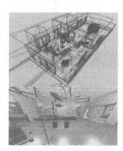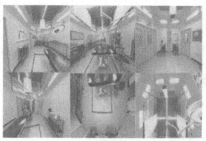

Fig. 2. We developed a virtual OR model complete with a fully detailed Virtual Patient that may be combined with Panoramic Video imagery obtained in the OR

4 Anatomically Guided Ultrasound System Using AR

Using the CyberCare system introduced above we have developed a prototype application for medical guidance and diagnosis. The basic setup of the compact anatomically guided Ultrasound system is shown in Figure 3. On the left, a medic is using the system to detect internal bleeding of a patient lying on the ground. The entire system is carried in a backpack on his back, his hands hold three outside components, namely the US probe, the reference cube for the tracking system, and the touch-sensitive computer screen which serves as the main interface to access the system's functions. On the right the HW elements packed tightly inside the backpack are shown. From left to right a Portable Ultrasound device (Sonosite C180 [7] is combined with a 6DOF, high precision tracker (Ascension Microbird [8]) to create a tracked sequence of US images. This information is transmitted to a small computer (Apple macMini), the heart of our Anatomical 3D Guidance solution, that combines this information with generic models of the human body, called virtual humans, and outputs guidance information to the medic's hand-held touch screen (or HMD if the field conditions permit). Figure 4shows the hand-held touch screen and its use during a field test, respectively. Specifically, The control interface allows the operator to:

- Calibrate the US probe to the injured body lying on the floor,
- Switch between views (in order all three visualization modes together, or 3D guidance, CT cross-section, or Ultrasound only) and control visualization parameters, such as guidance info for FAST exam.
- The navigation buttons on the left allow rotations of the 3D models up, down, left or right, as well as zooming in or out.

One of the key technical elements of our backpack Ultrasound guidance solution is a highly detailed digital and animatable representation of *the human body and its anatomy*. This representation comprises a generic 3D virtual human model as well as models of internal organs segmented from volumetric data representations. The purpose of this generic 3D model is to provide guidance to the operator showing major anatomical areas of interest when patient-specific data is not available. Guidance herein refers to showing regions inside the body in order to help medics properly move the US probe and thus obtain high quality US images. Guidance information is

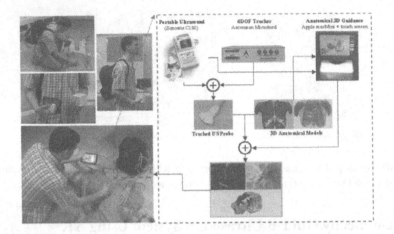

Fig. 3. Overall architecture of a "backpack" anatomical guidance solution

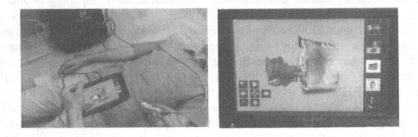

Fig. 4. Portable Augmented reality US guidance system to support FAST

also very important to the doctors reviewing the recorded US scans, as it provides 3-dimensional context information without which interpreting the US images would practically be impossible.

The visualization system was optimized for portable performance and it offers different methodologies for showing regions of interest to the operator. They all rely on the notion of *creating Anatomical Atlases* and use them later as reference for segmenting patient-specific CT's and visualizing target information. Instead of representing structures as polygonal objects, however, our atlas contains colored *image slices* combined with detailed *label maps*. Specifically, we focused our efforts on creating a complete model of the inside the torso section of the body and optimize it for real-time viewing and manipulation on a portable computational platform. As the first step in this process the torso segment from the volumetric data scans of the *Visible Human Male Data* set [9] was processed with an open-source segmentation and labeling tool, called *3D Slicer* [10]. *Slicer* provides a set of automated techniques to specify regions of interest in volumetric data sets and construct 3D polygonal surfaces. These organ models typically contain up to one million polygons each, thereby making them difficult to use in a real-time system. Figure 5 / Left shows examples of the named geometries including muscles, bone structure of the chest and spine, vascular structure of veins and arteries, and internal organs, (the entire model contains 478 identified anatomical structures in total.), while on the right, the same data structure is demonstrated encoded with the help of *label maps*.

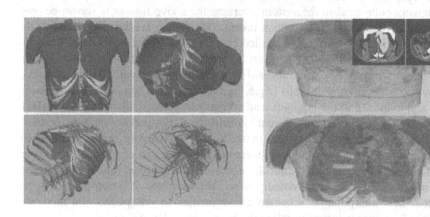

Fig. 5. Torso model of 478 elements shown as 3D geometry and labelmap-based visualization

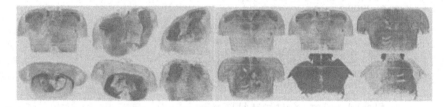

Fig. 6. Examples of visualizing internal anatomical structures at a constant rendering rate with the help of label maps and dynamic shading technology

The volumetric data set (MRI/CT) at the input of the visualization pipeline is defined as a stack of dynamic images (gray scale, color and/or label maps attached). In the first stage real-time image processing operators are used to automatically process all slices within a given volumetric object and implement the required preprocessing steps. These steps comprise of removing unwanted parts, image operators for noise reduction, contrast enhancement or substructure masking. Using the processed slices, a volumetric object is created and linked to an anatomical skeletal structure by an *object linking* mechanism. The resulting volume object then enters the rendering pipeline where it first passes through a vertex *shader* and subsequently in a pixel *shader*. The vertex *shader* implements *local shape deformations* (not used in this paper) while the *pixel shader* implements the algorithms required to highlight different internal structures inside the volume to help guide the US scanning process. The *pixel shader* can use gray scale images or color scheme for best viewing. More specifically, it can be programmed to color the pixels within a volume according to local image density, gray scale color or other algorithmically extractable features and its operation maybe directly controlled via label maps as well. The unit thereby offers an extended set of parameters to visualize anatomically important information a medic needs to scan. The key advantage of this approach is that it delivers high performance and constant visualization speed. Figure 6 demonstrates the power of shader-based visualization pipeline by showing the same structures with different settings.

The fragment code used in the system to create the above figures is shown below. The operation of the pixel shader which takes a 3D texture (*volumeTex*) as input is governed by a number of parameters, called constants all stored in registers (*baseRange, highlightColor, highlightDelta, massColor in c0 – c3*). These constants are four element vectors with x,y,z,w coordinates. For each voxel's output (*color*) the red, green, blue and transparency or alpha (*r,g,b, and a*) values are computed via the local algorithm and uploaded to the graphics card. When using this shader various constant settings (*c0 through c3*) refer to different visibility and transparency values for each pixel. The user interface of the system than allows for changing these constants to best fit the needs for showing internal structures. To take this concept even further these shader parameters can be dynamically uploaded and changed in real-time to best suite the needs of guidance and visualization. Different sets of parameters may be grouped together, interpolation schemed allow medics to interpolate and navigate these settings by a simple interface called the *Disc Controller* [5].

```
struct vertout
{
      float4 Pos : POSITION; float4 Col  : COLOR0; uvw :
TEXCOORD0;
};
sampler3D  volumeTex    : register( s0);
float4  baseRange    : register( c0);
float4  highlightColor : register( c1);
float4  highlightDelta : register( c2);
float4  massaColor   : register( c3);
float4 main( vertout IN) : COLOR
{
    float4 color = (float4)1;
    float4 texCol = tex3D(volumeTex, IN.uvw.xyz);
    color.rgb  = texCol.rgb;
    if ((texCol.a > baseRange.x) && (texCol.a < baseRange.y))
      color.a  = highlightColor.w;
    else
      color.a = 0;
    return color;
}
```

As stated above one of the key advantages of our proposed approach is to use volumetric representation in combination with label maps, a technique that delivers high performance and constant visualization speed even on portable computers. To test this assumption we measured the overall performance of the rendering algorithm on an Apple macMini computer (1.66GHz Intel Core Duo, 2GB 667 DDR2 SDRAM) we used in our "backpack" ultrasound guidance system. The speed evaluation comprised of two steps. First we used the polygonal models of increasing complexity in terms of polygon counts and recorded the overall rendering speed in frames-per-second (fps). Real-time performance requires a minimum of 15 fps update rate for the ultrasound operator to see smooth motion and perceive the system's reaction time as seamless. As shown in the figure below even with relatively small 3D polygonal models the Apple macMini did not reach this performance level. This is largely due to the relatively slow performance of the built-in graphics chip that is quite significantly slower than a high-end graphics card would be. In the second test the same anatomical structures are visualized using the label-map volume algorithm to compare the two methodologies. Our findings are summarized in Figure 7.

The graph shows the *rendering speed* (i.e. how fast the computer reacts and up-dates images on the screen during anatomical guidance) as a function of scene *com-plexity* (i.e. how many visual elements are shown). The blue line is the performance curve for 3D models. A typical guidance system shows a few major landmarks, bones, lungs, liver, kidney, vascular structure, etc. The blue curve demonstrates that more structures are shown the slower frame rate becomes, eventually reaching only two frames per seconds (fps). On the other hand the *labelmap-based shading algo-rithm* delivers much higher speeds (30fps) on the same hardware and a constant per-formance even when hundreds of internal structures are shown.

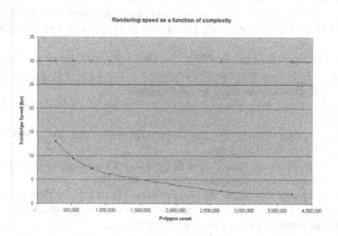

Fig. 7. Comparisons of rendering performance of polygon-based with our new. labelmap-based shading algorithms, the later providing constant visualization rate.

5 Conclusion

In this paper we described a *compact anatomically ultrasound system* that employs high fidelity 3D digital human models in compination of virtual- and augmented-reality techniques to provide medics with minimal training the capability to take highly accurate ultrasound scans. We discussed the benefits of using ultrasound as the only currently available imaging technology to detect internal hemorrhage, and showed that 3D guidance significantly increases the accuracy of diagnostic capabili-ties of novice and expert users alike. To fit the needs of creating a portable and low-cost AR visualization engine we introduced a novel methodology to display large numbers of complex anatomical structures for 3D guidance purposes. Specifically, our solution replaced polygonal models with colored volumetric representation com-bined with pre-segmented label maps. To test our approach we used a detailed 3D models segmented from the torso section of the NIH Visible Male data set and experimentally showed that our algorithm delivers high performance and constant speed visualization outperforming traditional polygon-based methods on the same portable computer hardware. The visualization method described herein was successfully integrated into an advanced ultrasound guidance framework and used to aid operators to find anatomical structures and obtain high quality ultrasound image sequences. Future work involves constructing reference data sets for the entire volume data made available and generalization of our algorithms to handle multiple volumes in parallel. We argue that these advanced capabilities in the future will allow for better patient care and medical response, as well as will help save the lives of many future accident victims or patients.

References

1. Elsmere, J., Stoll, J., Rattner, D., Brooks, D., Kane, R., Wells III, W., Kikinis, R., Vosburgh, K.: A Navigation System for Augmenting Laparoscopic Ultrasound. In: Ellis, R.E., Peters, T.M. (eds.) MICCAI 2003. LNCS, vol. 2879, pp. 184–191. Springer, Heidelberg (2003)
2. Boctor, E.M., Viswanathan, A., Pieper, S., Choti, M.A., Taylor, R.H., Kikinis, R., Fichtinger, G.: CISUS: An Integrated 3D Ultrasound System for IGT Using a Modular Tracking API. In: SPIE Proceedings, vol. 5367, p. 27 (2004)
3. Jones, R.A., Welch, R.D.: Ultrasonography in Trauma: The FAST Exam. ACEP Publishing (2003)
4. Kennedy, J.E.: High-intensity Focused Ultrasound in the Treatment of Solid Tumours. Nat. Rev. Cancer 5(4), 321–327 (2005)
5. Takacs, B., Kiss, B.: Virtual Human Interface: a Photo-realistic Digital Human. IEEE Computer Graphics and Applications 23(5), 38–45 (2003)
6. Takacs, B.: Special Education and Rehabilitation: Teaching and Healing with Interactive Graphics. IEEE Computer Graphics and Applications 25(5), 40–48 (2005)
7. Sonosite Inc. (2008), http://www.sonosite.com
8. Ascension Technology Corp. (2008), http://www.ascension-tech.com
9. National Library of Medicine, Visible Human Data Set, http://www.nlm.nih.gov/research/visible/getting_data.html
10. 3D Slicer, http://www.slicer.org

A Navigation System for Brain Surgery Using Computer Vision Technology

Jiann-Der Lee[1], Chung-Wei Lin[1], Chung-Hsien Huang[1], Shin-Tseng Lee[2], and Chien-Tsai Wu[2]

[1] Department of Electrical Engineering, Chang Gung University, Tao-Yuan, Taiwan
[2] Medical Augmented Reality Research Center, Chang Gung Memorial Hospital, Tao-Yuan, Taiwan
jdlee@mail.cgu.edu.tw

Abstract. In this paper, a surgical navigation system based on stereo-vision has been proposed. With the help of a projector, surface point data of a patient are firstly captured from two cameras by using the stereo-vision technique. Next, these point data is then registered by another surface point data obtained from the patient's pre-stored CT images using Feature-added ICP algorithm. For surgical navigation, a stereo-vision-based tracker is also designed in this system. In this manner, the anatomical information obtained from CT is fused on the images captured by the cameras and the tracker can be mounted to any surgical device for further surgical applications. Compared to conventional image guided surgeries, the proposed system has the advantage of fusing the visual and anatomical information such that it is more accurate and convenient.

Keywords: Stereo-vision, navigation system, ICP registration.

1 Introduction

Nowadays, the stereotactic surgery is widely applied in the brain surgery. The stereotactic surgery fixes a stereotactic frame on a patient's head to localize the nidus and then surgeons insert surgical instruments toward the nidus for advanced treatment. For example, in [1-2] surgeons performed brain surgery by consulting contiguous sequential CT or MRI and a Brown-Roberts-Wells (BRM) stereotactic system to localize positions of brain tissues for functional neurosurgery.

In order to replace the stereotactic frame, an alternative is using screw fiducials or skin markers. Surgeons choose at least three pairs of corresponding points from pre-stored patient's CT or MRI and on the patient lying on an operation platform, respectively. Then the transformation consisting three translations and three rotations, which brings the coordinate of CT onto the coordinate of surgery instrument, can be computed. In [3-5], the Polaris measurement system made by NDI is widely used as a navigation tool among medical navigation systems. In [6], due to its considerable measurement errors caused by disturbing fields, only few navigation systems adopt the aurora system for surgical applications. In [7-8], point clouds extracted from brain surface and feature points selected from bone markers are utilized to connect patient's

T. Dohi, I. Sakuma, and H. Liao (Eds.): MIAR 2008, LNCS 5128, pp. 289–299, 2008.

CT data and surgical instruments by using the weighted geometrical feature (WGF) and iterative closest point (ICP) registration algorithm.

Although these methods could obtain the transform which registers patient's CT data to the related patient, a significant drawback is that they all need to contact the patient and may make the patients' soft tissue deformed and even cause anatomical damage. During the registration, soft tissue deformation will decrease the data accuracy and lead the registration error. Therefore, in order to make non-contact registration possible, we take advantage of stereo-vision, which replaces the contact tracking device, to register pre-stored patient's CT to his/her physical location.

In this approach, we propose a navigation system dealing with the registration of pre-stored patient's CT data and the patient by using the stereo-vision techniques with the help of a projector for frameless brain surgery. The proposed algorithm is based on ICP but a new distance metric replaces the cost function of the traditional ICP. Before registration, neurosurgeons select at least three corresponding points at each data set. These corresponding points can be skin markers or feature points such as nose tip, corners of eyes or corners of mouth. Although the face features picked from the figures often have uncertainty more or less, it could be used as initial value. As a result, those roughly selected points should not be highly matched but they are still a cue for an initial alignment. The proposed algorithm brings this idea into the cost function of ICP. First, we give higher weight to these roughly selected points in order to obtain a good initial pose. In each iteration, we gradually decrease the weights of those selected points and increase the weights of the surface point cloud until a preset condition occur. That is, the final registration result is obtained.

2 The Proposed System

2.1 Frameless Brain Surgery System

With the help of surface registration, a frame-mounted stereotactic surgery can be preformed without using the stereotactic frame, called frameless brain surgery. It takes the advantage of registering two facial point data sets, one is captured from a patient's head directly using stereo-vision scanning equipment and the other is obtained from the patient's prestored CT images. The flowchart of the frameless brain surgery is shown in Fig. 1.

As shown in Fig. 1, our method for image guided surgery involves the following steps.

1) Before the registration, the two stereo cameras are calibrated to obtain the intrinsic and extrinsic camera parameters.

2) After obtaining the parameters, we manually select 3 feature point matches on each produced images. Mainly each feature point pairs must be visible.

3) With the parameters, we can create stereo cameras module and calculate these 6 point (2D) matches to produce 3 points (3D) based on stereo vision technology.

4) Also select 3 matching feature points (3D) on pre-stored CT data based on data coordinates.

5) Using the two pair of 3 feature points to perform coarse registration. After coarse registration process, an initial transfer matrix is obtained.

6) Combining the calibrated cameras and the projector, the point cloud of patients' surface based on the world coordinate of intra-operation could be obtained.

7) With the initial transfer matrix and the point cloud of patients' surface, Feature-added ICP Registration will be applied for the Fine Registration.

8) Use the stereo vision, surgery tools can be tracked directly or indirectly.

9) Finally, the fine transfer matrix and the tracker tracking could then be used for brain surgery navigation.

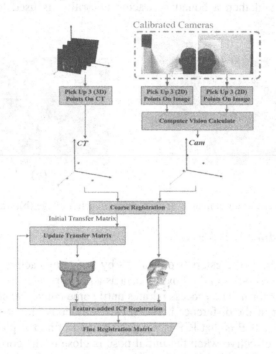

Fig. 1. The flowchart of the proposed system

2.2 Feature Points Dataset and Surface Points Dataset

The first step of this approach is to capture point-data required. Two facial point data sets are used here, one is captured from a patient's head directly using the stereo-vision technology and the other is obtained from the patient's pre-stored CT images. Next, three pairs of feature points are selected from the patient's CT and dual images captured by camera, respectively. These points could be the surface features or visible markers. The feature points could be artificial markers or natural features such as nose tip, eye corners or any discriminative points on the patient's head. The registration process is then performed. The proposed surface registration algorithm is robust since it combines the information of global coarse feature points and local fine curves into the cost function of ICP. The registration results in three translation and three rotation parameters, and then further processes such as stereo displaying, surgical target track-ing and other advanced surgery purposes can be achieved.

In additions, in capturing the point-data with calibrated camera, several single ap-proximately vertical thin lines are projected onto the surface of patient surface by using a projector. Fig. 2 shows the captured images of each camera. Using the charac-teristic of epi-polar line, each point on project line could find a compared point on the line of the other image. After repeating the calculation, the floating point data set could capture onsite from a patient lying on an operation table. The reference point data are extracted from patient's pre-stored CT images according to grayscale values. A threshold, which makes the head true and the background false, is applied to binary the CT image, and then a boundary tracing algorithm is used to obtain the facial points.

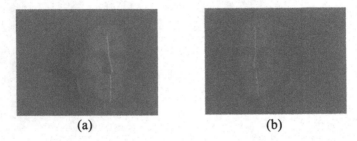

(a)   (b)

Fig. 2. Captured images of each camera, (a)left image (b)right image

2.3   Feature-Added ICP Algorithm

The ICP algorithm [9] registers two data sets by assigning each point in the reference data with its closest point in the floating data as a correspondence and then computing the aligning transform. The process iterates until some convergence criterions such as iteration number or the difference between two consecutive iterations is reached. The main limitation of ICP is that ICP is not guaranteed to find the global optimum. As a result, it is only effective when the initial pose is close to the correct pose. Since the initial pose of the floating data is the primary limitation of an effective ICP process, we take the advantage of using face features, resulting to not only obtain a good initial pose but also limit the solution space of searching the globally optimal solution. Fig. 3 shows the flowchart of the proposed Feature-added ICP Registration algorithm which is embedded into a coarse-to-fine registration framework. The detailed steps are de-scribed as follows:

1. The reference point data set $D_r = \{d_i^r \mid i = 1,2,...,n_r\}$ are extracted by a boundary tracing algorithm and the reference features $M_r = \{m_1^r, m_2^r, m_3^r\}$ are selected by mouse from patient's pre-stored CT data. The floating point data set $D_f = \{d_i^f \mid i = 1,2,...,n_f\}$ and the floating features $M_f = \{m_1^f, m_2^f, m_3^f\}$, which are corresponded to the reference features, are captured on the pair images by mouse.

2. Apply an initial transform T on the floating points and features. The transform T is the result of computing the best geometry match of the selected three features, M_r and M_f.

3. Set the weighting parameters W_1 and W_2. First, give weighting parameter W_2 of the coarsely selected features a higher value in order to obtain a good initial pose. After some iterations, we decrease W_2 and increase the weighting parameter W_1 of the fine selected surface points in order to obtain a reliable registration result.

4. Find the data set of the closest neighbor points $\overline{D_r} = \{\overline{d_i^r} \mid i = 1, 2, ..., n_f\}$ of the reference data D_r to the floating data transformed $T(F_f)$, i.e.

   $d(T(d_k^f), \overline{d_k^r}) = \min d(T(d_k^f), D_r)$.

5. Calculate the cost function which is defined as the following equation.

$$C = w_1 \cdot DistP + w_2 \cdot DistM,$$
$$0 \le w_1 \le 1, w_1 + w_2 = 1 \tag{1}$$

Where

$$DistP = \sum_{i=1}^{n_f} \sqrt{\left(\overline{d_i^r} - T(d_i^f)\right)^2} \tag{2}$$

$$DistF = \sum_{j=1}^{3_f} \sqrt{\left(f_j^r - T(f_j^f)\right)^2} \tag{3}$$

6. The transform T keeps updating until the cost function indicates reaching an optimum via an optimization algorithm.

7. If the optimization process is converged, then the registration process goes back to Step 3 to re-weight the weighting parameters W_1 and W_2.

8. If W_1 reaches one, it means the features no longer influence the registration. At the moment, we end the registration process and export the final transform matrix T_{FINAL}.

The proposed system can calculate the tracker tip point directly using the stereovision. The advantage of the method is to decrease the man-made error. On the other hand, environmental effect of light characteristic is the unavoidable drawback, which will cause the system unstable even the confused error. Fig. 4 shows the flowchart of the direct tracking which is embedded into a coarse-to-fine registration framework. Different navigation system will be used according to the different kinds of the brain surgical operation. For example, the cerebral endovascular surgery needs the electromagnetic tracker system. In fact, the proposed system has the ability to localize any kinds of tracker system. In additions, we also propose the indirectly method to combine the tracker system and our stereo-vision system. Fig. 5 shows the flowchart of the indirect tracking which is embedded into another coarse-to-fine registration framework.

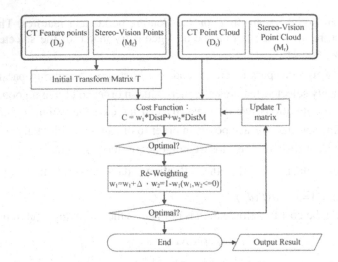

Fig. 3. Flowchart of the Feature-added ICP Registration algorithm

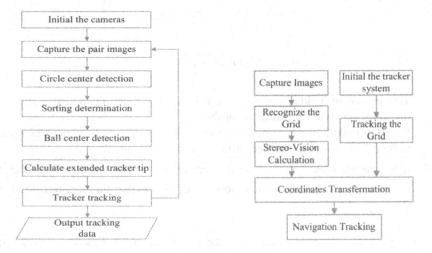

Fig. 4. Flowchart of direct tracking system   **Fig. 5.** Flowchart of indirect tracking system

3 Experimental Results

In the first experiment, the phantom is attached with five skin markers, Target1 (T1), Target2 (T2),…, and Target5 (T5), which are regarded as the ground truth for the accuracy evaluation of the registration algorithms. Three point pairs of the natural features, right eye corner Feature1 (F1), left eye corner Feature3 (F3), point between eye corners Feature2 (F2)and nose tip Feature4 (F4), were selected from CT as the reference features M_r and captured from the phantom as the floating features M_f.

Table 1 shows the surface features and markers used for accuracy test.

Table 1. Surface features and the coordinates of target markers

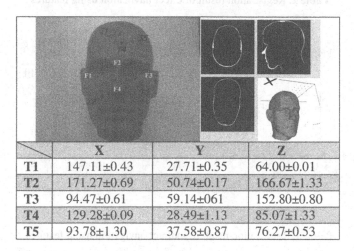

	X	Y	Z
T1	147.11±0.43	27.71±0.35	64.00±0.01
T2	171.27±0.69	50.74±0.17	166.67±1.33
T3	94.47±0.61	59.14±061	152.80±0.80
T4	129.28±0.09	28.49±1.13	85.07±1.33
T5	93.78±1.30	37.58±0.87	76.27±0.53

Target registration error (TRE), defined as Eq. (4), is utilized to evaluate the accuracy of the registration algorithms.

$$TRE = P_n^r - T\left(P_n^f\right) \tag{4}$$

where T is the transform obtained by the registration algorithm, P_n^r is the feature Point n of the reference dataset and P_n^r is the feature Point$_n$ of the floating dataset, respectively.

Fig. 6 shows the coarse registration using surface features. Table 2 shows the registration results of direct navigation tracking, which only use the surface features. Table 3 shows the registration results of indirect navigation tracking, which also use the surface features. Two operators performed the above procedure 10 times individually and then we computed the mean and the SD of errors. The results show that both of the navigation method could appear the same accuracy.

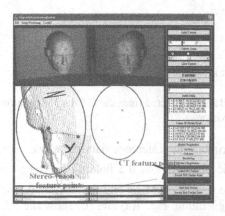

Fig. 6. Coarse registration using surface features

Table 2. Registration result of direct navigation using features

Feature Registration TRE(Ball Tracker) (mm)				
target	X	Y	Z	error
T1	147.6±5.35	22.2±3.58	67.5±1.26	6.40
T2	173.3±3.07	51.6±3.61	167.9±2.79	3.06
T3	97.9±3.87	60.1±5.23	153.3±5.07	3.97
T4	130.6±4.33	25.6±2.50	90.1±1.16	6.56
T5	96.9±7.06	33.8±2.80	79.7±1.98	6.71

Table 3. Registration result of indirect navigation using features

Feature Registration TRE(NDI Tracker) (mm)				
target	X	Y	Z	error
T1	155.9±1.67	27.4±0.4	64.5±1.67	8.90
T2	173.0±53.88	59.6±0.7	165.7±4.0	3.24
T3	92.7±1.28	56.9±0.3	153.9±1.6	7.50
T4	135.7±1.34	27.3±0.4	86.6±1.82	7.32
T5	99.0±1.04	30.6±0.4	75.7±2.06	8.76

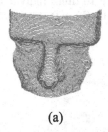
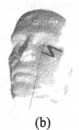

(a)   (b)

Fig. 7. (a)The reference dataset extracted from the CT data of phantom (b) the floating dataset captures by using stereo-vision

In the second experiment, the reference dataset D_r was extracted from pre-stored CT images of a plastic phantom and the floating dataset D_f was captured from the phantom's surface. The reference dataset and the floating dataset was used to perform Feature-added ICP Registration. Fig. 7(a) and (b) show the reference dataset and the floating dataset, respectively. Fig. 8 shows the registration result using surface

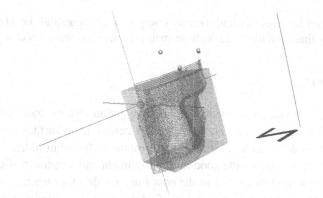

Fig. 8. (a)The reference dataset extracted from the CT data of phantom (b) the floating dataset captures by using stereo-vision

Table 4. Registration result of direct navigation using features-added ICP algorithm

target	\multicolumn{4}{c}{Feature-added ICP Registration TRE(Ball Tracker) (mm)}			
target	X	Y	Z	error
T1	173.0±0.61	49.1±0.33	166.0±0.6	**2.45**
T2	95.0±0.22	56.0±0.32	154.3±0.4	**1.34**
T3	128.5±0.44	30.5±0.34	84.5±0.50	**1.56**
T4	146.4±0.24	28.4±0.41	63.2±0.91	**1.61**
T5	146.4±0.24	28.4±0.41	63.2±0.91	**1.35**

Table 5. Registration result of indirect navigation using features-added ICP algorithm

target	\multicolumn{4}{c}{Feature-added ICP Registration TRE(NDI Tracker) (mm)}			
target	X	Y	Z	error
T1	144.8±5.01	26.3±2.20	64.2±3.22	**2.56**
T2	170.8±3.11	48.1±2.27	167.0±4.6	**2.41**
T3	96.2±0.82	59.9±1.89	153.8±2.2	**2.25**
T4	127.8±3.17	28.7±2.15	86.0±1.73	**1.60**
T5	97.3±0.72	38.6±2.30	78.0±1.80	**4.82**

features. Table 4 shows the registration results of direct navigation tracking, which only use the surface features. Table 5 shows the registration results of indirect navigation tracking, which also use the surface features. Two operators performed the above procedure 10 times individually and then we computed the mean and the SD of errors. The results show that both of the navigation methods have the same accuracy.

4 Conclusions

Since the primary drawback of brain surgery navigation system most comes from man-made error, we proposed a system combined stereo-vision surface scanning and Feature-added ICP registration algorithm. The proposed algorithm utilizes three corresponding features which provide good initial alignment and a coarse-to-fine strategy is embedded to re-weight two terms in the cost function. In other words, the Feature-added ICP algorithm takes the information of global coarse feature points and local fine point cloud into account to avoid the local optimum problem of ICP. In addition, the algorithm is integrated to a frameless surgical system which replaces the heavy head frame of traditional stereotactic surgery by registering two surface datasets, one is from the patient's pre-stored CT data and the other is from the patient's head stereo scanning. As a result, the anatomical information obtained from CT can be fused on the images captured by the cameras; the tracker can be mounted to any surgical device for further surgical applications. The navigation accuracy could be about 1~2mm. Compared to conventional image guided surgeries, the proposed system takes advantage of fusing the visual and anatomical information and has two features: without using markers and without contacting patient.

References

1. Askura, T., Uetsuhara, K., Kanemaru, R.: An applicability study on a CT-guided stereotactic technique for functional neurosurgery. Appl. Neurophys. 48, 73–76 (1985)
2. Nowinski, W.L., Yang, G.L., Ywo, T.T.: Computeraided stereotactic functional neurosurgery enhanced by the use of multiple brain atlas database. IEEE Trans. Med. Imag. 19(1), 62–69 (2000)
3. Bruyant, P.P., Gennert, M.A., Speckert, G.C., Beach, R.D., Morgenstern, J.D., Kumar, N., Nadella, S., King, M.A.: A Robust Visual Tracking System for Patient Motion Detection in SPECT: Hardware Solutions. IEEE Transaction. Nuclear Science 52(5), Part 1, 1288–1294 (2005)
4. Buzung, T.M., Hering, P., Bongartz, J., Ivanenko, M.: A Novel Navigation Principle in Computer-assisted Surgery. In: Proceedings of the 26th Annual International Conference of the IEEE EMBS, pp. 3132–3135 (2004)
5. Bartz, D.: Visual Medicine: Ppart Two-Advanced Applications of Medical Imaging. In: Tutorial 3 of IEEE Symposium on Information Visualization (2005)
6. Kneissler, M., Hein, A., Miitzig, M., Thomale, U.W., Lueth, T.C., Woiciechowsky, C.: Concept and clinical evaluation of navigated control in spine surgery. In: Proceedings of the 2003 IEEWASME International Conference on Advanced Intelligent Mechatronics, vol. 2, pp. 1084–1089 (2003)
7. Maurer, C.R., Aboutanos, G.B., Dawant, B.M.: Registration of 3-D images using weighted geometrical features. IEEE Transactions on Medical Imaging 15, 836–849 (1996)

8. Maurer, C.R., Maciunas, R.J., Fitzpatrick, J.M.: Registration of head CT images to physical space using a weighted combination of points and surfaces. IEEE Transactions on Medical Imaging 17, 753–761 (1998)
9. Besl, P.J., McKay, N.D.: A method for registration of 3D shapes. IEEE Transactions on Pattern Analysis and Machine Intelligence 14(2), 239–256 (1992)

Computer-Aided Delivery of High-Intensity Focused Ultrasound (HIFU) for Creation of an Atrial Septal Defect in Vivo

Hiromasa Yamashita[1], Tetsuko Ishii[1], Akihiko Ishiyama[1],
Noriyoshi Nakayama[1], Toshinobu Miyoshi[1], Yoshitaka Miyamoto[1],
Gontaro Kitazumi[1], Yasumasa Katsuike[1], Makoto Okazaki[2], Takashi Azuma[3],
Masayuki Fujisaki[4], Shinichi Takamoto[4], and Toshio Chiba[1]

[1] Department of Strategic Medicine, National Center for Child Health and Development.
2-10-1, Okura, Setagaya-ku, Tokyo, Japan
{yamashita-h,ishii-t,ishiyama-a,nakayama-n,chiba-t,kitazumi-g,
katsuike-y}@ncchd.go.jp, {tmiyoshi,ymiyamoto}@nch.go.jp
http://www.ncchd.go.jp/
[2] Infinity Medicalsoft Co.,Ltd. 2120-6-102, Higashi-naganuma, Inagi-shi, Tokyo, Japan
mokazaki@inf-medicalsoft.co.jp
http://www.inf-medicalsoft.co.jp/
[3] Central Resarch Laboratory, Hitachi Ltd. 1-280, Higashi-koigakubo, Kokubunji-shi,
Tokyo, Japan
takashi.azuma.sa@hitachi.com
http://www.hqrd.hitachi.co.jp/crl/index.cfm
[4] Department of Cardiothoracic Surgery, Graduate School of Medicine, University of Tokyo.
7-3-1, Hongo, Bunkyo-ku, Tokyo, Japan
masafujicardio@yahoo.co.jp, takamoto-tho@h.u-tokyo.ac.jp
http://ctstokyo.umin.ne.jp/

Abstract. In recent years, several fetal cardiac malformations have been increasingly treated before birth with gradually improved outcome, although the technique is still demanding and invasive. We newly developed a computer-aided system for energy delivery of high-intensity focused ultrasound (HIFU) to correct cardiac morphologic abnormalities *in vivo* much less invasively. The HIFU system could be controlled in real-time by a computer-based analysis of 2D-sonographic left ventricular images for optimal triggering off HIFU. Using beating heart of two anesthetized adult rabbits, the system successfully achieved a non-touch gross ablation of the atrial septum in one animal, and in the other HIFU energy was inadvertently mistargeted on the posterior wall of the left atrium with a resultant small transmural opening. We believe that the HIFU system will be introduced with pinpoint accuracy to minimally invasive treatment of fetal cardiac abnormalities that have intact or highly restrictive atrial septum.

Keywords: Fetal cardiac intervention, Computer-aided HIFU energy delivery, Real-time sonographic image analysis.

1 Introduction

Several fetal cardiac malformations have been increasingly treated before birth. Fetal cardiac intervention targets an in utero correction of simple intracardiac abnormalities

T. Dohi, I. Sakuma, and H. Liao (Eds.): MIAR 2008, LNCS 5128, pp. 300–310, 2008.

that potentially progress to complex heart diseases in utero, such as fetal critical aortic stenosis that might advance to hypoplastic left heart syndrome (HLHS) and HLHS with restrictive atrial septum leading to irreversible pulmonary vascular damages ([1]-[3]). Current fetal procedures for correction of restrictive atrial septum with an atrial decompression are still invasive because they, percutaneously and through both the uterine and fetal chest walls, require ultrasound-guided maternal puncture into the pulsating cardiac cavity of tiny fetal hearts and to create interatrial communications. Accordingly, these procedures have been reportedly accompanied by serious complications including profound bradycardia, bleeding and hemopericardium, intracardiac thrombus formation, and recurrent in utero closure of the created atrial septal defects.

Instead, to accomplish our goal of establishing fetal interatrial communications with minimal adverse effects, we developed an entirely new approach with the use of high-intensity focused ultrasound (HIFU). HIFU is an acoustic modality using ultrasound energy (cavitation or coagulation or both) focused to operate on an internally targeted tissue without damaging overlying and/or underlying tissues. Accordingly, HIFU has been employed predominantly for non-touch treatment of tumors including prostate cancer and uterine fibroids ([4], [5]). Unlike an extensive ablation of stationary tumors, the HIFU ablation to a pulsating narrow area in the beating and tiny fetal heart requires a pinpoint accuracy based on computer-aided target autotracking capacity. We originated a precise HIFU delivery device coupled with a real-time computer-aided 2D ultrasound image analysis. In this article, we report the outcome of our feasibility study for atrial septal defect creation using the beating heart of anesthetized adult rabbits.

2   Material and Methods

2.1   System Configuration

The system configuration of the computer-aided HIFU energy delivery system consists of predominantly 4 parts (Fig. 1). The first one is a HIFU energy delivery device which comprises a monocoque spherical shaped piezo transducer (PZT) and a diagnostic 2D-US imaging probe. The tomographic images of the latter include the focal point of the former. Radius of the PZT curvature is 40 mm, and the focal point is elliptical in shape (0.6-mm wide, 5.0-mm long). Focal point is located 40-mm apart from the PZT edge face. The second part is a diagnostic 2D-US imaging equipment (EnVisor C HD, Philips, Andover. MA) to drive a 2D-US imaging probe (s12, Philips, Andover. MA) and to do sector scanning of a cardiac four-chamber view. The equipment outputs grayscale NTSC-video data (640x480 pixels) into the workstation with 30 frames/sec. The third part is a signal generator (Agilent 33220A, Agilent technologies, Santa Clara, CA) and RF power amplifier (AG1012, T&C power Conversion Inc., Rochester, NY) to drive the PZT with a 3.3-MHz sine-wave. Input voltage into the PZT is about 160 Vpp from and temporal average intensity of the continuous-wave spatial peak is 6.5 kW/cm^2. The fourth part is a workstation (HP xw8200, OS:WindowsXP Pro SP2, CPU:Intel Xeon 3.8 GHz, Memory:2 GB, GPU:NVIDIA Quadro FX3450) to analyze input 2D-US tomographic image of cardiac four-chamber with our original real-time HIFU energy delivery control algorithm. A capture board (MTPCI-DC2,

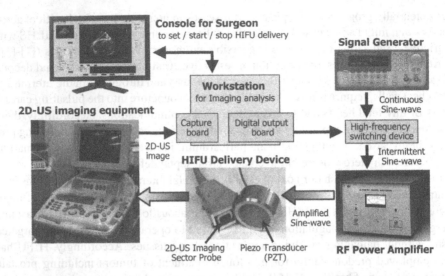

Fig. 1. System configuration of the computer-aided HIFU energy delivery

MICRO-TECHNICA, Tokyo, Japan) rasterizes the 2D-US image with an image-processing sub-system (Image-Pro. Plus. MediaCybernetics, Inc., Bethesda, MD) to analyze a cardiac beating cycle of the target. According to the analysis outcome, a digital I/O board (PIO-16/16L(LPCI)H, Contec CO., Ltd., Osaka, Japan) outputs the trigger signals for HIFU energy delivery into the high-frequency switching device to switch HIFU energy delivery ON/OFF.

2.2 Control of HIFU Energy Delivery

We developed an algorithm to recognize a cardiac beating cycle and to control a computer-aided HIFU energy delivery to an atrial septum based on prediction of its proper timing. Although cardiac beating motion is spatial, the atrial septum is not so moved spatially in the beating heart but contracted and stretched in sync with the cardiac beating motion. So with 2D-US tomographic image including the atrial septum, our system decides HIFU energy delivery timing. This software works with the following sequence.

1. Setting the position of HIFU energy delivery device
2. Accumulating cardiac beating cycle to recognize the optimal timing of HIFU energy delivery by 2D-US tomographic image
3. Computer-aided HIFU energy delivery to the atrial septum
4. Confirmation of an interatrial communication by color Doppler US
5. Repeat HIFU energy delivery to achieve an interatrial communication

Initial setting of the HIFU energy delivery system. Firstly, an operator positions the HIFU energy delivery device to scan the four-chamber view sighting the PZT focal point on the atrial septum. The HIFU energy beam should be directed perpendicular to the atrial septum as much as possible. Resolution for image analysis of the captured

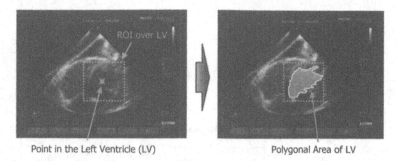

Point in the Left Ventricle (LV)   Polygonal Area of LV

Fig. 2. Region of interest is set by the operator to extract a polygonal area of the left ventricle in the captured 2D-US four-chamber view

2D-US sector view is 0.2 mm in the beam direction which depends on display resolution, and 0.5-mm in the angular orientation which depends on sector angle and depth of region of interest (ROI).

Secondly, the operator sets a suitable rectangle ROI surrounding the left ventricle (LV) on the 2D-US images and indicates a single position within the LV. The system binarizes and extracts the polygonal area of LV (total number of pixels) (Fig. 2). In the animal experiments, the LV area includes the target's high-frequency cardiac beating (CB) element and low-frequency respiration element. The latter is controlled to be 20 cycles/min by an artificial respiration (AR). In order to separate the AR element from the CB element, we use a running average of the LV area for a low-pass filter with a small calculation amount. Where the time is t, the LV area is $S_{LV}(t)$ and the AR element is $S_{AR}(t)$, $S_{AR}(t)$ is shown in the equation (1) with sampling time Δt and a running average of $S_{LV}(t)$. N is sampling number to get the running average. According to Fourier transformation, when the running average is with sampling number six, only the AR element can be extracted from the LV area.

$$S_{AR}(t) = \frac{1}{N} \sum_{n=0}^{N-1} S_{LV}(t - n\Delta t) \qquad (1)$$

Accordingly the CB element $S_{CB}(t)$ is shown in the equation (2) without high-frequency noise (more than 15 Hz) by averaging a current value $S_{LV}(t)$ and an adjacent value $S_{LV}(t - \Delta t)$ (Fig. 3).

$$S_{CB}(t) = \frac{S_{LV}(t) + S_{LV}(t - \Delta t)}{2} - S_{AR}(t) \qquad (2)$$

Furthermore, with the calculation of an average cardiac beating cycle T_{CB}, maximum and minimum values of $S_{CB}(t)$ (MAX_{CB} and MIN_{CB}) and of $S_{AR}(t)$ (MAX_{AR} and MIN_{AR}) can be registered automatically.

Timing determination of HIFU energy delivery. Duration of each HIFU energy delivery is set 1/3 of the average time of cardiac beating cycle and the delivery should

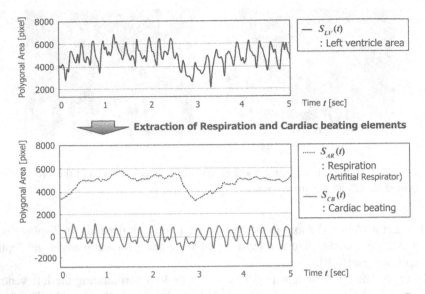

Fig. 3. Extraction of the respiration element ($S_{AR}(t)$) and the cardiac beating element ($S_{CB}(t)$) from the left ventricle polygonal area ($S_{LV}(t)$)

be triggered off from the moment when $S_{CB}(t)$ becomes a local minimal value in systolic period, or when the atrial septum is most stretched. The HIFU energy delivery is performed in real time (more than 25 frames/sec), although there is a certain time delay (total 69 ms) in the sequence of 2D-US image input (30 ms), rasterizing and image analysis (30 ms), and HIFU energy delivery signal output (9 ms). Therefore, the system needs a predictive control to cancel this time delay, which is shown by D. To estimate the HIFU energy delivery timing, which is shown by t_P, the system uses the moment t_M when $S_{CB}(t)$ achieves around the local maximal value. To determine the moment t_M, with a sampling interval of Δt, a current value $S_{CB}(t)$ and a difference value $\Delta S_{CB}(t)$ between $S_{CB}(t)$ and $S_{CB}(t - \Delta t)$ are used (Fig. 4). Next, t_P is estimated as $t_M + T_{CB}/2$ and HIFU energy delivery can be triggered from the moment $t_P - D$.

Furthermore, to avoid inadvertent HIFU deliveries caused by abnormal cardiac rhythms, unexpected target behavior, false recognitions in imaging analysis and so on, the HIFU energy delivery timing is constrained strictly by two boundary conditions with the tolerance range T_{CB} for $S_{CB}(t)$ and the tolerance range T_{AR} for $S_{AR}(t)$ (Fig. 5). In this study, T_{CB} is set $(MAX_{CB} - MIN_{CB}) \times 20\%$, and T_{AR} is set $(MAX_{AR} - MIN_{AR}) \times 30\%$.

3 Animal Experiments

All animal experiments were performed according to the institutional animal ethics guidelines, based on the guidelines of the National Institute of Health, USA[7].

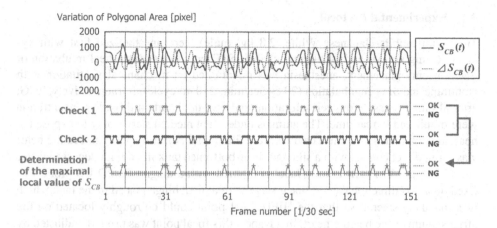

Fig. 4. Determination whether $S_{CB}(t)$ achieves around local maximal value or not. If $S_{CB}(t)$ comes close to MAX_{CB} enough (for example $S_{CB}(t) > MAX_{CB} \times 50\%$) (Check 1 is "OK") and if $\Delta S_{CB}(t)$ comes to 0 enough (for example $| \Delta S_{CB}(t) | < (MAX_{CB} - MIN_{CB}) \times 30\%$) (Check 2 is "OK"), that moment t is determined t_M.

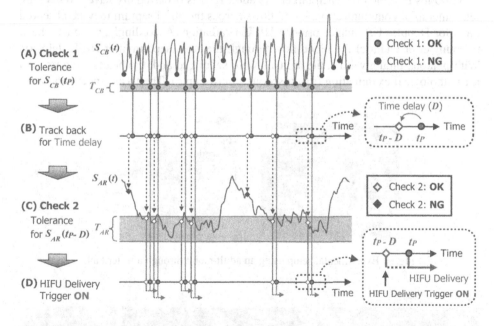

Fig. 5. Prevention of inadvertent HIFU energy delivery by means of two boundary conditions. (A) Check 1 for $S_{CB}(t_P)$: Whether $S_{CB}(t_P)$ falls in the tolerance range T_{CB} or not, that is $MIN_{CB} \leq S_{CB}(t_P) \leq MIN_{CB} + T_{CB}$. (B) If Check 1 is cleared, the moment $t_P - D$ is considered. (C) Check 2 for $S_{AR}(t_P - D)$: Whether $S_{AR}(t_P - D)$ falls in the tolerance range T_{AR} or not, that is $MIN_{AR} \leq S_{AR}(t_P - D) \leq MIN_{AR} + T_{AR}$. (D) If Check 2 is cleared, the HIFU energy delivery is triggered at the moment of $t_P - D$.

3.1   Experimental Protocol

Two adult rabbits (Japanese White, 2.8 kg, male) were anesthetized first with xy-lazine (5 mg/kg IM) and isoflurane inhalation. Then, after endotracheal intubation or tracheostomy placement, anesthesia was maintained on mechanical ventilation with isoflurane and oxygen inhalation (20 cycles/min, 240 ml/cycle). Intraoperatively, ECG, arterial blood pressure/oxygen saturation, and end-tidal carbon dioxide concentration were monitored in real time. The animals underwent median sternotomy to expose the heart and, on both sides, chest cavities were filled with buffering gel. The beating heart was set in direct contact with a silicone sheet-bottomed tank filled with degassed water (37°C) (Fig. 6). A HIFU transducer combined with a diagnostic 2D-US probe was fixed on a two-directional (x-y) linear stage with a pivot hinge placed in the tank which was manually steered so that the HIFU focal point could be roughly located on the atrial septum of the beating heart. In advance, this focal point was properly adjusted by simulated polymer-coated rubber irradiation using the same system (Acoustic standoff, Eastek Corporation, Tokyo, Japan). Fig. 7 shows the coagulated ellipsoid focal point (5-mm long, 2-mm wide) along with its focal length of 30-mm. Both could be visualized on the 2D-US images and marked in the console. HIFU energy delivery time amounted to 3,000 ms in a total for each target. As adult rabbits occasionally have a remaining fetal interatrial communication, blood flows across the atrial septum may be observed on color Doppler US images prior to HIFU irradiation. Accordingly, we must check the number or width of the blood flow through the atrial septum after HIFU delivery. With pentobarbital given IV, the animals were sacrificed and, the hearts were excised for pathological examination (macroscopic, microscopic). The tissue specimens were

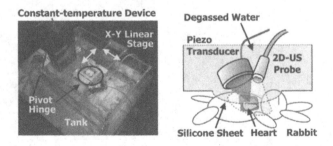

Fig. 6. Experimental setup using an adult rabbit through a water tank

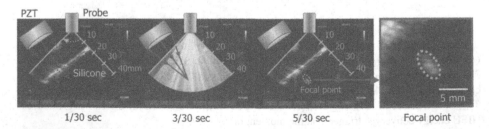

Fig. 7. The focal point is adjusted with a test HIFU energy delivery to the polymer-coated rubber

fixed with 10% neutral formalin and embedded in paraffin. Thereafter, sections of 10 μm thickness were stained with hematoxylin-eosin (HE) for microscopic studies.

3.2 Results

In the first animal, HIFU was delivered in a total of 26 times with each delivery time of 115 ms over a total of 23 seconds for treatment. Due to an inadvertent mistargeting, the atrial septum failed to be ablated and, instead, a small opening was made in the posterior wall of the left atrium with a blood flow through there was visualized with color Doppler US during the experiment. Fig. 8 shows the gross appearance of the ablated portion. Based on the microscopic study (B) of the stained section (C), we confirmed that a small area was definitely coagulated with a resultant small transmural opening. The opening was located just behind the atrial septum along the assumed axial direction of the HIFU beam and its focal point. In the second animal experiment, 23 HIFU deliveries were carried out for a total of 57 seconds with each delivery time of 130 ms. Although the pulsating atrial septum could be autotracked and targeted precisely by our system, the atrial septum apparently remained non-penetrated with mere transmural

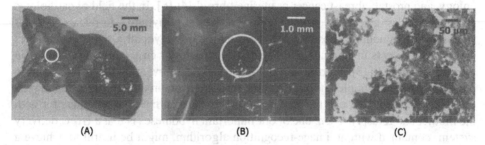

Fig. 8. Heart specimen ablated with HIFU (first animal). (A) Gross appearance of the inadvertent ablation with an opening. (B) Magnification of the area opened by HIFU irradiation. Both pictures (A, B) represent the opening of the left atrial posterior wall. (C) Microscopic findings of the ablated area (H-E stain). Coagulation changes are seen unlike the surrounding normal area.

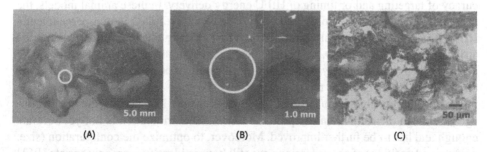

Fig. 9. Heart specimen ablated with HIFU (second animal). (A) Gross appearance of the inadvertent ablation with an opening. (B) Magnification of the area opened by HIFU irradiation. Both pictures (A, B) represent just transmural coagulation changes of the targeted atrial septum. (C) Microscopic findings of the ablated area (H-E stain). Coagulation changes are clearly found.

coagulation changes on gross appearance. It is suggested that the HIFU energy transfer was somehow reduced because it took longer to finish HIFU delivery than in the first one. When interval time of each HIFU delivery was too long, heated tissue at the focal point might be cooled down by intracardiac blood flow. Macroscopic view of the excised tissue is shown in Fig. 9. Assumingly, improvements in HIFU delivery parameters will settle the problems because a precise autotargeting was successfully achieved in our study.

4   Discussion

In this report, we demonstrated that our computer-aided HIFU delivery system, coupled with a newly developed real-time image-recognition algorithm, could create defects in the pulsating tissues of within beating hearts of anesthetized adult rabbits. Furthermore, the procedure could be expected to affect just a restricted targeted area without impairing adjacent tissues. Then, we believe that the computer-aided HIFU delivery system will contribute to developing minimally invasive correction of intracardiac abnormalities including those of fetal and pediatric patients.

In recent years, HIFU has been explored as a therapeutic modality in urology, oncology, and prostatic/breast cancer or uterine fibroids[4]-[6]. In the field of cardiology, HIFU was investigated as a promising device to treat arrhythmia, to release valvular stenosis and to ameliorate obstructive hypertrophic cardiomyopathy. HIFU also enables us to create defects in cardiac tissues such as ventricles or cusp of the aortic valve *in vitro* or *ex vivo*[8]-[13]. Worthy of note, fetal cardiac intervention has been shown to potentially prevent simple fetal cardiac abnormalities from in utero progression to serious heart diseases, although the procedure still remains an invasive technique for both the mother and fetus[1]. Then, one of our important hypotheses is that a HIFU delivery system, combined with an image-recognition algorithm, might be useful to achieve a safer, faster, and less expensive fetal procedure.

We conducted our HIFU experiment to affect intracardiac structures *in vivo* using two adult rabbits and their microscopic examination showed that all areas irradiated with HIFU presented with restricted coagulation changes with or without making a transmural opening. Our results of the experiment are not yet satisfactory in terms of accuracy of targeting and/or timing of HIFU energy delivery. In these animal models, the heart might have been malpositioned (or rotated) which resulted in non-perpendicular HIFU irradiation to the atrial septum or the HIFU focal point inadvertently set at the atrial free wall. Accordingly, we believe that creation of atrial septal defects could be accomplished more precisely with careful device/animal positioning and adjusting the direction of HIFU delivery more appropriately. For this purpose, we developed the image-recognition algorithm/software based on real-time 2D sonographic cardiac images, although the estimation of optimally timed HIFU irradiation is not yet accurate enough and has to be further improved. Moreover, to optimize the configuration (size, volume and position) of ablated lesions, we still have to identify more appropriate HIFU delivery parameters including HIFU frequency, focal depth, ratio between aperture size and focal depth, size or shape of focal point, and duration of HIFU irradiation[12]. In fact, Zhen et al. suggested that the ablation should be better performed by pulsed ultrasound. Strickberger et al. reported that ECG-triggered HIFU delivery could effectively treat experimental arrhythmia[13]. In addition about accurate positioning of the focal point, Koizumi et al. presented HIFU irradiation with a pair of 2D-US imaging probes and XYZ positioning mechanism for 3D-tracking system[14].

In our experiment, another prospective biological limitation is that the experimental animals had normal hearts. In pathological conditions with intracardiac abnormalities, the cardiac structure including the atrial septum is occasionally hypertrophied. Accordingly, before employing the HIFU for clinical intervention, it is necessary to test the effects of HIFU using pathologic animal models.

In conclusion, the HIFU irradiation, combined with newly developed computer-aided algorithm/software, is expected to be feasible for correcting intracardiac abnormalities in beating hearts. This outcome suggests that even the current fetal cardiac intervention is likely to further advance to much less invasive one employing an integrated and sophisticated HIFU system.

Acknowledgments. A part of this work is supported by Grant Program for Child Health and Development "Minimally Invasive Techniques for Fetal Surgery (16-3)" administrated by Ministry of Health, Labour and Welfare of Japan.

References

1. Kohl, T., Sharland, G., Allan, L.D., Gembruch, U., Chaoui, R., Lopes, L.M., Zielinsky, P., Huhta, J., Silverman, N.H.: World experience of percutaneous ultrasound-guided balloon valvuloplasty in human fetuses with severe aortic valve obstruction. Am. J. Cardiol. 85, 1230–1233 (2000)
2. Marshall, A.C., van der Velde, M.E., Tworetzky, W., Gomez, C.A., Wilkins-Haung, L., Benson, C.B., Jennings, R.W., Lock, J.E.: Creation of an atrial septal defect in utero for fetuses with hypoplastic left heart syndrome and intact or highly restrictive atrial septum. Circulation 110, 253–258 (2004)
3. Makikallio, K., McElhinney, D.B., Levine, J.C., Marx, G.R., Colan, S.D., Marshall, A.C., Lock, J.E., Marcus, E.N., Tworetzky, W.: Fetal Aortic valve stenosis and the evolution of hypoplastic left heart syndrome patient selection for fetal intervention. Circulation 113, 1401–1405 (2006)
4. Rebillard, X., Gelet, A., Davin, J.L., Soulie, M., Prapotnich, D., Cathelineau, X., Rozet, F., Vallancien, G.: Transrectal high-intensity focused ultrasound in the treatment of localized prostate cancer. J. Endourol. 19(6), 693–701 (2005)
5. Chan, A.H., Fujimoto, V.Y., Moore, D.E., Martin, R.W., Vaezy, S.: An image-guided high intensity focused ultrasound device for uterine fibroids treatment. Med. Phys. 29(11), 2611 (2002)
6. Hengst, S.A., Ehrenstein, T., Herzog, H., Beck, A., Utz-Billing, I., David, M., Felix, R., Ricke, J.: Magnetic resonance tomography guided focused ultrasound surgery (MRgFUS) in tumor therapy?anew noninvasive therapy option. Radiologe 44(4), 339–346 (2004)
7. U.S. Department of Health and Human Services, Public Health Service, National Institutes of Health. Guide for the care and use of laboratory animals, pp. 85-23. NIH Publication (1985)
8. Otsuka, R., Fujikura, K., Hirata, K., Pulerwitz, T., Oe, Y., Suzuki, T., Sciacca, R., Marboe, C., Wang, J., Burkhoff, D., Muratore, R., Lizzi, F.L., Homma, S.: In vitro ablation of cardiac valves using high-intensity focused ultrasound. Ultrasound in Med. & Biol. 31(1), 109–114 (2005)

9. Fujikura, K., Otsuka, R., Kalisz, A., Ketterling, J.A., Jin, Z., Sciacca, R.R., Marboe, C.C., Wang, J., Muratore, R., Feleppa, E.J., Homma, S.: Effects of ultrasonic exposure parameters on myocardial lesions induced by high-intensity focused ultrasound. J. Ultrasound Med. 25, 1375–1386 (2006)

10. Lee, L.A., Simon, C., Bove, L.E., Mosca, R.S., Ebbini, E.S., Abrams, G.D., Ludomirsky, A.: High intensity focused ultrasound effect on cardiac tissues: Potential for Clinical application. Echocardiography 17(6), 563–566 (2000)

11. Xu, Z., Ludmirsky, A., Eun, L.Y., Hall, T.L., Tran, B.C., Fowlkes, J.B., Cain, C.A.: Controlled ultrasound tissue erosion. IEEE transactions on ultrasonics, ferroelectrics, and frequency control 51(6), 726–736 (2004)

12. Kluiwstra, J.U.A., Tokano, T., Davis, J., Strickberger, S.A., Cain, C.A.: Real time image guided high intensity focused ultrasound for myocardial ablation: In Vivo study. In: IEEE Ultrasonics Symposium, vol. 1327 (2007)

13. Strickberger, S.A., Tokano, T., Kluiwstra, J.U.A., Morady, F., Cain, C.: Extracardiac ablation of the canine atrioventricular junction by use of high-intensity focused ultrasound. Circulation 100, 203–208 (1999)

14. Koizumi, N., Ota, K., Lee, D., Yoshizawa, S., Ito, A., Kaneko, Y., Yoshinaka, K., Matsumoto, Y., Mitsuishi, M.: Feed-forward controller for the integrated non-invasive ultrasound diagnosis and treatment. J. Robotics and Mechatronics 20(1), 89–97 (2008)

Basic Study on Real-Time Simulation Using Mass Spring System for Robotic Surgery

Kazuya Kawamura, Yo Kobayashi, and Masakatsu G. Fujie

2-2 03C201 Wakamatu-cho, Shinjuku-ku, Tokyo, Japan
{kazuya_k.fmr, you-k}@fuji.waseda.jp, mgfujie@waseda.jp

Abstract. Medical technology has advanced with the introduction of robot technology, making previous medical treatments that were very difficult far more possible. However, operation of a surgical robot demands substantial training and continual practice on the part of the surgeon because it requires difficult techniques that are different from those of traditional surgical procedures. So we focused on a simulation technology based on the physical characteristics of organs as an intra-operative assistance for a surgeon. In this research, we proposed the development of surgical simulation, using a physical model, for intra-operative navigation. In this paper, we describe the design of our proposed system, in particular our organ deformation calculator. We performed two experiments with pig liver and silicone model to evaluate the accuracy of the calculator. We obtained adequate experimental results of a target node at a nearby point of interaction, because this point ensures better accuracy for our simulation model.

Keywords: robotic surgery, real-time simulation, organ deformation, MSD.

1 Introduction

Robots have been introduced into the medical domain to make operations more precise and reduce the burden on patients. Medical technology has advanced with the introduction of this robot technology, making it possible to use previously difficult or impossible medical treatments. In clinical cases, the latest medical technologies, such as da Vinci® surgical system and Zeus® (Intuitive Surgical Inc.), have been indispensable. Applying these surgical robots in the medical domain has allowed doctors to achieve the aim of reducing the burden on patients.

However, operating a surgical robot demands substantial training and continual practice for the surgeon because it requires difficult techniques that differ from traditional surgical procedures. This problem adds to the surgeon's already heavy workload during surgery. In addition, during minimally invasive surgery, the visual and tactile information of organs that surgeon obtained directly during traditional surgery is restricted. So an assisting system is required to overcome this restriction.

In recent years, assisting systems have been developed that depend on simulation technology with a computer. The latest enhancements of information technology have improved computer capability and have allowed reproduction of a surgical

T. Dohi, I. Sakuma, and H. Liao (Eds.): MIAR 2008, LNCS 5128, pp. 311–319, 2008.

environment in virtual space. This virtual surgical environment can be applied to find new ways of training surgeons in surgical tasks. Because of the configurability and repeatability of a surgical environment, this assisting system in virtual space on a computer is most appropriate for this training. These simulation technologies enable corroboration with medical imaging diagnostic systems such as MRI. So this simulation also can be applied to pre-operative planning.

2   Motivation

In robotic surgery, information of the conditions of target organs such as stress state is indispensable because minimum invasive surgery using a robot is required of a surgeon. A simulation applicable to medical domains allows estimating the conditions of target organs. Therefore, the surgical simulation enables the presentation of intra-operative information in real time to a surgeon and a surgical assisting robot. However, surgical procedures most often entail modifying a patient's macroscopic tissue structure. Cutting, tearing, and carving are some of the most common tasks that surgeons perform in both traditional surgery and robotic surgery.

A surgical simulation that presents intra-operative information must accommodate the change in the conditions of target organs based on such surgical tasks during surgery. While the ability to quickly simulate and accommodate the change in a target's condition such as a deformation of soft tissue is important, a system that does not include the capability to modify the simulated tissue has limited utility. So, we focused on a simulation technology using the physical characteristics of organs. In this research, our purpose was to develop a surgical simulation system based on a physical model for a surgeon's intra-operative navigation (Fig.1).

In this paper, we will describe the design of our system, in particular our organ deformation calculator. Section 3 presents the design of our surgical simulation system. Section 4 discusses organ deformation architecture and one experiment. Section 5 explains another evaluation of the calculator. And Section 6 gives a summary and our plans for future work.

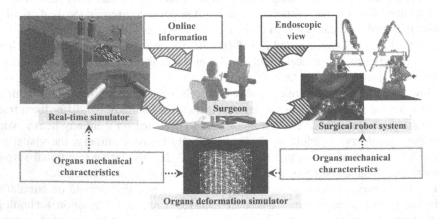

Fig. 1. Concept overview

3 Design of Surgical Simulation System

3.1 Simulation System Concept

Surgical simulation is a graphical application that requires real-time interaction with deformable objects. The surgical environment depends on surgical tools, characteristics of target organs, and individual difference in the physical properties of organs. In addition to incorporating these aspects of the surgical environment, a surgical assisting system also must allow the surgeon to interact with virtual soft tissue. Therefore, a requirement for developing efficient models of soft tissues is that realistic simulation of tool–tissue interaction can be performed in real time.

Among the potential applications of deformable objects, soft tissue modeling is one of the most demanding because of the complexity of tissue mechanics. From a purely mechanistic point of view, soft tissues exhibit complex material properties. They are nonlinear, anisotropic, visco-elastic, and non-homogeneous. Soft tissues deform considerably under the application of relatively small loads. In addition, it is quite difficult to obtain material properties of tissues in vivo. Pre-operative procedures such as surgical planning are required to reproduce tissue properties as accurately as possible to predict a surgery's exact outcome; the computation time is a negligible factor. In intra-operative surgical simulation, however, a tradeoff has to be considered. Computational issues should be examined to allow physical simulation in real time; on the other hand, the model must be realistic enough to allow practitioners to acquire relevant surgical skills.

The most commonly used methods to simulate organ deformation are the mass-spring system and the finite element model. The mass-spring system is allows calculating the displacement and reaction force of organs with low computational effort. The mass-spring system can achieve online calculation but cannot accurately calculate the precise behavior of organs because it cannot use such tools as the coefficient of elasticity and Poisson's ratio[1-2]. A finite element model allows the rendering of the mechanical properties for calculating the behavior of organs, but it requires high computational effort [3-10]. Some researchers have used unique models [11-14]. Our group have reported several research efforts for organ modeling and some applications, for example, material properties of the liver [15-16], identification of material parameter of an organ model using FEM and EKF [17], positional control of a deflected needle tip[18], stress control method using an FEM based stress observer[19], stress evaluation of the brain for surgical navigation using a 2D-Finite Element Method (FEM) organ model [20], an MSS based organ model for intra-surgical navigation [21].

In this research, we aimed to construct an information assist system for presenting the intra-operative condition of organs in real time. Therefore, we first focused on not accurate but real-time calculation. Thus, we employed a mass-spring system as the method of organs deformation. Before the development of this real-time simulator, we constructed the virtual tools for real-time interaction with a deformable object.

3.2 Virtual Slave Simulator

A slave simulator that is moved with a material master manipulator in real time was initially constructed to verify the control methods suited for robotic surgery and to reproduce surgical tools such as forceps. Specifications and the configuration of this simulation system, as well as an overview of the simulator, are shown in Fig. 2.

3.3 Organs Deformation Calculator

An organ deformation simulation requires real-time calculation to support a time-oriented environment. In this research, to obtain more real-time quantitative calculations than possible with FEM, the Mass-Spring-Damper (MSD) method was adopted as a calculation technique for reproducing dynamic characteristics such as deformation of internal organs. A three-element model was adopted as a model to represent visco-elasticity (the dynamic character of the organs) with the MSD method, and a lattice-shaped model was developed as the prototype simulator (Fig.3). The prototype model includes 196 nodes and 897 edges.

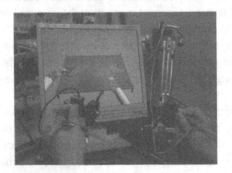
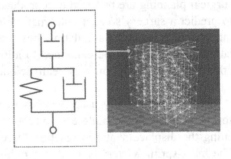

Fig. 2. Virtual slave manipulator [21-22]   **Fig. 3.** Simulation Model

4   Organ Deformation Calculation

In our research, we developed a real-time simulation using the physical properties of organs, to obtain the intra-operative conditions of organs such as deformation and stress state. This prototype model uses the MSD method to simulate deformation. This method enables us to make calculations in real-time and to apply those calculations to a broad range of surgical interactions such as gripping and cutting.

4.1 Organs-Deformation Model

Mass-spring systems are one of the physical based methods that have been proven effective for modeling deformable objects. In our research, the target was modeled as a collection of point masses connected by a three-element model in a lattice structure (Fig. 3). This model is a Voigt model and a damper model connected in series. In addition, this model demonstrates the creep characteristics of visco-elastic objects. In a dynamic system, Newton's second law governs the motion of a single mass point in the lattice:

$$m_i \ddot{x}_i = \sum f_{internal} + f_{external} \tag{1}$$

$$\sum f_{internal} = -\gamma_i \dot{x}_i - k_i x_i \tag{2}$$

where m_i is the mass of the point, x_i is its position, and $f_{internal}$ is the force exerted on mass i by three-element model between mass i and j, and $f_{external}$ is the sum of other external forces. The $f_{internal}$ is the sum of the force of elasticity and viscosity Each parameter of viscosity γ_i and elasticity k_i was provided from the results of characteristics measured with a rheometer.

4.2 Evaluation of the Calculator

In our research, we aimed to develop an assisting system for surgeons during robotic surgery. A surgeon uses various procedures for treatment purposes depending on the situation. Surgical procedures consist of gripping, cutting, tearing, and so on. In our research, we focused on the gripping motion since it is the most commonly used motion during surgery. Gripping consists of indentation and tension motion. Therefore, in our research, we performed an indentation experiment and a tension experiment to evaluate the performance of our simulator. In this paper, we present the indentation experiment.

4.3 Experimental Conditions

Using an organ deformation calculator, we performed an indentation experiment using silicone, because of its well-known deformation characteristics. We evaluated the results of displacement and reaction force of both the silicone and the deformation model. In this experiment, the silicone and simulation model were compressed by a slave manipulator (Fig.4). During this experiment, the deformation of the silicone was measured using a pattern-matching method, and the reaction force was measured using a force sensor on the tip of the slave manipulator.

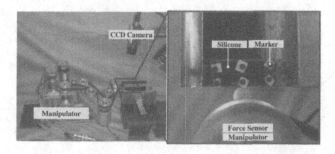

Fig. 4. Experimental conditions using slave manipulator[21]

4.4 Experimental Result and Discussion

In surgery, the interaction area between surgical tools and target organs is the most important area. A target node at a nearby interaction point has a large deformation, and a target node far from an interaction point has a small deformation. The deformation volume becomes smaller that farther the target node is from an interaction point. So, we focused on the neighborhood of an interaction point to evaluate the deformation (Fig. 5). The result of node displacement is in Fig. 6, and the result of reaction force is in Fig.7. Displacement overshoot was confirmed by the external load when the deformation of the simulation model followed a silicone model. This result demonstrated that the elasticity of the simulation model has greater influence than the silicone on the deformation. The graphs in Fig. 6 and Fig. 7 show that there is a slight overshoot in both node displacement and reaction force between the simulation results and the experimental results. These results were seen as adequate in this research, because the nearby point of interaction ensures better accuracy in the simulation model in terms of the error from the reference value. Before simulating the interaction between tools and organs for online information, we showed the validity of the action in the nearby interaction area. A little overshoot was confirmed, but we dealt with it by adjusting a coefficient to set up in the model and a model-type. Therefore, we demonstrated that the prototype simulation model in this research is adequate to use as a presentation method of intra-operative information.

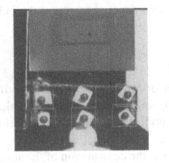
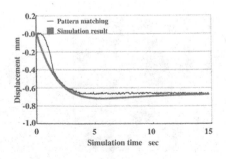

Target point of evaluation

Fig. 5. Experiment overview and target model scale

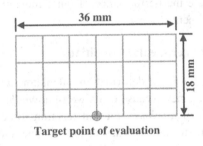
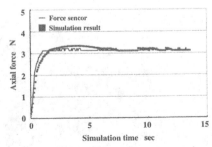
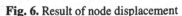

Fig. 6. Result of node displacement   **Fig. 7.** Result of reaction force

5 Experiment the Calculator with Pig Liver

5.1 Experimental Method and Condition

We performed a tensile experiment with a pig liver to evaluate the organ deformation calculator. The experimental condition of this tensile experiment is under the constant velocity using a linear motor (Fig.8 and Fig.9). We evaluated the results of reaction force of the pig liver and deformation model. During this experiment, the deformation of the pig liver is measured using pattern matching method and reaction force is measured using force sensor on the tip of the linear motor. In this experiment, we set the pig liver to edge face ("A" in Fig.8).

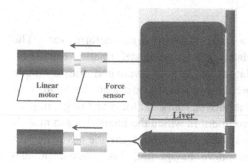
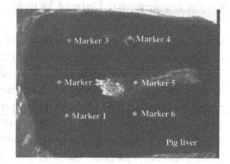

Fig. 8. Experimental Tool and Condition   **Fig. 9.** Marker layout

5.2 Experimental Results and Discussion

The results of the tensile experiment with pig liver are shown in Fig.10 and Fig.11. In Fig.10, Vertical axis is displacement of the marker and horizontal axis is simulation time. In Fig.11, Vertical axis is reaction force from the pig liver and horizontal axis is simulation time. In surgery, the interaction area between surgical tools and target organs is the most important area. A target node at a nearby interaction point has a large deformation, and a target node far from an interaction point has a small deformation. The deformation volume becomes smaller that farther the target node is from an interaction point.

Compared to the result of force sensor, this simulation could simulate the reaction force within the range of small deformation. But the reaction force was confirmed the difference between force sensor and simulation within the range of large deformation. This result demonstrated that non-linearity of the pig liver has greater larger than the simulation model. In this experiment, we dealt with it by adjusting a coefficient to set up in the model and a model-type. Therefore, we demonstrated that the prototype simulation model in this research is adequate to use as a presentation method of intra-operative information even in the case of the pig liver.

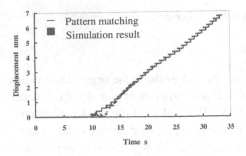

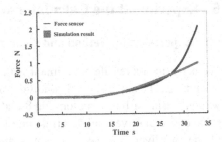

Fig. 10. Comparison of displacement   **Fig. 11.** Comparison of force

6 Summary and Future Work

We presented our simulation system for a basic study of organ deformation. The system consists of a virtual slave manipulator and an organ deformation calculator. The accuracy of our three-element simulation model was evaluated with a simple indentation test. As a result of these experiments, we demonstrated the validity of model accuracy at a nearby interaction point between surgical tools and target organs. The next step is to focus on a surgical environment in which the internal organ models could be integrated into a slave simulation system. This would provide advantages in force feedback, surgical training, intra-operative navigation, risk assessment, and other aspects.

Acknowledgement. This work was supported in part by "the robotic medical technology cluster in Gifu prefecture," Knowledge Cluster Initiative, Ministry of Education, Culture, Sports, Science and Technology, was supported in part by the 21st Century Center of Excellence (COE) Program "The innovative research on symbiosis technologies for human and robots in the elderly dominated society", Waseda University, Tokyo, and was (partly) supported by "Establishment of Consolidated Research Institute for Advanced Science and Medical Care", Encouraging Development Strategic Research Centers Program, the Special Coordination Funds for Promoting Science and Technology, Ministry of Education, Culture, Sports, Science and Technology, Japan.

References

1. Bielser, D., Gross, M.H.: Open surgery simulation. In: Proceedings of Medicine Meets Virtual Reality 2002 (January 2002)
2. Suzuki, N., Hattori, A., Kai, S., Ezumi, T., Takatsu, A.: Surgical planning system for soft tissues using virtual reality. In: MMVR5, pp. 159–163 (1997)
3. Costa, F., Bakaniuk, R.: LEM -An approach for real time physically based soft tissue. In: Proceedings 2001 IEEE International Conference on Robotics and Automation, pp. 2337–2343 (2001)

4. Hutter, R., et al.: Mechanical modeling of soft biological tissues for application in virtual reality based laparoscopy simulators. Technol. Health Care 8(1), 15–24 (2000)
5. Gladstone, H.B., et al.: Virtual reality for dermatologic surgery. Virtually a reality in the 21st century. J. Am. Acad. Dermatol. 42(1 pt 1), 106–112 (2000)
6. Liu, W., et al.: A mechanical model to determine the influence of masses and mass distribution on impact force during running. J. Biomech. 33(2), 219–224 (2000)
7. Miller, K.: Constitutive modeling of abdominal organs. J. Biomech. 33(3), 367–373 (2000)
8. Cotin, S., et al.: Real-time elastic deformations of soft tissues for surgery simulation. IEEE Transaction Visual Computer Graphics 5(1), 62–73 (1999)
9. Delingette, H., et al.: Efficient linear elastic models of soft tissues for real-time surgery simulation. Study Health Technology Information 62, 100–101 (1999)
10. Berkley, J., et al.: Fast finite element modeling for surgical simulation. In: MMVR7, pp. 55–61 (1999)
11. Suzuki, N., et al.: Performing virtual surgery with a force feedback system. In: The eight international conference on artificial reality and telexistence, pp. 182–187 (1998)
12. Marwscaux, J., et al.: Virtual reality applied to hepatic surgery simulation. The next revolution Ann. Surg. 228(5), 627–634 (1998)
13. Gibson, S., et al.: Simulating surgery using volumetric object representations, real-time volume rendering and haptic feedback. Medical Image Analysis 2(2), 121–132 (1998)
14. Cotin, S., et al.: Geometric and physical representations for a simulator of hepatic surgery. Health Care in the Information Age, pp. 139–151 (1996)
15. Kobayashi, Y., et al.: Physical Properties of the Liver for Needle Insertion Control. In: IEEE International Conference on Intelligent Robotics and Systems, pp. 2960–2966 (2004)
16. Kobayashi, Y., et al.: Physical Properties of the Liver and the Development of an Intelligent Manipulator for Needle Insertion. In: IEEE International Conference on Robotics and Automation, pp. 1644–1651 (2005)
17. Hoshi, T., Kobayashi, Y., Kawamura, K., Fujie, M.G.: Developing an Intraoperative Methodology Using the Finite Element Method and Extended Kalman Filter to Identify the Material Parameter of an Organ Model. In: 29th conference of IEEE Engineering in Medicine and Biology Society (2007)
18. Kobayashi, Y., Onishi, A., Hoshi, T., Kawamura, K., Fujie, M.G.: Viscoelastic and Nonlinear Organ Model for Control of Needle Insertion Manipulator. In: 29th Conference of IEEE Engineering in Medicine and Biology Society (in press, 2007)
19. Kobayashi, Y., Hoshi, T., Kawamura, K., Fujie, M.G.: Control Method for Surgical Robot to Prevent Overload at Vulnerable Tissue. In: IEEE International Conference on Robotics and Automation (2007)
20. Yoshizawa, A., Okamoto, J., Yamakawa, H., Fujie, M.G.: Robot Surgery based on the Physical Properties of the Brain-Physical Brain Model for Planning and Navigation of a Surgical Robot. In: IEEE International Conference on Robotics and Automation, pp. 916–923 (2005)
21. Kawamura, K., Kobayashi, Y., Fujie, M.G.: Development of Real-time Simulation for Workload Quantification in Robotic Tele-surgery. In: Proceedings of the 2006 IEEE International Conference of Robotics and Biomimetics, pp. 1420–1425 (2006)
22. Toyoda, K., Umeda, T., Oura, M., Iwamori, Y., Kawamura, K., Kabayashi, Y., Okayasu, H., Okamoto, J., Fujie, M.G.: Dexterous master-slave surgical robot for minimally invasive surgery-Intuitive interface and interchangeable surgical instruments. In: Proc. of the 20th International Congress and Exhibition, Computer Assisted Radiology and Surgery CARS 2006, pp. 503–504 (2005)

A Precise Robotic Ablation and Division Mechanism for Liver Resection

Florence Leong[1,*], Liangjing Yang[1], Stephen Chang[2], Aun Neow Poo[1], Ichiro Sakuma[3], and Chee-Kong Chui[1]

[1] Department of Mechanical Engineering, National University of Singapore, Singapore
g0700886@nus.edu.sg
[2] Department of Surgery, National University Hospital, Singapore
[3] Department of Precision Engineering, The University of Tokyo, Tokyo, Japan

Abstract. Radiofrequency Ablation (RFA) assisted liver resection results in lesser blood loss during liver resections. It involves a time consuming and error prone process of alternating coagulation and cutting until the line of transaction is completed to finally divide the liver. We proposed a new robotic mechanism to automate the ablation and division process. The robotic device comprises a 2-link manipulator, an x-y translator, a flexi-arm as well as a liver ablation and division device. The process of precise linear motion ablation and cutting has been integrated with the guidance of a robotic mechanism to uniformly coagulate and slit areas of the parenchymal. A prototype of the robotic device has been evaluated on its ability to uniformly target a large region.

Keywords: Surgical robot, RF ablation, needle insertion, liver division, liver.

1 Introduction

Liver cancer is one of the leading sources of cancerous death around the world, ranking at the fourth place. As reported by The World Health Organization, in year 2002, there were approximately 618,000 deaths for one million new cases of patients with liver cancer [1]. Much research has been done over the past few decades to seek suitable interventions and cures. Hepatic or liver resection is a preferred treatment world wide [2]. There are however several problems with liver resections. Bleeding during liver division is the most significant problem.

The ablation technologies comprising radiofrequency (RF) ablation or RFA, microwave ablation, and laser coagulation therapy have recently been the preferred option for many liver resection cases [3]. The RFA process has the advantage over the others as tissue can be coagulated at the needle insertion area [4]. The RFA technique can be performed during open surgery, during laparoscopy, or percutaneously through a small incision in the skin [3, 5, 6]. RFA involves the use of high-frequency alternating currents which produce ionic agitation flowing through the needles attached to the probes. When the liver tissue heats up, coagulation necrosis occurs [6]. RF ablation can also be used to assist in liver resection because of its ability to create an avascular

---

[*] Corresponding author.

T. Dohi, I. Sakuma, and H. Liao (Eds.): MIAR 2008, LNCS 5128, pp. 320–328, 2008.

plane. In RF ablation assisted liver resection; the liver parenchyma is first coagulated with RF ablation. The surgeon then uses a separate cutting mechanism to cut within the coagulated tissue to divide the liver. This alternating coagulation and cutting step is continued until the line of transaction is completed to finally divide the liver. There is a need to ensure that there will be no void space between successive ablations. The liver parenchyma is thick, and cannot be completely coagulated in a single attempt. It is also difficult to estimate how deep the avascular plane is after coagulation. The laborious process of coagulation and cutting is prone to error and time consuming. Hence, there is a need for a medical robotic device to assist the surgeon in performing the task. As to further assist the liver resection process, the development of a single bio-electromechanical instrument to coagulate and cut ablated liver tissue is desirable. This will help eliminate the risk of bleeding due to over cutting, and time loss due to re-ablation of coagulated areas.

This paper describes a robotic mechanism designed to perform the alternating ablation and cutting process. Section 2 elaborates on the robotic ablation and division mechanism developed with an overview on the kinematics studies, while Section 3 briefly describes the proposed integration of RFA and the division mechanism into a single device. Section 4 presents the experimental methodology and a brief discussion on the results obtained. Lastly, a review of future work is provided in Section 5 in addition to the summary of this paper.

2 Robotic Ablation and Division Mechanism

The positioning mechanism of the robotic device proposed here is a 7 DOF (degrees-of-freedom) articulated arm that consists of three components: a 2-link structure, an x-y linear translator and an octopus-flexi arm. Figure 1(a) shows the computational 3-dimensional solid CAD (Computational-Aided Design) model and Figure 1(b) is a prototype of the robotic device constructed according to this model. It is a passive device. We are developing a second prototype that will enable all the joints to be locked in position with a single tightening action.

The robotic mechanism can be attached to the operating table via a base clamp. The x-y linear translator at the proximal end of the 2-link structure is used to provide precise and very fine translational motion. The octopus-flexi arm is connected to the adapter piece fixed onto the x-y translator assembly. The end-effector of the robotic mechanism holds a guiding plate which in turn holds the RFA needle for RFA assisted liver resection, as well as our proposed instrument for combined ablation and division. Insertion and cutting is done by a motorized module.

Figure 1(c) is an illustration of the operation of the robotic device. After a line of division is identified, the manipulator inserts the RFA needle into the liver organ. After ablation, the RFA needle is withdrawn and moved to the next ablation location. This precise movement is achieved via the x-y translator assembly. After the line of division is ablated, the RFA needle is replaced by a knife. The knife is inserted into the liver organ at the end of division line and cuts the organ along the ablated division line in the reverse direction.

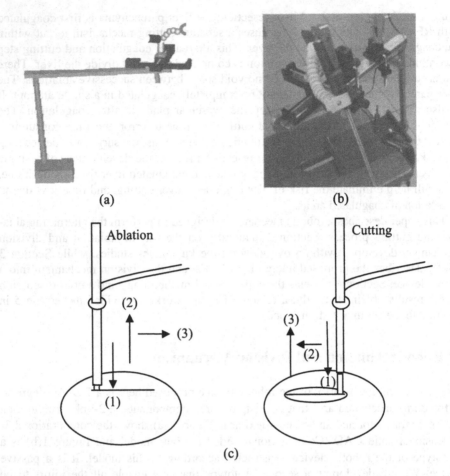

Fig. 1. Overview of robotic device for ablation and cutting: (a) 3 dimensional CAD model of the positioning mechanism, (b) prototype robotic device, (c) illustration of robotic device operation. The numbers in parenthesis indicate the operation sequence.

2.1 Kinematic Analysis

A conservative estimate of the workspace for RFA treatment sufficient to cover the entire liver will be a planar area of 180 mm by 180 mm assuming the insertion trajectory to be vertical. The prototype device described above can cover a circular plane of radius 350 mm for vertical insertions. Hence, any point on the liver organ can theoretically be reached by the device. The kinematics of the manipulator can be represented by a transformation matrix. The link parameters are tabulated in Table 1. Frames and link parameters are assigned based on the Denavit-Hartenberg (D-H) convention.

With reference to the schematic diagram of the robot-guided mechanism depicted in Figure 2, Frame 0 being the base of the passive robot links, the transformation is extended till Frame 5, which is the x-y translator adapted with the octopus flex arm.

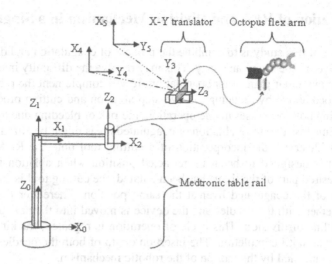

Fig. 2. Schematic diagram of the robot guided mechanism

Table 1. D-H parameters derived from the schematic diagram

	θ	r	d	α
$^0T_1$	0	l_1	0	0
$^1T_2$	0	0	l_2	0
$^2T_3$	q_3	0	0	90
$^3T_4$	90	t_1	0	90
$^4T_5$	0	t_2	0	0

The parameters of the robotic mechanism are as shown in the D-H parameter table in Table 1 in which l_1 and l_2 are the lengths of Link 1 and Link 2 respectively, and t_1 and t_2 are the movement of the x- and the y-axis of the x-y translator respectively. This information is required in deriving the kinematic transformation matrix, from the base to the end-effector, for structure manipulation analysis. The corresponding lengths, heights and angles are as listed, with the restrain of the X-Y translator at -50 mm < t_1 < 50 mm and -50 mm < t_2 < 50 mm in the horizontal and vertical directions respectively.

The transformation matrix is given by

$$^0T_5 = \begin{bmatrix} 0 & s_{12} & c_{12} & t_2c_{12}+t_1s_{12}+l_2c_1 \\ 0 & -c_{12} & s_{12} & t_2s_{12}-t_1c_{12}+l_2s_1 \\ 1 & 0 & 0 & l_1 \\ 0 & 0 & 0 & 1 \end{bmatrix}. \tag{1}$$

where c_i and s_i are the cosines and sines, respectively, of angle rotations of Link i of the robotic mechanism.

For any given values of the angles and lengths, the location of the octopus-flexi arm alongside with the RFA and cutting device which holds onto it can be determined.

3 Integration of RFA and Division Mechanism in a Single Device

An objective of this study is to combine the process of coagulation and division of the unwanted liver tissue simultaneously. This may resolve the difficulty in estimating the depth of the avascular plane after coagulation. It will complement the robotic manipulator described above by reducing the two-step ablation and cutting process into one. By combining both processes in one operation, the risk of bleeding due to over-cutting as well as time loss due to re-ablation of coagulated areas might be eliminated.

Figure 3 illustrates the incorporation of a cutting tool onto the RFA device. The cutting tool is designed to be in its retracted position when ablation is performed. After the desired part of the tissue has been ablated, the cutting tool is extended to cut the portion of the coagulated liver at the same position. Thereafter the cutting tool retracts together with the needles and the device is moved into the next position along the desired line of division. This cycle of operation is repeated, tracking the desired line of division until completion. The insertion depth of both the needles and the cutting tool is controlled by the motion of the robotic mechanism.

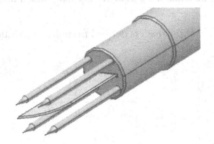

Fig. 3. RFA device with mounted cutting tool

The flow chart in Figure 4 describes the algorithm for robotic tissue ablation and division using the proposed device. After the line of division is identified by the surgeon, the proposed RFA device, held by the octopus-flexi arm end effector, will be positioned above this line and locked into place. At this point, the cutting device is in its retracted position. The two pairs of RFA needles will first be driven with a servo motor into the liver organ to the depth specified by the surgeon. This is followed by RF ablation and, thereafter, cutting by the embedded knife. The needles and the knife are both then retracted by the servo motor and the device positioned to the next position along the line of division. This process repeats until the line of division is completely ablated and cut. In order to avoid cutting the liver tissue when it has not been fully ablated, a force sensor is built into the device. A fully ablated tissue is significantly harder than a normal tissue due to water loss from tissue and denaturalization [7, 8]. From the stress-strain curve, the stress at 20% strain is about 1,000 Pa and 2,000 Pa for liver tissues ablated at 37 degree C and at 60 degree C respectively. At an ablation temperature of 80 degree C, the stress is about 20,000 Pa. This stiffness and the sensed compressive force information during cutting of the ablated tissue are used to determine the appropriateness of the coagulated regions to be divided. If the

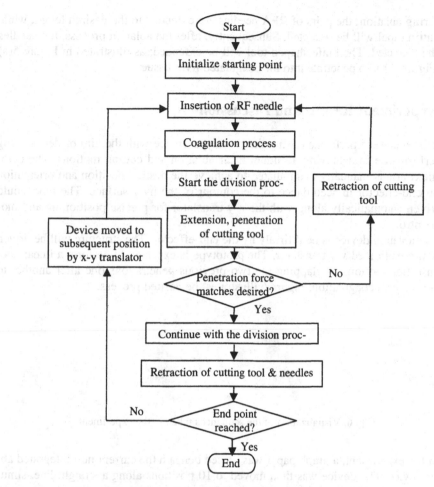

Fig. 4. Flow chart on the ablation/cutting process

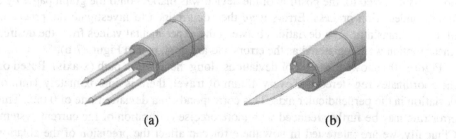

(a)   (b)

Fig. 5. (a) RFA device with cutting tool retracted, (b) RFA device with cutting tool extracted while needles retracted

sensed force feedback information indicates that the tissue has not been properly coagulated, re-ablation can then be immediately repeated in the same area before further cutting.

During ablation, the pairs of RFA needles are extended to the desired length while the cutting tool will be retracted. Subsequently, after the ablation process, the needles will be retracted. The knife shaped tool will be extended; as illustrated in Figure 5(a) and Figure 5(b), to penetrate into the coagulated liver tissue.

4   Experiment Results and Discussion

Experiments were performed using the prototype device with the aim of determining its performance in achieving accurate linear ablation and cutting motions. The octopus-flexi arm is manually manipulated to achieve the desired position and orientation of the end-effector in accordance to the contour of the liver surface. The links could be driven automatically along with the x-y translator for precise positioning and motion control.

The ablation device is held firmly by the end-effector. The structure will be driven using the motorized x-y translator. The prototype is expected to perform a linear needle insertion motion, overlapping the two previous penetrations one after another to ensure uniform coagulation. Figure 6 illustrates the desired process.

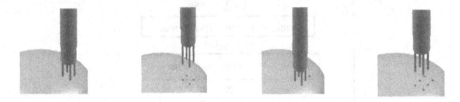

Fig. 6. Visualization of the sequences taken in the experiment

In the experiment, a graph paper was placed beneath the current non-integrated ablation device. The device was then moved to 10 positions along a straight line, simulating what would be needed for ablation. It was then moved back to the same 10 positions, simulating what is needed for the cutting operation. At each of these 20 positions it moved to, the position of the device was marked onto the graph paper by a simple indentation process. Errors were then determined to investigate the precision of the x-y translator. The deviations between the experimental values from the desired linear motion were registered as the errors and are as shown in Figure 7(b).

Figure 7(b) shows the trend of deviations along the ablation path (x-axis). Based on the coordinates registered, for every 45mm of travel, there is approximately 1mm of deviation in the perpendicular axis. This corresponds to a deviation rate of 0.022. This error rate may be further reduced with more precise calibration of the current system. Clinically, we are interested in how the error can affect the precision of the ablation and cutting process. The maximum magnitude of error registered was less than 1.5mm for a travel path as long as 45mm. This suggests that needle ablation using the proposed device can be achieved with an error within what is normally required, or within 5% assuming an ablation of 30mm in diameter.

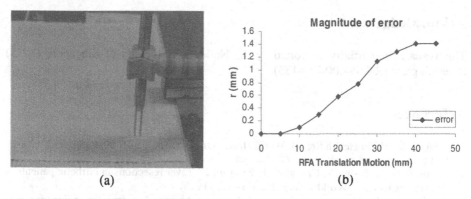

Fig. 7. Experimental results: (a) Experimental setup, (b) Positioning errors

The precision of the current prototype is limited by its low cost DC motor. A better model of motor will improve the precision. The proposed integrated ablation and division device with simultaneous ablation and cutting will further improve the accuracy and effectiveness of this system.

5 Conclusion and Future Works

The concept of integrating robotics with an RF ablation and division mechanism for liver resection is proposed, and its feasibility has been demonstrated. With a single integrated device for both ablation and resection, greater accuracy and speedier hepatic resections can be achieved and this should lead to higher success rates in this operation. This integration will greatly aid in reducing blood loss during resection surgery. Prior to the implementation of an overall medical robotic device in the actual medical environment, a more efficient and advanced computer guided or robotic manipulator is desired. The mechanism of higher dexterity will be preferred for better maneuverability of the end-effector.

Future works will focus on improvement of the robotics mechanism control and also the means to more precisely drive its automated segments. Force analysis of the liver tissue is also vital prior to the development of the division tool as compression and elongation of the liver varies at differing temperatures [7, 8]. Thus, subject on modeling of the liver tissue will be investigated. Experiments to study the subjects of interest, as well as to test the applicability of the overall robotics mechanism, will be performed on fresh porcine livers. Experiments on pig in-vivo will also be performed following the approval of the animal use protocol. The mechanical properties of a pig's liver are similar to that of a human's [9]. More precise and accurate motor will be incorporated with appropriate sensors along with suitable control schemes. These models and processes will greatly aid in the development of the precise robotic mechanism. More advanced designs of the robotic mechanisms will also be explored; for example the use of a platform integrated above the operating bed, will also be considered for future implementations.

Acknowledgement

This research is partially supported by the National University of Singapore (NUS) research grant (R-265-000-270-133).

References

1. WHO: The World Health Report. World Health Organization, ISBN 92 4 156265 X (2002), http://www.who.int/whr/2002/en
2. Bismuth, H., Houssin, D., Ornowski, J., Merrigi, F.: Liver resections in cirrhotic patients: a Western experience. World J. Surg. 10, 311–317 (1986)
3. Haemmerich, D.: Hepatic radiofrequency ablation - An overview from an engineering perspective. In: IEEE EMBS, San Francisco, CA, USA, p. 5433 (2004)
4. Rhim, H., Dogg III, G.D.: Radiafrequency Thermal Ablation of Liver Tumors. Journal of Clinical Ultrasound 27, 221–229 (1999)
5. Haemmerich, D., Wright, A.W., Mahvi, D.M., Lee Jr., F.T., Webster, J.G.: Hepatic bipolar radiofrequency ablation creates coagulation zones close to blood vessels: a finite element study. Medical and Biological Engineering and Computing 41, 317–323 (2003)
6. Steven, B.C., Fred, T.L., Gregory, D.K., Cynthia, C., Christopher, D.J., Thomas III, C.W., Thomas, F.W., David, M.M.: Effect of Vascular Occlusion on Radiofrequency Ablation of the Liver: Results in a Porcine Model. AJR 200 176, 789–795
7. Sakuma, I., Chui, C.K.: Methods in Combined Compression and Elongation of Liver Tissue and Their Application in Surgical Simulation. In: Biomechanical System Technology. Computational Methods, vol. 1, p. 56. World Scientific, Singapore (2007)
8. Deshan, Y., Mark, C.C., David, M.M., John, G.: Measurement and Analysis of Tissue Temperature during Microwave Liver Ablation. IEEE Transactions on Biomedical Engineering 54, 150–155 (2007)
9. Chui, C.K., Kobayashi, E., Chen, X., Hisada, T., Sakuma, I.: Combined compression and elongation experiments and non-linear modeling of liver tissue for surgical simulation. Medical and Biological Engineering and Computing 42, 787–798 (2004)

Fast Image Mapping of Endoscopic Image Mosaics with Three-Dimensional Ultrasound Image for Intrauterine Treatment of Twin-to-Twin Transfusion Syndrome

Hongen Liao[1,2], Masayoshi Tsuzuki[1], Etsuko Kobayashi[1], Takeyoshi Dohi[3], Toshio Chiba[4], Takashi Mochizuki[5], and Ichiro Sakuma[1]

[1] Graduate School of Engineering, The University of Tokyo
[2] Translational Systems Biology and Medicine Initiative, The University of Tokyo
[3] Graduate School of Information Science and Technology, The University of Tokyo
[4] National Center for Child Health and Development, Japan
[5] Aloka Co., LTD., Japan
7-3-1 Hongo, Bunkyo-ku, Tokyo 113-8656, Japan
liao@bmpe.t.u-tokyo.ac.jp

Abstract. This paper describes a fast image mapping system that integrates endoscopic image mosaics with three-dimensional (3-D) ultrasound images for assisting intrauterine treatment of twin-to-twin transfusion syndrome (TTTS) by laser photocoagulation. Endoscopic laser photocoagulation treatment has a good survival rate and a low complication rate for twins. However, the small field of view and lack of surrounding information makes the identification of vessels anastomosis difficult. We have developed an extended placenta visualization system with the fusion of endoscopic image mosaics with a 3-D ultrasound-image placenta model. Fully automatic and fast calibration is used for endoscope calibration in fluid. The 3-D spatial position of the endoscopic images and the ultrasound image are tracked by a 3-D position tracking device. The mosaiced endoscope images are registered to the surface of the 3-D ultrasound placenta model by using a fast GPU-based image rendering method. Experimental results show that the system may provide an improved and efficient way of planning and guidance in laser photocoagulation TTTS treatment.

1 Introduction

Twin-to-twin transfusion syndrome (TTTS) is a disease of the placenta that affects identical twins or higher multiple pregnancies where two or more fetuses share a common (monochorionic) placenta [1-2]. The syndrome occurrs in the vascular communications between the fetuses in a monochorionic gestation. Although each fetus uses its side of the placenta, the blood vessels connecting the twins allow blood to pass from one twin to the other. This serious condition occurs when the shared placenta contains abnormal blood vessels that connect the twins, resulting in an imbalanced blood between the twins. The implication of this condition is that one fetus (the recipient) may get too much blood, thereby overloading his or her cardiovascular

T. Dohi, I. Sakuma, and H. Liao (Eds.): MIAR 2008, LNCS 5128, pp. 329–338, 2008.

system, while the other fetus (the donor) may experience an inadequate supply of blood. If not treated, TTTS may be life-threatening to both the fetuses, and those who survive may suffer from many serious health problems.

Several techniques have been developed for treatment of TTTS. Surgical treatments include amniotic septostomy, amnio reduction, and laser photocoagulation. Obliteration of the vessels can halt the pathophysiologic process. Laser photocoagulation is a useful method, which has a good survival rate and a low complication rate [3]. In this method, a laser fiber and an endoscope are inserted into the uterus. With the guidance of ultrasound and direct video, specific vessels that cause the blood-sharing problem are coagulated using a laser light beam to stop the imbalanced flow of blood between the twins [4]. Thus precision in laser treatment requires the accurate vessels position information.

Advances in ultrasound and endoscopic techniques and devices have aided the identification and treatment of this potentially lethal condition. In laser photocoagulation treatment, the connecting vessels are identified by visual measurement based on endoscopic images. However, the small field of view, as well as the lack of image depth and surrounding information make it difficult for the surgeon to grasp the whole information of the placenta and decide whether the blood vessel being observed is one of the connecting vessels or not. As a result, surgical success relies on the surgeon's ability to memorize the blood vasculatory system on the placenta surface, a task that leaves the risk of missing some connecting vessels. Quintero *et al.* compared the selective laser photocoagulation with non-selective laser photocoagulation [5]. The selective laser photocoagulation of communicating vessels is a valuable application of minimally invasive endoscopic intrauterine surgery.

The fusion of intra-operative endoscopic images and pre- or intra- operative three-dimensional (3-D) data has the potential to lead to minimally invasive fetal surgery. Dey *et al.* described the automatic fusion of endoscopic images to the surface of a 3-D model derived from pre-operative data [6]. Szpala *et al.* demonstrated the real-time fusion of endoscopic views with dynamic 3-D cardiac images [7] and Reeff *et al.* developed a mosaicing method for endoscopic placenta images [8]. To improve the safety and accuracy of laser photocoagulation treatment for TTTS, we have developed an image mapping system for the intra-operative fusion of endoscopic images to a 3-D placenta model derived from ultrasound data. Our system provides an easy and fast way to obtain an intra-operative overall image of the placenta and enables the surgeon to identify connecting vessels three-dimensionally. Experimental results show that this image mapping system will give a promising support to surgeons performing laser photocoagulation treatment.

2 System and Methods

2.1 Procedure and Requirements of Laser Photocoagulation Treatment of TTTS

In the treatment of TTTS, the placenta is inspected with a very thin endoscope, which is commonly called a "fetoscope". With expectant mother under general anesthesia, the scope is placed into the uterus through a tiny hole in the abdomen. The small connecting blood vessels can then be visualized and "coagulated" using laser light from a small optic fiber passed inside or outside of the scope. The connecting blood vessels on the surface of the placenta are closed by the precision-guided laser light so that the fetuses' blood is no longer shared with each other (Fig.1). The procedure of laser photocoagulation treatment of TTTS is as follows.

1) Insert the fetoscopic instrument into the uterus (womb) through a small incision at a suitable position relative to that of the fetuses and placenta under the guidance of ultrasound. 2) Locate the recipient twin first and then the donor twin or "stuck twin", which is enveloped by a membrane. 3) Search the placenta for communicating (shared) vessels and identify vascular anatomoses. 4) Map the placenta for the abnormal vessels with a guiding light and use a laser to coagulate the vessels. 5) After a review of all of the lasered vessels, finish the treatment and exit the uterus.

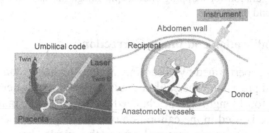

Fig. 1. Laser photocoagulation treatment for TTTS

The procedure for identifying the abnormal connections is not so easy. The endoscope has a small field of view and the obtained images with severe lens distortions suffer from weak visibility in the amniotic fluid. This makes it difficult for the surgeon to ensure that all the abnormal vascular connections have been found and treated accordingly. Precision in laser treatment requires the accurate 3-D position information, as well as the ability to view the placenta and the corresponding vessels panoramically.

2.2 System Configuration

Our image mapping system consists of an endoscope, an ultrasound device, a 3-D position tracking system, and a computer (Fig.2). The endoscope captures images of the placenta surface, and the ultrasound is used to obtain images of the intra-operative placenta. The 3-D position tracking system (POLARIS Vicra, NDI, Canada) provides the position and orientation of the endoscope and the ultrasound probe. Optical tracking markers are attached to the shaft of the endoscope and the ultrasound probe.

The position and orientation of the probe are used to estimate the position and orientation of placenta model. The image distortion is corrected to make the endoscope images to be mapped without distortion. The corresponding positions of points on image data and placenta model are calculated to map the images onto the placenta. The mapping results of endoscopic images and 3-D object model can be displayed three-dimensionally.

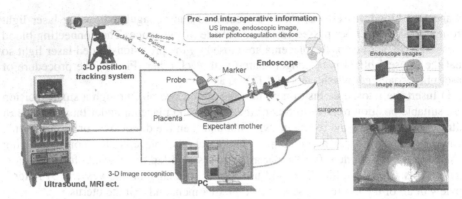

Fig. 2. System configuration for mapping endoscopic image mosaic with 3-D placenta model derived from ultrasound images

2.3 Endoscope Calibration and Image Correction

Camera calibration is performed by observing an object whose geometry in 3-D space is known with good precision. The calibration is performed in water simulating amniotic fluid since the focal length will be changed by the refractive index of the medium. A test pattern image is used in the calibration of endoscope. Correction of endoscope images is performed only to the captured area with a circle shape. We use an active contour method [9] to extract the image area. Since the active contour is greatly affected by image noise, we pass the image through a low-pass filter of fast Fourier transformation (FFT) and then apply a Gaussian filter onto the image to blur the image to reduce the noise influence.

The fish-eye lens in the endoscope's camera produces a barrel-type spatial distortion due to its wide-angle configuration. Compensation for the distortion of the image is required in image mapping to enable accurate measurement and registration [10]. To correct the image distortion, we calculate the positions of point where lines intersect on the captured image with those on a test pattern image and find the equation that describes the relationship between them. The position of each point on the captured image is measured from the optical center, which is found with the use of a low-power laser beam. The camera parameters and equations that describe the relationship of the calibration are used to correct the position of every point on the captured endoscopic image.

2.4 Ultrasound Image Calibration and Surface Extraction

To map the mosaics of endoscopic images with the surface of the object, we first acquire 3-D intra-operative data from the ultrasound device (ProSound α 10, Aloka Co., LTD.). We use a 3-D ultrasound probe with the volume data acquisition rate of 2 volumes per second. Coordinate transformation and image enhancement are performed as 3-D data preprocessing. To track the position and orientation of the ultrasound images with respect to transmitter reference coordinate system, we mount an optical position-tracking tool on the ultrasound probe. The 3-D spatial position of ultrasound data is calibrated with a set of metal balls which can be observed clearly with the ultrasound device. We calibrate the position of the metal balls in the ultrasound images. Their exact positions are measured with the same optical tracking system. Consider the coordinates of a set of N corresponding points (balls) in two different coordinate spaces. The objective is to determine a geometric transformation that associates the two coordinate spaces. The relationship of the ultrasound coordinate and the mounted optical tracking tool can thus be derived from the corresponding transformation. An interpolation profile is used to improve coordinate transformation performance.

We implemented a 3-D diffusion stick filter for speckle suppression to enhance image quality. The surface of the placenta is extracted from the 3-D ultrasound data with 3D Slicer based software and the surface configuration is converted to polygon triangle patches by using VTK and polygon reduction algorithms.

2.5 Registration of Endoscopic Image onto 3-D Ultrasound Model

After obtaining the endoscopic image area and correcting the image distortion, we map the image data onto the placenta model. Image mapping is typically used to map 2-D images to the surface of 3-D objects [11]. To map an image to a surface, the correct image coordinates for the vertex of each polygon must be computed. The relationships of the coordinates are shown in Fig. 3. For image mapping, the calibration and registration process is as follows.

For calibration of an ultrasound image, we achieve the relationship between the ultrasound probe and the coordinate of the volume data:

1) Register 3-D ultrasound image data to reproduce the reconstruction volume for placenta model representation with the coordinate system of C. Calculate the positions of metal balls in ultrasound images, producing transformation ${}^B_C T$.

2) Calibrate the rigid body of the optical position markers attached to the ultrasound probe, R_0, relative to the optical tracking system, P_0, by ${}^{R_0}_{P_0} T$. Mark the fiducial markers (metal balls), B, with a tracked pointer to indicate their position with respect to the physical space of metal balls, producing transformation ${}^{P_0}_{B} T$. Then we can get the relationship between the metal balls and the ultrasound probe ${}^{R_0}_{B} T$ as shown in Fig. 3. The ultrasound probe and the coordinate of the volume data is therefore given by ${}^R_C T = {}^B_C T\, {}^{R_0}_B T = {}^B_C T\, {}^{P_0}_B T\, {}^{R_0}_{P_0} T$.

For ultrasound images, a real-time tracking of the optical markers mounted on the ultrasound probe give the following transformations:

3) Calculate the rigid body motion of the optical position markers attached to the ultrasound probe, R, relative to the optical tracking system, P, by ${}^P_R T$. Then we can get the transformation ${}^P_C T = {}^P_R T\, {}^R_C T$

For endoscope images, we attach another set of optical position markers to the shaft of the endoscope and calculate the position and orientation of the camera lens:

4) Using transformation ${}^E_P T$, calculate the rigid body motion of the optical position markers attached to the endoscope, E, relative to the optical tracking system, P.

5) Calculate the position and the six degrees of freedom of the endoscope's pinhole camera using the transformation $_E^V T$, the tracking position markers attached to the endoscope and the coordinates associated with the endoscope lens.

For the image mapping, we can project the endoscope image onto the 3-D ultrasound model and map the image to the corresponding polygon triangle patches:

6) The projection image of the endoscope for mapping is therefore given by

$$I_V = {}_E^V T\, {}_P^E T\, {}_C^P TC = {}_E^V T\, {}_P^E T\, {}_R^P T\, {}_C^R TC$$

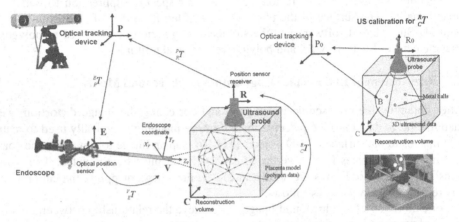

Fig. 3. Geometrical framework for mapping 2-D endoscopic images to 3-D model

2.6 GPU-Based Fast Image Mapping

Once we know the relationship between the focal point of the endoscope and the corresponding projected polygon triangle patches on the placenta model, we map every pixel in the image data onto the triangle patches through the focal point of the endoscope, assuming the endoscope can be represented as a pinhole camera model. To map every image pixel, first we calculate the vector between the focal point and pixel position. Using this vector, we calculate the position of every image pixel on the plane of a triangle patch and check whether the position is inside the triangle patch or not. If the position is inside the triangle patch, we check whether the vector comes to the front or back of the triangle patch. The corresponding position of the image pixel on the placenta model is found when the vector comes to the front of the triangle patch.

Tiling multiple images is a viable way to build a high-resolution and wide-area imaging system. However, aligning and synthesizing a seamless image become a challenge when the endoscopic images are used. For alignment, the endoscopic images for mapping are projected onto the surface of the placenta model with a panoramic image mosaic [12], and seamless processing is accomplished by geometrical correction and color modulation [13]. Coordinate transformation, median filtering, and mapping is implemented with GPU acceleration using Compute Unified Device Architecture (CUDA). Image process for mapping an endoscopic image onto the surface of the ultrasound 3-D model takes less than 10 milliseconds.

3 Experiments and Results

3.1 Ultrasound Calibration

We used a Polaris Vicra optical position tracking system to track the position of the endoscope and the probe of the ultrasound. The system includes a computer for integrating the position information of the captured endoscopic image and the 3-D ultrasound data of the object. In order to establish transformation of the coordinate of the ultrasound probe and the volume data described in subsections 2.4 and 2.5, we manufactured a phantom with four metal balls set in different planes and calibrated the positions both of the ultrasound image and physical space. For image acquisition, an optical pointer pivoted to obtain an accurate estimate of the desired 3-D point was used to collect 3-D points of each metal ball for offline processing. The transformation matrices were derived from the relative transformations between the balls of the calibration phantom with a positional offset on the basis of the pixel coordination of the phantom in the acquired ultrasound image.

3.2 Accuracy Measurement of Image Calibrations and Image Mapping

We used a phantom with a set of test pattern lattices. The phantom includes a grid of several crossing threads with different colors for identification of the endoscopic images and the accurate measurement of image mapping. Each thread is placed and intersected to be a check-pattern with an interval of 2 cm. An agar mixed with graphite, which can be observed by ultrasound clearly, was closely placed under the thread grid. The check-pattern thread phantom was placed in a water container (Fig. 4a). The 3-D structure of the phantom (Fig. 4b) was acquired with the ultrasound device and generated a 3-D model with polygon triangle patches (Fig. 4d) using the algorithms mentioned in subsection 2.4. The image of the phantom was also captured by the endoscope (Fig. 4c).

We first evaluated the accuracy of the ultrasound image by measuring of the positions of the intersecting thread in ultrasound images. The average error for 36 (6x6 threads) measured points was about 2 mm. Next, we mapped the corrected endoscopic images to the surface model of the phantom. The image mapping system was evaluated by calculating the intersected point of the threads both in the ultrasound model and the endoscope mapping results. The average error for 36 points was 2.8 mm and the standard deviation was 1.51 mm. The experimental results showed that the image mapping system is effective for providing a high-precision large-scale image of the endoscope image mapping 3-D model.

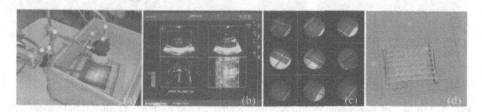

Fig. 4. Experimental devices and test pattern phantom: (a) Experimental setup. (b) Ultrasound image. (c) Endoscope images. (d) Surface model of phantom.

3.3 Placenta Model Experiment

We used a placenta model with red and blue vessels simulating veins and arteries to test our placenta mapping system. The placenta model was placed into a container simulating a uterus. The image of the placenta was captured by the endoscope (Fig. 5).The structure of the placenta was acquired by ultrasound image (Fig. 6a) and a 3-D model with polygon triangle patches was generated (Fig. 6b). We corrected the captured endoscope images and performed image mapping onto the 3-D placenta model. The adjacent image maps onto the model were overlaid each other (Fig. 7a). The image could not be observed smoothly without correction. We mosaiced the endoscope images and used alignment information, geometric correction and color modulation so that the image looked seamless, as if projected from a single source (Fig. 7b). The procedure for mapping five endoscope images to the 3-D surface model took less than 50 milliseconds.

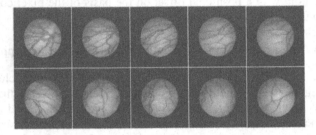

Fig. 5. Captured endoscopic images

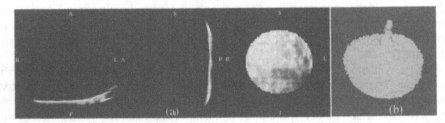

Fig. 6. (a) Ultrasound images and (b) 3-D model generated from ultrasound images

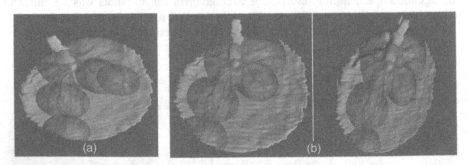

Fig. 7. Mosaics of panoramic endoscope image are mapped on the 3-D ultrasound model. (a) Without seamless processing. (b) With seamless processing; the extended endoscopic-image-mapped 3-D placenta is viewed from different directions.

The image mapping results show that the developed image mapping system can generate a large-scale high-quality 3-D placenta and help surgeon to get the information in convenient way, which could provide the overall image of placenta and help the surgeon in performing identification of connecting vessels.

4 Discussion and Conclusion

We developed an image mapping system for automatically creating a 3-D structure of the entire placenta with high-quality and panoramic endoscopic image surface mapping. We demonstrated that the system can provide significantly enlarged view of the placenta, which would be very useful for surgeons to identify connecting vessels and execute laser photocoagulation treatment. The image mapping system can provide 3-D images of the entire placenta, which enables surgeons to observe the vessels on the placenta of twins without any need for memorization.

The image mapping accuracy was 2.8 mm on average, which could be improved by increasing the tracking accuracy of the ultrasound probe and the endoscope. One solution would be to calibrate the position and the orientation of the endoscope lens by using another tracking system, such as an electromagnetic measurement system. Since the position of the placenta can change during the image acquisition, how to reduce the influence of the movement in intra-operative measurement of the placenta is another challenge. Our future work includes improving the accuracy of the image mapping and the quality of the resultant images. The quality of mapped image could be improved by image enhancement techniques to get a clearer endoscopic image and by color-shading correction for the inhomogeneous light distribution of the light source. We plan to test the system in an in-vivo experiment and improve the speed of placenta segmentation from ultrasound images, which will be especially important in the clinical implementation.

In conclusion, we developed a placenta mapping system for the treatment of TTTS. The image mapping system can provide 3-D large-scale images of the placenta surface, which enables surgeon to observe the vasculatory system of the twins without any need for memorizing it. This can reduce the risk of missing important vessels in the treatment. With the improvement of the image mapping accuracy and image quality, the system should be of practical use in laser photocoagulation TTTS treatment.

Acknowledgment

This work was supported in part by Health and Labor Sciences Research Grants of Ministry of Health, Labor and Welfare in Japan, Special Coordination Funds for Promoting Science and Technology commissioned by the Ministry of Education, Culture, Sports, Science and Technology in Japan, and Grant for Industrial Technology Research of New Energy and Industrial Technology Development Organization, Japan.

References

1. Bruner, J.P., Rosemond, R.L.: Twin-to-twin transfusion syndrome: A subset of the twin oligohydramnios-polyhydramnois sequence. Am. J. Obstet. Gynecol. 169, 925–930 (1993)
2. Bruner, J.P., Anderson, T.L., Rosemond, R.L.: Placental pathophysiology of the twin-to-twin transfusion syndrome. Placenta 19, 81–86 (1996)
3. Hecher, K., et al.: Endoscopic laser surgery versus serial amniocenteses in the treatment of severe twin-twin transfusion syndrome. Am. J. Obstet. Gynecol. 180, 717–724 (1999)
4. Lia, J.E.D., Cruikshank, D.P., Keye, W.R.: Fetoscopic neodymium: YAG laser occlusion of placental vessels in severe twin-twin transfusion syndrome. Obstetrics & Gynecology 75, 1046–1053 (1990)
5. Quintero, R.A., Comas, C., Bornick, P.W., Allen, M.H., Kruger, M.: Selective verus non-selective laser photocoagulation of placental vessels in twin-twin transfusion syndrome. Ultrasound Obstet Gynecol. 16, 230–236 (2000)
6. Dey, D., Gobbi, D.G., Slomka, P.J., Surry, K.J.M., Peters, T.M.: Automatic fusion of free-hand endoscopic brain images to three-dimensional surfaces creating stereoscopic panoramas. IEEE Trans. Medical Imaging 21(1), 23–30 (2002)
7. Szpala, S., Wierzbicki, M., Guiraudon, G., Peters, T.M.: Real-Time Fusion of Endoscopic Views with Dynamic 3-D Cardiac Images: A Phantom Stugy. IEEE Trans. Medical Imaging 24(9), 1207–1215 (2005)
8. Reeff, M., Gerhard, F., Cattin, P., Székely, G.: Mosaicing of Endoscopic Placenta Images. GI Jahrestagung (1), 467–474 (2006)
9. Williams, D., Shah, M.: A fast algorithm for active contours and curvature estimation. CVGIP: Image Understanding 55, 14–26 (1992)
10. Shah, S., Aggarwal, J.K.: A Simple Calibration Procedure for Fish-Eye (High Distortion) Lens Camera. In: IEEE Intl. Conference on Robotics and Automation, vol. 4, pp. 3422–3427 (1994)
11. Heckbert, P.: Survey of texture mapping. IEEE Computer Graphics and Applications, 56–67 (1986)
12. Szeliski, R.: Video Mosaics for Virtual Environments. IEEE Computer Graphics and Applications (March 1996)
13. Liao, H., Iwahara, M., Koike, T., Hata, N., Sakuma, I., Dohi, T.: Scalable high-resolution integral videography autostereoscopic display by use of seamless multi-projection. Applied Optics 44(3), 305–315 (2005)

Non-rigid 2D-3D Registration Based on Support Vector Regression Estimated Similarity Metric

Wenyuan Qi[1], Lixu Gu[1,*], and Jianrong Xu[1,2,*]

[1] Computer Science, Shanghai Jiaotong University,
800 Dongchuan Road, Shanghai 200240, China
[2] Shanghai Renji Hospital, Shanghai
{jimmyqwy,gu-lx}@sjtu.edu.cn

Abstract. In this paper, we proposed a novel non-rigid 2D-3D registration framework, which is based on Support Vector Regression (SVR) to compensate the disadvantages of generating large amounts of Digitally Rendered Radiographs (DRRs) in the stage of intra-operation for radiotherapy. It is successfully used to estimate similarity metric distribution from prior sparse target metric values against different featured transforming parameters of non-rigid registration. Through applying the appropriate selected features and kernel of SVR solution to our registration framework, experiments provide a precise registration result efficiently in order to assist radiologists locating the accurate positions of radiation surgery. Meanwhile, a medical diagnosis database is also built up to reduce the therapy cost and accelerate the procedure of radiotherapy in the case of future scheduling of multiple treatments.

Keywords: 2D-3D Registration, Non-rigid, Support Vector Regression, DRR, Registration Framework, Radiotherapy.

1 Introduction

Nowadays, non-rigid registration [1] algorithm is widely employed into many kinds of modern surgery, diagnosis and operation planning in order to combine and enhance the information of two or several different modality data sets at different times. Especially, in the field of radiation surgery [2], most radiologists traditionally diagnose diseases through viewing 2D X-ray film only. It is very hard for a radiologist to imagine the complex 3D shapes of tissue or organ various from different patients and difficult for them to locate the surgical position accurately. To this point, during radiotherapy, we should introduce information of a 3D model reconstructed from pre-operative data obtaining by CT or MRI machine into 2D X-ray image to aid radiologists to diagnose various diseases and locate the surgical position easily and accurately in real time [3]. Because many surgical objects are soft tissues, we have to develop the non-rigid registration to reach the above goal.

---

* Corresponding authors.

T. Dohi, I. Sakuma, and H. Liao (Eds.): MIAR 2008, LNCS 5128, pp. 339–348, 2008.
© Springer-Verlag Berlin Heidelberg 2008

Our target is to utilize an effective 2D-3D registration algorithm [4,5] to decide the physical space position of 3D model for matching the intra-operative 2D X-ray image with deformation as accurately as possible. Scholars had engaged into developing many effective, highly evaluated, deeply proved and widely used cutting-edge non-rigid 2D-3D registration algorithm. Few of them involve the area of matching the intensities between 3D data sets and X-ray images in elasticity deformation by minimizing a similarity measure to reach the goal of registration. On the other hand, Voxel-based registration [4] had been widely used for its simplicity and robustness. As the key technology in this kind of 2D-3D registration, generation of digitally rendered radiographs (DRRs) [7], however, becomes a bottleneck of whole registration routine. Among steps of optimization [1], large amounts of intra- operative 2D DRRs had to be generated from the 3D data sets, which used to be compared with X-Ray image in order to obtain best similarity metric mapping the parameters of transform to match the 3D data sets with 2D X-ray image. Due to the tremendous number of iteration and reduplicated computation during optimization, generation of intra-operative 2D DRRs is very time-consuming, which could not be tolerated by the radiologist during operation. Although lots of accelerated DRR generation method [7] had been rushed out in the past several years, few real-time virtual surgery applications appeared by means of current 2D-3D registration methods.

Aiming at the above two points, we engaged into changing the workflow of traditional registration framework in order to avoid generating intra-operative DRRs and combining with the technology of free-form deformation [1] to realize the non-rigid registration effectively. Among that, a novel intensity based 2D-3D registration method using Support Vector Regression (SVR) [8] was employed into our platform of virtual surgery. It is constructed from the relationship between parameters of non-rigid transformation for 3D volume data sets and sparse offline metric distribution, which evaluates the similarity of X-ray image and pre-operative DRR images of 3D data sets. Because of the characteristics of SVR, it could estimate the real similarity metric during operation and avoid generating intra-operative DRRs during optimization steps. In this way, we could naturally compensate the disadvantage of time-consuming calculation of DRR generation and finally boost up the performance of 2D-3D registration algorithm.

The rest of the paper is organized as follows: in Section 2, the theoretical concept of SVR is briefly reviewed followed by the non-rigid application, based on which a novel registration framework is figured out in section 3, while the merits of the registration algorithm are also demonstrated in this section. Section 4 presents the implementation and some experimental results respectively. Finally, Section 5 summarizes our current work and leads to outlook on further work.

2   Support Vector Regression in Non-rigid 2D-3D Registration

2.1   Support Vector Regression

It is well-known that Support Vector Machine (SVM) [9] was developed from statistical learning theory [10]. It could be applied to solve classification problems [11] and had also been extended to solve lots of regression problems [10], named Support Vector Classification (SVC) and Support Vector Regression (SVR) respectively. SVM is very suitable for estimating values based on non-uniform sampling data sets, which would form a sparse distribution in the input space. Furthermore, SVR has advantages to estimate continuously and smoothly from the discrete data distribution through various kinds of kernel function.

As mentioned above, our target is to estimate the similarity metric without generating intra-operative DRRs to approach real metric distribution depending on sparse pre-operative DRRs as accurately as possible. This problem could be demonstrated as follows:

Given a training data set $\{(x_i, y_i)\}_{i=1}^{l}$, minimizes the empirical risk

$$\arg \min_{f \in H_n} R_{emp}[f] \tag{1}$$

$$R_{emp}[f] = \frac{1}{l} \sum_{i=1}^{l} L(y_i, f(x_i)) \tag{2}$$

Where, H_n is hypothesis space, x_i (feature element) is the parameters of non-rigid transformation in the registration method, y_i is the real similarity value between pre-operative DRR image from 3D data and 2D X-Ray image with the current parameter x_i of transform and f is a non-linear evaluation function to estimate similarity metric. Here, the L is anε- insensitive loss function. This problem is equivalent to the regression problem using *SVR* method [10]:

$$\min_{w,b,\xi_i,\xi_i^*} \frac{1}{2} w^T w + C \sum_{i=1}^{l} \xi_i + C \sum_{i=1}^{l} \xi_i^* \tag{3}$$

subject to

$$f(x_i) - y_i \leq \varepsilon + \xi_i,$$
$$y_i - f(x_i) \leq \varepsilon + \xi_i^*, \tag{4}$$
$$\xi_i, \xi_i^* \geq 0, i = 1,...,l.$$

Where ε, C are both customized, ξ_i, ξ_i^* are slack variables, we assumed that $f(x)$ is composed of several non-linear basic functions $\{\varphi_j(x)\}$ as follows:

$$f(x) = w^T \varphi(x) \tag{5}$$

After introducing Lagrange function, the above optimization problem could be converted into its dual problem, which is easy to be realized by means of computer programming.

$$w = \sum_{i=1}^{l} (\alpha_i - \alpha_i^*) \varphi(x_i) \tag{6}$$

α_i, α_i^* are Lagrange multiplier. $\mathbf{\alpha} = \{\alpha_i\}, \mathbf{\alpha}^* = \{\alpha_i^*\}$. And

$$K(x_i, x_j) \equiv \varphi(x_i)^T \varphi(x_j) \tag{7}$$

$K(x_i, x_j)$ is the Kernel function. In our paper, we choose exponential radial basis function to satisfy the special characteristic of similarity metric in 2D-3D registration. Finally, we find appropriate Lagrange multipliers to construct the approximate function, which could estimate the metric value without generating intra-operative DRR image in a reasonable time. The approximate function is like:

$$\sum_{i=1}^{l} (\alpha_i^* - \alpha_i) K(x_i, x) \tag{8}$$

2.2 Non-rigid Registration

Refer to the soft tissues to be registered, our SVR involved registration method ought to be enhanced with a non-rigid resolution. We use free-form deformation (FFD) model [9] to solve the non-rigid deformation part of registration. The basic idea of FFD is to deform an object by manipulating an underlying mesh of control points. The deformation of the inset mesh controls the shape of the object or image that we want to deform to match another object or image.

Given an image with resolution ρ and spacing Δ, the control mesh with resolution σ, we can get the spacing of control grid:

$$\delta = \Delta/(\sigma - 1) \tag{9}$$

The deformation at any position X of the image is interpolated using a cubic B-spline convolution kernel:

$$D(X) = \sum_{i=-1}^{2} \beta^{(3)}((X - \phi_{i+n})/\delta) \tag{10}$$

Where, $n = \lfloor X/\delta \rfloor$, ϕ_j denotes the displacement of the *jth* control point of the mesh, $\beta^{(3)}(X)$ is a differentiable convolution kernel given by the product of B-spline kernel function in each dimension.

In FFD deformation, each control point presents three deformation coefficients for 3D data set, which scanned before operation during routine check. Furthermore, these coefficients should be treated as the features vector of the training data set for SVR method. The high resolution of control mesh can offer more flexible local deformations while also introduce a larger number of coefficients, which makes the optimization procedure much more time-consuming. Fortunately, the above procedure and training process are both implemented before in-line operation. And we only choose those active control points deform the control mesh while those passive ones not. Through which, this method can speed up the algorithm while contain the same deformations that we concern.

3 Novel Non-rigid 2D-3D Registration Framework

3.1 Novel Non-rigid 2D-3D Registration Framework Using SVR

As mentioned above, we introduce SVR method to estimate similarity metric between 3D data sets and 2D X-Ray image without the help of generating intra-operative DRR images in every optimization step for non-rigid registration. We could utilize the promising empirical performance of SVR to predict the similarity metric value by means of sparse training data sets. To this point, the SVR separate the traditional calculation of similarity metric into two parts. One is the offline sparse similarity distribution in real condition, the other one is the online estimated continuous similarity distribution. The latter could be calculated out by the promising empirical performance of SVR method without generating any DRRs. Theoretically speaking, it could boost up the efficiency of the process of registration in the aspect of the intra-operative operation.

The framework of our effective non-rigid 2D-3D registration algorithm is depicted as the following figure:

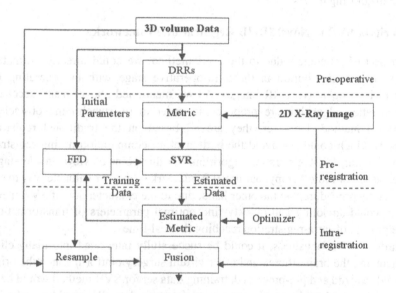

Fig. 1. Novel 2D-3D Registration Framework using SVR

Through which we could build up an evaluation metric function of similarity for optimizer in registration method to find the optimal parameters of transformation to match 3D data sets with 2D X-Ray perfectly. Note that the feature vector of the training data of SVR method is carefully selected from the parameters of control points of FFD transformation in the non-rigid transformation. Furthermore, the kernel function of SVR method is also the most suitable function for the non-rigid registration after various experiments.

We could also figure out that the above flow chart illustrate that our novel 2D-3D registration has three indispensable stages including pre-operative, pre-registration and intra-registration, which comes from the SVR method.

In detail, in the *pre-operative* stage, a 3D model reconstructed from CT or MRI machine when doing the routine check of patient. We just generate a little number of pre-operative DRR images on the key position of each degree of freedom separately as training data according to the 3D model. The second stage called *pre-registration* is responsible for generating the training data constructed from the information of DRR images and the intra-operative X-Ray images. The features of training data for SVR method are the parameters of active control points of FFD transformation. The outputs of training data for SVR method are the real sparse similarity metric value between the pre-operative DRR images and the intra-operative X-Ray images. The third stage called *intra-registration* is responsible for searching the optimal parameters in the estimated space built up in the previous stage. There is no need to generate the DRR image comparing with the intra-operative fluoroscopic X-Ray image. Finally optimal multi-parameters could be obtained until the convergence of optimizer. With the help of these optimal parameters, complicated information of pre-operation 3D data could be fused into intra-operative 2D X-Ray image to assist radiologists in making surgery plan and diagnosing disease.

3.2   Merits of SVR in Novel 2D-3D Registration Framework

In the aspect of efficiency, due to the SVR method, we could directly estimate the similarity metric distribution in the intra-operative stage without generating large number of intra-operative DRR images. As we mentioned above, many accelerated DRR generation algorithm are proposed in order to overwhelm the obstacles of conventional method. However, they are all based on the traditional registration framework, which could not avoid the bottleneck of computation during registration even accelerating DRR generation algorithm. To this point of view, in the stage of intra-operation for radiotherapy, our novel framework is another valuable way to speed up the therapy procedure. On the other hand, due to the characteristic of SVR method, optimizer could smoothly and quickly find optimal parameters of transformation to help the process of intra-registration reaching the real-time.

Regarding to its robustness, it could be successfully integrated into many clinical cases including the brain, thorax and other virtual surgery platform. Once the original data are normalized and pre-processed, training data set for SVR method would be kept stable, which would be insensitive to noise of source data. We could also find that optimizer on the estimated similarity metric between the pre-operative DRR images and 2D image data would be free of local minima, which could increase the robustness and result in good convergence.

The expansibility of our new registration framework is very obvious. We utilize the feature of the training data of SVR method to realize the non-rigid registration. That is to say, the pre-operative DRR images could be generated according the adjustment of different parameters of transforms. There is no need to replace or re-design the other part of our framework. And it could also build up the database classified by each different patient, which services for the future multi-treatments.

4 Experimental Results

We evaluated our non-rigid 2D-3D registration methods with preoperative 3D volume data sets and intra-operative fluoroscopic X-Ray image. In order to test the robustness and universality of our novel registration framework, our source data cover different modalities and different typical thorax area in the human body. The experiments are performed on a PC with Core-T2400 1.83GHz, 1GB RAM.

A Brain Case

Once most suitable SVR is decided and the estimated searching space is acquired, we could adopt our optimizer to search the space finding the optimal parameters. At first, an experimental result of registration for 3D MRI Brain data set and 2D X-Ray image is illustrated in Fig. 2. The format of 3D T1-MRI data is 181×217×181, slice thickness is 1mm. 2D X-Ray image is simulated by 3D MRI using DRR method, its size is 220×250.

In order to evaluate the results of our proposed registration method, Table.1 summarized some attributes in order to compare our proposed registration method with the conventional one, which uses Mutual Information [12] as similarity metric and calculates large number of intra-operative DRRs at each optimization step for searching the optimal parameters of free form transformation.

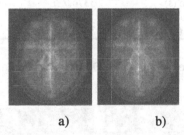

a)   b)

Fig. 2. Registration between 3D MRI data and simulated X-Ray image. (Brain Case) a) 2D X-Ray image with contours (wire frames) of DRR image from initial 3D volume data. The initial position of 3D volume data is minus ten degree rotated against Z axis with some deformation. b) 2D X-Ray image with contours of DRR image from registered 3D volume data by our proposed registration method.

Table 1. Evaluation of our proposed method compared with conventional method. (Brain Case)

Features	Our Proposed Method	Conventional Method
DRR generation times	218(pre-operative)	435 (intra-operative)
Time consuming (s)	376.7	930.1
Squared Sum Difference	0.1713	0.2033

B Thorax Cases

Four thorax cases of volunteers had been experimented to validate the effective and robustness of our registration framework. Here, the direction of DRR image is along the Y axis. The format of 3D T1-MRI data is listed in Table 2 and the size of intra-operative 2D X-Ray image is 500×500. The control points of FFD for non-rigid transformation, the total consuming time and accuracy of registration results are also illustrated in Table 2.

Table 2. Evaluation of our proposed method under four thorax data sets

Our Proposed Method	3D Volume Size	Control points	Time consuming (s)	Squared Sum Difference (SSD)
Data #1	233×233×138	18×18×11	2928.5	0.1056
Data #2	482×482×128	12×12×10	3197.1	0.1641
Data #3	522×522×138	13×13×11	2778.1	0.0189
Data #4	600×600×128	15×15×10	3289.7	0.0718

In order to evaluate the results of our proposed registration method, Table.3 gives the comparison results between our proposed method and conventional method, which had been mentioned in Table.1. The data provided here are the average results of all the thorax cases.

Table 3. Evaluation of our proposed method compared with conventional method. (Thorax Cases)

Features	Our Proposed Method	Conventional Method
DRR generation times	313 (pre-operative)	473 (intra-operative)
Squared Sum Difference (SSD)	0.1951	0.2118
Offline Calculation Time (s)	3374.7	--
Online Calculation Time (s)	0.60	3048.5
Total Time consuming (s)	3375.3	3048.5

Experimental result of registration for 3D MRI thorax data sets and 2D X-Ray image is illustrated in Fig.3.

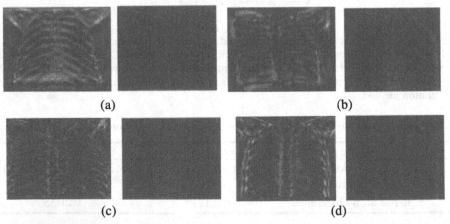

(a)   (b)

(c)   (d)

Fig. 3. Registration between 3D MRI data and simulated X-Ray image. (Four Thorax Cases (a-d)). First Column of each case shows the difference image of 2D X-Ray image and DRR image of 3D volume at an initial position. Second Column of each case shows the difference image of 2D X-Ray image and DRR image of 3D volume at a final position by our proposed registration method. (a) is the registration between 2D X-Ray image and 3D volume data with ten degree rotated against X axis with some deformation. In (b), the initial position of 3D volume data is minus ten degree rotated against Y axis with some deformation. Similarly, ten degree rotated against Z axis with deformation in (c) and twenty mm offset against Z axis with deformation in (d).

5 Conclusion

This paper proposed a novel non-rigid 2D-3D registration framework using Support Vector Regression with free form deformation. We estimated the similarity metric efficiently and avoid generating time-consumed intra-operative DRR images successfully. The experiments also reveal that our method has a satisfying performance comparing with the conventional registration method.

Our future work will be focus on the multi-resolution non-rigid registration. It would be promoted to apply for the large scale data sets. The selection of feature vector of training set should be changeable during registration. The main challenges are efficiency and accuracy.

Acknowledgements

The authors would like to thank to all the members in the image-guided surgery and therapy laboratory in Shanghai Jiaotong University. We are also grateful to ITK members for their warm suggestion and enthusiastic help. And thanks to Shanghai ShuGuang Hospital for providing some volunteers' clinical data. This research is partially supported by Chinese Nature Science Foundation 60571061, Chinese 863 High Technique Research Project 2007AA01Z312, Chinese 973 Key Research Foundation 2007CB512700-1 and 2006CB504801.

References

1. Rohde, G.K., Aldroubi, A., Dawant, B.M.: Adaptive freeform deformation for inter-patient medical image registration. In: Sonka, M., Hanson, K.M. (eds.) Proc. SPIE Medical Imaging: Image Processing, vol. 4322, pp. 1578–1587. SPIE Press, Bellingham (2001)
2. Adler Jr., J., Murphy, M., Chang, S., Hancock, S.: Image-guided robotic radiosurgery. Neurosurgery 44(6) (1999)
3. Wein, W.: Intensity Based Rigid 2D-3D Registration Algorithms for Radiation Therapy. Ph.D. thesis (2003)
4. Gocke, R., Weese, J., Schumann, H.: Fast Volume Rendering Methods for Voxel-based 2D-3D Registration – A Comparative Study. In: International Workshop on Biomedical Image Registration 1999, Bled, Slovenia, August 30-31 (1999)
5. Weese, J., Penney, G.P., Desmedt, P., Buzug, T.M., Hill, D.L.G., Hawkes, D.J.: Voxel-Based 2-D/3-D Registration of Fluoroscopy Images and CT Scans for Image-Guided Surgery. IEEE transactions on information technology in biomedicine 1(4) (1997)
6. Rueckert, D., Sonoda, L.I., Hayes, C., et al.: Nonrigid registration using free-form deformations: application to breast MR images. IEEE Transactions on Medical Imaging 18(8), 712–721 (1999)
7. Lacroute, P., Levoy, M.: Fast Volume Rendering Using a Shear-Warp Factorization of the Viewing Transform. In: Computer Graphics Proceedings, Annual Conference Series (1994)
8. Christopher, J.C.B.: A Tutorial on Support Vector Machines for Pattern Recognition, pp. 1–43. Kluwer Academic Publishers, Boston (1998)

9. Cortes, C., Vapnik, V.: Support-vector network. Machine Learning 20, 273–297 (1995)
10. Vapnik, V.: Statistical Learning Theory. Wiley, New York (1998)
11. Hsu, C.-W., Lin, C.-J.: A comparison of methods for multi-class support vector machines. IEEE Transactions on Neural Networks 13(2), 415–425 (2002)
12. Pluim, J.P.W., Maintz, J.B.A., Viergever, M.A.: Mutual-Information-Based Registration of Medical Images: A Survey. IEEE Transactions on Medical Imaging 22(9), 986–1004 (2003)

Real-Time Autostereoscopic Visualization of Registration-Generated 4D MR Image of Beating Heart

Nicholas Herlambang[1], Hongen Liao[2,3], Kiyoshi Matsumiya[1], Ken Masamune[1], and Takeyoshi Dohi[1]

[1] Graduate School of Information Science and Technology,
[2] Graduate School of Engineering,
[3] Translational Systems Biology and Medicine Initiative,
The University of Tokyo, Japan
{nicholas,liao}@atre.t.u-tokyo.ac.jp,
{masa,takdohi}@i.u-tokyo.ac.jp

Abstract. This paper presents a real-time autostereoscopic visualization system using the principle of Integral Videography(IV). We develop MIP and composite volume ray casting method for IV volume rendering, and implemented the algorithm on GPU to achieve real-time rendering. The system was used to visualize 4D MR image that was generated from registration of 3D MR image and 4D ultrasound image. The registration scheme consists of inter-modality rigid registration between 3D MR image and 3D ultrasound image and intra-modality non-rigid registration between 3D ultrasound images. Registration processes were also implemented on GPU. Evaluation of processing speed showed that GPU processing time was 48x, 13x, 21x faster than CPU processing time for IV volume rendering, rigid registration, and non-rigid registration respectively. We also enabled real-time user interactivity for IV visualization system. In the future, We plan to use this system to develop intra-operative surgery navigation system for intra-cardiac surgery on beating heart.

Keywords: Integral Videography, rigid registration, non-rigid registration.

1 Background

In order to realize intra-cardiac surgery without cardio-pulmonary bypass, intra-operative navigation is required. Especially as the surgery targets intra-cardiac organs, the surgery needs to be navigated by medical images with see-through capability such as CT, MRI, or ultrasound. And also, performing surgery without cardio-pulmonary bypass means that the surgery has to be performed on a beating heart, and therefore real-time navigation is required. Although medical image acquisition technologies advanced rapidly in recent years, it is still a trade-off between image quality and image acquisition speed. Ultrasound is

T. Dohi, I. Sakuma, and H. Liao (Eds.): MIAR 2008, LNCS 5128, pp. 349–358, 2008.

the only method that can acquire 3D data in real-time manner, but lacks image quality. On the other hand, methods that produce superior image quality such as CT and MRI lack speed. In this paper, we are trying to address that issue by proposing a method that combine data acquisition speed of ultrasound and image quality of MRI. We develop a method to generate 4D MR image from 3D MR image and 4D ultrasound image through image registration.

Moreover, doing image-quided intra-cardiac surgery on beating heart means that there is no direct vision onto the target. This kind of surgery will be very difficult to perform without a superior depth perception of the image. Surgery navigation with stereoscopic visualization is one of the solution. Among stereoscopic visualization methods, Integral Videography (IV)[1,2] is one that has many advantages over other methods. IV is an autostereoscopic visualization method that use the combination of high resolution LCD display and micro convex lens array to project the lights from LCD display onto 3D space in front of the display. IV does not need glasses or other viewing devices, is spatially accurate, and allows multiple observers at the same time, so that we believe IV is the suitable method for use in clinical situation. However, IV volume rendering, creating an IV image from 3D data, is a computationally heavy process, and for that reason current IV technology see iso-surface rendering as the only feasible approach. In this research, we would like to bring real-time processing and a more robust rendering methods such as composite volume rendering into IV.

Also, targetting intra-operative surgery navigation, we realize the importance of fast calculation not only for IV visualization but also for image registration. Therefore, we implement our algorithms on Graphic Processing Unit (GPU) for fast calculation.

The purpose of this paper is to develop a real-time auto-stereoscopic visualization system using IV for future intra-cardiac surgery navigation system. In details, We develop a fast and robust volume rendering method for IV and a method to generate 4D MR image by registration, then we apply our methods to visualize registration-generated 4D MR image of volunteer's beating heart data.

2　Materials and Methods

We developed a real-time IV volume rendering and a 3D-4D registration methods, which will be explained in the following subsections. Then we implemented our algorithms on GPU computing and introduced real-time user interactivity for IV visualization system which will be discussed in implementation issues.

2.1　IV Direct Volume Rendering

Current IV volume rendering method is based on iso-surface ray tracing algorithm. This method only provides surface information, which is not enough for surgical navigation where information of inner organs is also required. Therefore,

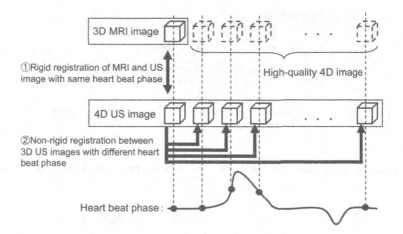

Fig. 1. Registration scheme: 4D MR image generation from 3D MR image and 4D ultrasound registration

we developed a new IV direct volume rendering method using Maximum Intensity Projection(MIP) rendering and composite rendering[3]. In MIP rendering the value of each pixel is assigned to the maximum intensity along the light ray. In composite rendering, using color and alpha transfer function, value of each pixel was calculated by taking the integral value of voxels passed by the ray until a certain opacity value is reached. We also enabled the combination of iso-surface rendering and composite rendering or iso-surface rendering and MIP rendering which proportion defines transparency level.

2.2   Registration Scheme

We have developed a method to generate 4D MR image by image registration between 3D MR image and 4D ultrasound image[4]. The registration scheme consists of rigid registration between 3D MRI and 3D ultrasound image with the same heart beat phase, and non-rigid registration between 3D ultrasound images with different heart beat phases (Fig 1). Rigid registration aligned the position and orientation of 3D MRI and corresponding 3D ultrasound image. Then from non-rigid registration, deformation field of each 3D ultrasound image relative to the one used in rigid registration was obtained. Applying the deformation fields of the 4D ultrasound image to 3D MR image, we can produce a set of 4D MR image.

Intra-modality Rigid Registration. Rigid registration is performed using mutual information as similarity measure and Powell optimization method (Fig.2). We defined 3D MR image as the reference image and 3D ultrasound image as the target image because 3D ultrasound image has lower resolution and therefore has lower computational cost to apply transformation. As the result of rigid registration, linear transformation operator R_{rigid} was obtained.

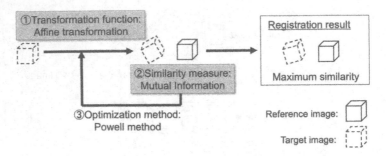

Fig. 2. Rigid registration method. Grey box indicate processes implemented on GPU.

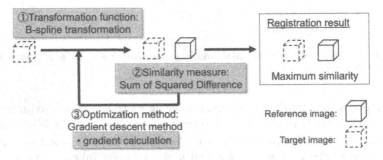

Fig. 3. Non-rigid registration method. Grey box indicate processes implemented on GPU.

Applying R_{rigid} on ultrasound image will align the ultrasound image to the MR image. R_{rigid} is reversible, so the reverse transformation operator can be defined as R_{rigid}^{-1} so that applying R_{rigid}^{-1} on the 3D MR image will align the 3D MR image to the 3D ultrasound image.

Inter-modality Non-rigid Registration. As non-rigid registration method, we used B-spline based registration[5]. In B-spline based registration, both image and deformation field are represented in smooth B-spline functions. We chose B-spline based non-rigid registration because of its relatively low calculation cost and its ability to cover a wide range of deformation. We used Sum of Squared Differences (SSD) as the similarity measure and gradient descent method as the optimization method (Fig. 3). As the result of non-rigid registration, non-rigid registration operator $R_{non-rigid}$ was obtained. Applying $R_{non-rigid}$ on target image will elastically deform target image to match reference image.

4D MR Images generation. 4D MR image was generated by combining both registration results. In 4D image generation, it is important to keep the resolution of MR image while applying deformation field of ultrasound images. For calculation simplicity reason, elastic transformations were performed in ultrasound coordinate system rather than in MRI coordinate system. Using resulted rigid registration operator R_{rigid} and non-rigid registration operator $R_{non-rigid}$, 4D MR image generation was performed as follows:

1. Align the position and orientation of the MR image using the inverse rigid registration operator R_{rigid}^{-1} so that it matched the US image.
2. Apply non-rigid registration operator $R_{non-rigid}$ on the aligned MR image.
3. Move the deformed MR image using rigid registration operator R_{rigid} so that it is back to its original position.

2.3 Implementation Issues

GPU Implementation on CUDA Platform. We implemented IV rendering and registration tasks on GPU. We used Compute Unified Device Architecture (CUDA)[6] platform for GPU programming platform. We used NVIDIA GeForce 8800GTX (128 processors at 1.35 GHz) as the GPU. Optimization was performed by maximizing paralelism of the calculation tasks. In volume rendering, ray tracing from one pixel was set as a single calculation task, which was calculated parallelly on Single Program Multiple Data (SPMD) execution model of CUDA platform.

For rigid and non-rigid registration, we implement each process of registration process on GPU. In rigid registration, affine transformation and mutual information calculation were implemented on GPU, and in non-rigid registration, B-spline transformation, SSD calculation, and SSD gradient calculation were implemented on GPU.

User Interactivity. Implementing IV rendering on GPU computing, we expected the IV rendering to be real-time, so it is possible to put multiple volume rendering cycles in between data inputs (Fig. 4). By adjusting rendering parameters before each rendering cycle, real-time manipulation became possible. Interactive user interface was realized using a 3D mouse with 6 DOF and 2 input buttons (SpaceNavigator, 3dconnexion). In this system, we realized real-time

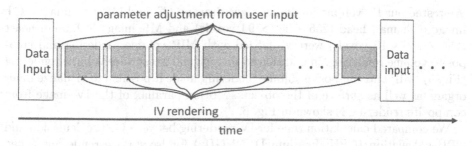

Fig. 4. Fast IV volume rendering will enable multiple rendering cycles in between data input, and thus allow user interactivity

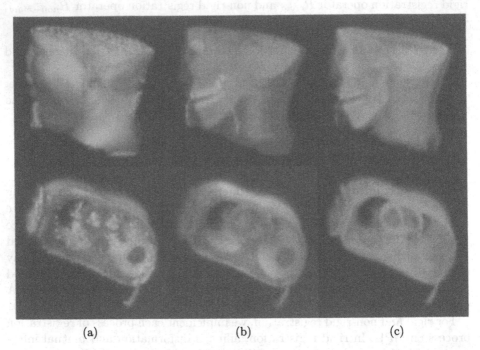

(a)   (b)   (c)

Fig. 5. Various IV rendering result on CT image (above) and MR image (below). (a) iso-surface rendering (b) MIP rendering (c) composite rendering.

translation, rotation, data slicing, threshold adjustment, and opacity control for maximum user experience. Users are also able to switch between IV volume rendering methods.

3   Results

3.1   IV Volume Rendering

We tested our IV volume rendering algorithms on CT and MR test images. CT image of human head ($256 \times 256 \times 94$ voxels) and MR image of human heart ($256 \times 256 \times 19$ voxels) were visualized with MIP volume rendering and composite volume rendering, in addition to the original iso-surface volume rendering (Fig. 5). MIP and composite volume rendering made it possible to visualize inner organs as well as surface of the objects. Motion parallax of the IV image from composite rendering is shown in Fig. 6.

We compared calculation time for IV rendering between GPU calculation and CPU calculation (CPU: Pentium D 3.2 GHz) for iso-surface rendering. Then calculation time of various rendering methods were also evaluated (Table 1). The data used in this experiment was CT image of human heart with data size

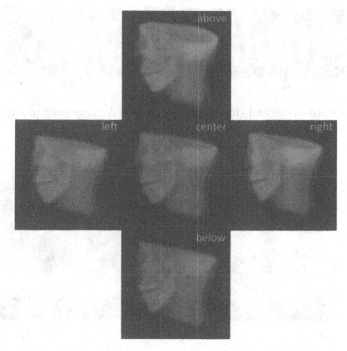

Fig. 6. Motion parallax of IV: the same IV image observed from 5 different eye positions

Table 1. Calculation time evaluation of IV volume rendering

Process	CPU(ms)	GPU(ms)	Δ
IV(iso-surface)[a]	3527± 312	73± 5	48x
IV(MIP)[a]	not implemented	66± 4	-
IV(composite)[a]	not implemented	85± 5	-

[a]data size256 × 256 × 256 voxels (n=100).

$256 \times 256 \times 256$ voxels. Calculation time on GPU is 48 times faster compared to that on CPU. MIP rendering was the fastest among the three rendering methods, but with unsignificant difference.

3.2 Visualization of Beating Heart

Then we use the real-time IV system to visualize a beating heart dataset. 3D MR image ($256 \times 256 \times 256$ voxels, $1.25 \times 1.25 \times 8.00$ cm) and 32 volumes of 3D ultrasound images ($63 \times 63 \times 63$ voxels) were acquired (Fig. 7). One of 3D ultrasound image was rigidly registered to 3D MR image, and the rest of 3D ultrasounds image were non-rigidly registered to the that registered 3D ultrasound image. As the result, 31 volumes of 3D MR images was generated (Fig. 8). Those generated 3D MR images, together with the original MR image was visualized

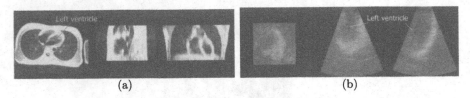

(a)   (b)

Fig. 7. (a) 3D MR image and (b) one of 3D ultrasound image used in registration. 3 cross-sections are shown.

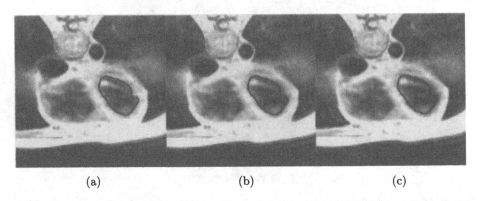

(a)   (b)   (c)

Fig. 8. Various IV rendering result on CT image (above) and MR image (below). (a) original MR image (b),(c) 2 of 31 generated MR images. Only one slice is shown here.

Table 2. Calculation time evaluation of image registration

Process	CPU(ms)	GPU(ms)	Δ
Affine transformation[b]	110±7	1.2±0.1	91x
MI calculation[b]	92±12	9.8±1.2	9.3x
B-spline transformation[b]	2600±230	24±1	110x
SSD calculation[b]	4.1±0.3	1.6±0.1	2.6x
SSD gradient calculation[b]	110000.0±13000	3025±40	36x
Registration process	**CPU(s)**	**GPU(s)**	Δ
Rigid registration[b]	238±52	18±5	13x
Non-rigid registration[b]	1897±302	88±13	21x

[b]data size 63 × 63 × 63 voxels (n=30).

in cycle, while user can change viewing parameters (translation, rotation, slicing, etc) interactively during visualization (Fig. 9). In this experiment, we also compared the processing time of registration process between GPU processing and CPU processing. Registrations on GPU were 13 and 21 times faster than registrations on CPU for rigid and non-rigid registration respectively (Table 2).

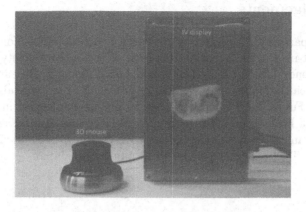

Fig. 9. Real-time autostereoscopic IV visualization system with user interactivity

4 Discussions

MIP volume rendering and composite volume rendering have enabled a wider range of visualization for IV autostereoscopic image visualization system. The capability of visualizing inner organs as well surfaces of the object would make it unnecessary to do segmentation prior to surgery. We successfully generated 4D MR image by registration, but only a small part of the heart movement can be reconstructed due to the narrow image acquisition range of ultrasound. It is also possible to reconstruct movement of a wider part of the heart by combining deformation fields from multiple ultrasound image acquisitions. Calculations on GPU have shown an impressive performace compared to CPU calculations. This is a promising technology to be applied to various medical image computings in the future, especially for applications where real-time processing is important, such as intra-operative surgery navigation systems.

5 Conclusion

We have developed GPU-accelerated IV volume rendering algorithms that enable real-time visualization of 3D/4D medical images. Using the real-time IV visualization system, we successfully visualized 4D MR image of human heart generated from image registration of 3D MR and 4D ultrasound images. Our implementation of the volume rendering and registration algorithms on GPU has shown superior performances compared to conventional CPU calculations. In the future, we plan to use this system for various surgical navigation systems, especialy for surgeries with large intra-operative organ deformation such as intra-cardiac surgery on beating heart.

Acknowledgements

This work is partially supported by Research Fellowships for Young Scientists and the Grant-in-Aid for Scientific Research of the Japan Society for the Promotion of Science (JSPS), and Health and Labor Sciences Research Grants of Ministry of Health, Labor and Welfare in Japan. H. Liao was also by Special Coordination Funds for Promoting Science and Technology commissioned by the Ministry of Education, Culture, Sports, Science and Technology MEXT) in Japan, and Grant for Industrial Technology Research (07C46050) of New Energy and Industrial Technology Development Organization, Japan.

References

1. Liao, H., Nakajima, S., Iwahara, M., Kobayashi, E., Sakuma, I., Yahagi, N., Dohi, T.: Intra-operative real-time 3D information display system based on integral videography. In: Niessen, W.J., Viergever, M.A. (eds.) MICCAI 2001. LNCS, vol. 2208, pp. 392–400. Springer, Heidelberg (2001)
2. Liao, H., Hata, N., Dohi, T.: Image-guidance for cardiac surgery using dynamic aurostereoscopic display system. In: Proc. of IEEE ISBI 2004, pp. 265–268 (2004)
3. Krueger, W.: The Application of Transport Theory to Visualization of 3D Scalar Data Fields. Computers id Physics, 397–406 (1994)
4. Herlambang, N., Liao, H., Matsumiya, K., Tsukihara, H., Takamoto, S., Dohi, T.: 4D Ultrasound and 3D MRI Registration of Beating Heart. Proc. of CARS 2007. Journal of CARS 2(1), 237–239 (2007)
5. Rueckert, D., Sonoda, L.I., Hayes, C., Hill, D.L.G., Leach, M.O., Hawkes, D.J.: Nonrigid registration using free-form deformations: application to breast mr images. IEEE Trans. Med. Imag. 18(8), 712–721 (1999)
6. CUDA Zone Home - NVIDIA (Retrieved February 22, 2008), http://www.nvidia.com/object/cuda_home.html

Realtime Organ Tracking for Endoscopic Augmented Reality Visualization Using Miniature Wireless Magnetic Tracker

Masahiko Nakamoto[1], Osamu Ukimura[2], Inderbir S. Gill[3], Arul Mahadevan[3], Tsuneharu Miki[2], Makoto Hashizume[4], and Yoshinobu Sato[1]

[1] Division of Image Analysis, Graduate School of Medicine, Osaka University, Japan
[2] Department of Urology, Kyoto Prefectural University of Medicine, Kyoto, Japan
[3] Cleveland Clinic, Cleveland, OH, USA
[4] Graduate School of Medical Sciences, Kyushu University, Japan

Abstract. Organ motion is one of the problems on augmented reality (AR) visualization for endoscopic surgical navigation system. However, the conventional optical and magnetic trackers are not suitable for tracking of internal organ motion. Recently, a wireless magnetic tracker, which is called the Calypso 4-D localization system has been developed. Since the sensor of the Calypso system is miniature and implantable, position of the internal organ can be measured directly. This paper describes AR system using the Calypso system and preliminary experiments to evaluate the AR system. We evaluated distortion error caused by the surgical instruments and misalignment error of superimposition. Results of the experiments shows potential feasibility and usefulness of AR visualization of moving organ using the Calypso system.

1   Introduction

Laparoscopic partial nephrectomy is a minimally invasive technique to remove a renal tumor. In order to remove the tumor completely and preserve healthy tissues as much as possible, augmented reality (AR) visualization of the CT image where the resection line is depicted would be useful because the boundary between healthy tissues and the tumor is not clear by endoscopic observation [1]. However, the surgeon holds up the kidney and changes its direction during resection of the tumor to confirm the resection line from several viewpoints. Therefore, realtime tracking of the kidney motion is required to superimpose the CT image onto live endoscopic images accurately.

Magnetic trackers are suitable to track objects inside the body. Conventional wired magnetic trackers have been used to track flexible tubular instruments like a catheter or a bronchoscope [2][3]. However, they have not been employed to track organ motion because it is necessary to pass the wire through the body. Recently, a wireless magnetic tracker, which is called the Calypso 4-D localization system (Calypso Medical Technologies, Inc., Seattle, WA, USA), has been developed and applied to tracking of the prostate motion during the radiation

T. Dohi, I. Sakuma, and H. Liao (Eds.): MIAR 2008, LNCS 5128, pp. 359–366, 2008.

therapy [4][5][6]. Three miniature magnetic sensors, which are called "transponders", are implanted into the prostate beforehand, and then their 3D positions are measured in realtime. Although the measurement and gating methods for internal organ motion caused by respiration were proposed [7][8][9][10], these methods assume periodical and regular motion. Since organ motion caused by surgical operation is not periodical and regular unlike the organ motion caused by respiration, the Calypso system is suitable for this purpose.

Our objective is to evaluate feasibility of endoscopic AR system using the Calypso system. We evaluate the Calypso system from two viewpoints: (1) Distortion error caused by metallic surgical instruments. (2) Accuracy of superimposition. The conventional magnetic trackers suffer from magnetic field distortion caused by metallic objects. Since the kidney is held by metallic surgical instruments during surgical operation, effects of metallic surgical instruments would not be negligible. Therefore, magnitude of the distortion error is an important factor for clinical application of the Calypso system. We also demonstrate superimposition of the CT image onto live endoscopic images, and thus accuracy and feasibility of the endoscopic AR system are evaluated.

2   Clinical Background

We demonstrated AR visualization for laparoscopic partial nephrectomy (Fig. 1) [1]. In order to assist determination of the resection line, the resection margin was visualized by colored areas. The kidney is divided to tumor, resection margin, resection and healthy tissue areas, and these areas are colored with red, yellow, green and blue (Fig. 1 left). The width of the resection margin and resection areas is 5 mm. If the surgeon resects the tumor along the green resection area, the resection margin of 5 mm or more can be kept. In order to maintain accurate superimposition, the kidney needed to keep staying at the same position and orientation as when the registration was performed because the kidney was not tracked. Since the kidney is moved by surgical operation practically, realtime tracking of the kidney is required.

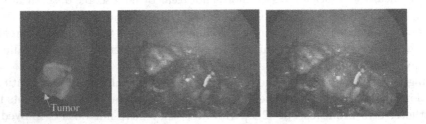

Fig. 1. Augmented reality visualization for laparoscopic partial nephrectomy. Left: 3D kidney model reconstructed from CT image. Middle: original laparoscopic image. Right: superimposed image.

3 Methods

3.1 System Overview

The AR system consists of the Calypso 4D Localization System, Polaris (Northern Digital Inc., Waterloo, Ontario, Canada), laparoscope (OTV-S5, Olympus, Japan) and PC. The Calypso system consists of the miniature implantable electromagnetic transponder, which is 8.5 mm in length (Fig. 2(a)), 4D electromagnetic array, which is a source of AC electromagnetic energy (Fig. 2(b)), and console. The Calypso system measures the position of the transponder in 3.3 frames per second. Measurement volume is 150 × 150 × 270 mm. Bias error and reproducibility are less than 0.4 mm and 0.6 mm, respectively [11]. Three transponders are attached to the organ to track position and orientation of a target organ. The Polaris is also employed to track the laparoscope.

Integration of the coordinate systems of both trackers and registration of the CT image are required to render superimposed images. Firstly, the matrix $T_{MT \to OT}$, which transforms the coordinate system from the Calypso system frame to the Polaris frame, is obtained by point matching algorithm described as the following:

$$T_{MT \to OT} = \arg \min_{T} \sum_{i=1}^{3} |T\mathbf{r}_i - \mathbf{p}_i|^2, \tag{1}$$

where $\mathbf{r}_i$ and $\mathbf{p}_i$ are positions of the transponder measured by the Calypso system and the Polaris, respectively. Secondly, the registration matrix between the CT and Polaris frames at time t, $T_{IMG \to OT,t}$, is obtained by point matching algorithm described as the following:

$$T_{IMG \to OT,t} = \arg \min_{T} \sum_{i=1}^{3} |TS\mathbf{q}_i - T_{MT \to OT}\mathbf{r}_{t,i}|^2, \tag{2}$$

where S is a diagonal matrix of which diagonal factors represent the voxel sizes of the CT image and $\mathbf{q}_i$ is a position of the transponder in the CT image.

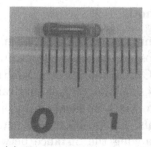
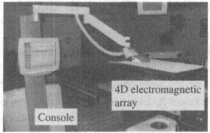

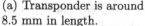

(a) Transponder is around   (b) Appearance of Calypso system.
8.5 mm in length.

Fig. 2. Calypso 4D localization system

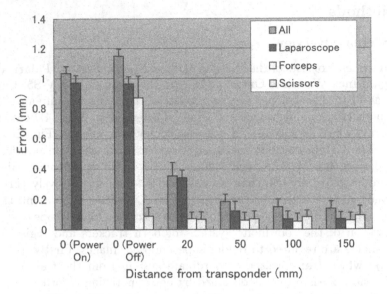

Fig. 3. Distortion error caused by surgical instruments

Finally, arbitrary position $\mathbf{q}_t = (x, y, z, 1)^t$ in the CT image is projected to $\mathbf{q}'_t = (sx', sy', s, 1)^t$ in the laparoscopic image by the following equation:

$$\mathbf{q}'_t = AT_{ext}T_{cam}^{-1}T_{IMG \rightarrow OT,t}S\mathbf{q}_t, \tag{3}$$

where A and T_{ext} are intrinsic and extrinsic camera parameters obtained by camera calibration, and $T_{cam,t}$ is a rigid transformation matrix measured by the Polaris.

Because the Calypso system is not connected to the PC in the current system, position data measured by the Calypso system is imported to the PC offline and then the superimposed images are rendered after the acquisition of positions and laparoscopic images.

3.2   Experimental Conditions and Methods

We evaluated effects of metallic surgical instruments on the position measured by the Calypso system. We employed the laparoscope, forceps (CLICKline Bowel grasper, KARL Storz, Germany) and scissors (CLICKline Sciccors, KARL Storz, Germany), which were commonly used in laparoscopic surgery, as surgical instruments. The transponder and the surgical instrument were fixed on the operating table which was made of non-metallic materials. The position of the transponder was measured around 50 times while changing the distance between the transponder and the instrument from 0 to 150 mm. We performed the measurements for each instrument and performed them for all three instruments. Powers of the laparoscope and the light source were turned off except when the distance was 0 mm. The powers of them were turned on and off when the

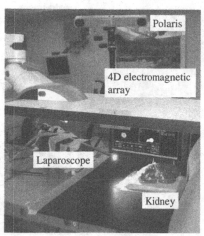

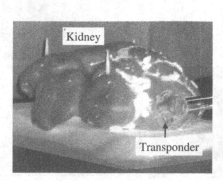

(a) Cow kidney with transponders.   (b) Arrangement of instruments.

Fig. 4. Experimental setup for augmented reality visualization

distance was 0 mm. Distortion error caused by the surgical instruments is defined as the difference of positions between with and without the surgical instruments.

We employed a cow kidney to demonstrate AR visualization. In order to simulate laparoscopic partial nephrectomy, a pseudo tumor was embedded in the kidney, and three transponders were attached around the pseudo tumor (Fig. 4(a)). The CT image of the kidney was acquired, and then the kidney and the pseudo tumor were segmented. The kidney and the laparoscope with optical markers were fixed on the operating table (Fig. 4(b)). A part of the kidney was grasped with the forceps and moved up and down, and then the pseudo tumor was resected with the scissors and lifted up and down. The above operation was divided into three sequences, and then superimposed images were rendered for each sequence. Misalignment error of superimposition at time t is defined as $\frac{1}{3}\sum_{i=3}^{3} |\mathbf{u}_{i,t} - \mathbf{v}_{i,t}|$, where $\mathbf{u}_{i,t}$ is a 2D position of the transponder given by transforming the position of the transponder in the CT image using equation (3), and $\mathbf{v}_{i,t}$ is a 2D position of the transponder in the laparoscopic image obtained by manual pointing.

4   Experimental Results

4.1   Distortion Error Caused by Surgical Instruments

Distortion error caused by the surgical instruments was around 1.0 mm when the distance between the transponder and the instrument was 0 mm, and 0.4 mm or less when the distance was 20 mm or more as shown in Fig. 3. The error when the powers were up was almost same as the error when the powers were down.

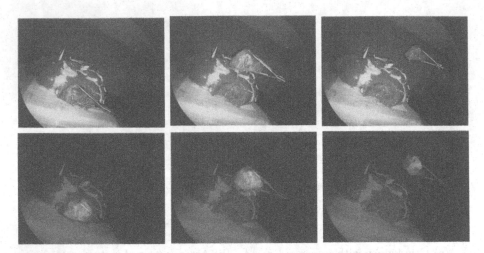

Fig. 5. Augmented reality visualization (third sequence). Upper row: original laparoscopic images. Lower row: superimposed images.

4.2   Accuracy of Superimposition

Superimposed images of the third sequence are shown in Fig. 5. Kidney tissue, pseudo tumor and transponder are depicted as blue, yellow and red part, respectively. Delay of a few frames were observed.

Average misalignment errors of three sequences were 10.7 ± 4.9, 14.0 ± 2.9, 16.7 ± 9.5 pixels, respectively. Since 1 pixel in the laparoscopic image was approximately equal to 0.33 mm in this condition, the average misalignment errors

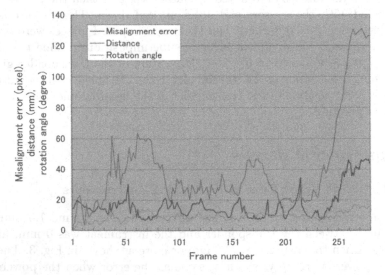

Fig. 6. Misalignment error of augmented reality visualization in third sequence

corresponded to around 3 to 5 mm. Fig. 6 shows time varying misalignment error, distance from the position of the initial frame and rotation angle from the orientation of the initial frame. Change of the distance means the resected part was lifted up three times in this sequence. Change of the rotation angle means change of the orientation of the resected part was moderate. When the resected part was far from the initial position in the last part of the sequence, the misalignment error increased greatly in proportion to the distance.

5   Discussion and Conclusions

We have described endoscopic AR visualization using the Calypso system. We evaluated distortion error caused by metallic surgical instruments. Since distortion error was 0.4 mm or less when the distance from the transponder to the instrument was 20 mm or more and around 1 mm even when the instrument made contact with the transponder, the error would be negligible without distortion correction in most cases.

In the experiment of AR visualization, we demonstrated that the colored 3D kidney model was superimposed onto the moving kidney in live laparoscopic images. The demonstration means potential feasibility and usefulness of the AR system using the Calypso system. Since the AR system is applicable to internal organs which can be assumed as a rigid body (i.e. prostate), this study would contribute to development and progress of the endoscopic surgical navigation system for the internal organs. Average misalignment error of superimposition was around 3 to 5 mm. Since the width of the resection margin in laparoscopic partial nephrectomy is 5 mm, the misalignment error is not small enough to clinical application. Delay of a few frames means there were some errors in temporary registration. The misalignment error which increased in proportion to the distance also means there were some errors in integration of the coordinate systems. Therefore, it is guessed that temporal and spatial misalignments between the Calypso system and the Polaris are main factors of the error.

Future work includes integration of the Calypso system into the AR system. Because the Calypso system can not control from the PC currently, complexity to deal with the Calypso system obstructs accurate registration. If the Calypso system is integrated, accuracy of temporal and spatial registration would be improved.

References

1. Ukimura, O., Nakamoto, M., Desai, M., Herts, B., Aron, M., Haber, G.P., Kaouk, J., Miki, T., Sato, Y., Hashizume, M., Gill, I.: Augmented reality visualization during laparoscopic urologic surgery: The initial clinical experience. In: The 102nd American Urological Association 2007 Annual Meeting, Anaheim, CA (2007)
2. Krueger, S., Timinger, H., Grewer, R., Borgert, J.: Modality-integrated magnetic catheter tracking for x-ray vascular interventions. Physics in Medicine and Biology 50, 581–597 (2005)

3. Mori, K., Deguchi, D., Akiyama, K., Kitasaka, T., Maurer Jr., C.R., Suenaga, Y., Takabatake, H., Mori, M., Natori, H.: Hybrid bronchoscope tracking using a magnetic tracking sensor and image registration. In: Duncan, J.S., Gerig, G. (eds.) MICCAI 2005. LNCS, vol. 3750, pp. 543–550. Springer, Heidelberg (2005)

4. Willoughby, T.R., Kupelian, P.A., Pouliot, J., Shinohara, K., Aubin, M., Roach III, M., Skrumeda, L.L., Balter, J.M., Litzenberg, D.W., Hadley, S.W., Wei, J.T., Sandler, H.M.: Target localization and real-time tracking using the Calypso 4D localization system in patients with localized prostate cancer. International Journal of Radiation Oncology Biology Physics 65, 528–534 (2006)

5. Kupelian, P., Willoughby, T., Mahadevan, A., Djemil, T., Weinstein, G., Jani, S., Enke, C., Solberg, T., Flores, N., Liu, D., Beyer, D., Levine, L.: Multi-institutional clinical experience with the Calypso System in localization and continuous, real-time monitoring of the prostate gland during external radiotherapy. International Journal of Radiation Oncology Biology Physics 67, 1088–1098 (2007)

6. Kupelian, P.A., Willoughby, T.R., Reddy, C.A., Klein, E.A., Mahadevan, A.: Hypofractionated intensity-modulated radiotherapy (70 gy at 2.5 gy per fraction) for localized prostate cancer: Cleveland clinic experience. International Journal of Radiation Oncology Biology Physics 68, 1424–1430 (2007)

7. Rohlfing, T., Maurer Jr., C.R., O'Dell, W.G., Zhong, J.: Modeling liver motion and deformation during the respiratory cycle using intensity-based nonrigid registration of gated MR images. Medical Physics 31, 427–432 (2004)

8. Olbrich, B., Traub, J., Wiesner, S., Wiechert, A., Feußner, H., Navab, N.: Respiratory motion analysis: Towards gated augmentation of the liver. In: Proceedings of Computer Assisted Radiology and Surgery (CARS 2005), Berlin, Germany, pp. 248–253 (2005)

9. von Siebenthal, M., Szekery, G., Gamper, U., Boesiger, P., Lomax, A., Cattin, P.: 4D MR imaging of respiratory organ motion and its variability. Physics in Medicine and Biology 52, 1547–1564 (2007)

10. Nakamoto, M., Hirayama, H., Sato, Y., Konishi, K., Kakeji, Y., Hashizume, M., Tamura, S.: Recovery of respiratory motion and deformation of the liver using laparoscopic freehand 3D ultrasound system. Medical Image Analysis 11, 429–442 (2007)

11. Balter, J.M., Wright, J.N., Newell, L.J., Friemel, B., Dimmer, S., Cheng, Y., Wong, J., Vertatschitsch, E., Mate, T.P.: Accuracy of a wireless localization system for radiotherapy. International Journal of Radiation Oncology Biology Physics 61, 933–937 (2005)

Fusion of Laser Guidance and 3-D Autostereoscopic Image Overlay for Precision-Guided Surgery

Hongen Liao[1,2], Hirotaka Ishihara[3], Huy Hoang Tran[3], Ken Masamune[3], Ichiro Sakuma[1], and Takeyoshi Dohi[3]

[1] Graduate School of Engineering, the University of Tokyo
[2] Translational Systems Biology and Medicine Initiative, the University of Tokyo
[3] Graduate School of Information Science and Technology, the University of Tokyo
7-3-1 Hongo, Bunkyo-ku, Tokyo 113-8656, Japan
liao@bmpe.t.u-tokyo.ac.jp

Abstract. This paper describes a precision-guided surgical navigation system for minimally invasive surgery using fusion of laser guidance technique and three-dimensional (3-D) autostereoscopic image overlay technique. The images superimposed onto the patient are created by employing an animated autostereoscopic image called integral videography (IV), which display geometrically accurate 3-D autostereoscopic images and reproduce motion parallax without the need for special viewing or tracking devices. To improve the insertion accuracy of surgical instrument, we integrated the image overlay system with laser guidance for visualization of insertion point and orientation of the surgical instrument. We designed and manufactured a laser guidance device and mounted it to the IV image overlay device. Accuracy evaluations showed that the system could guide a linear surgical instrument toward a target with an average error of 2.48 mm and standard deviation of 1.76 mm. Improvement in the design of the laser guidance device and the patient-image registration of the IV image overlay will make this system practical and its use will increase surgical accuracy and reduce invasiveness.

1 Introduction

Image-guided surgery is a means of navigation that guide the surgeon by indicating the location of a tracking device through a set of cross-sectional images, for example, X-ray computed tomography (CT) and/or magnetic resonance (MR) images, or three-dimensional (3-D) anatomical models reconstructed from such images. By localizing the targeted lesion and the critical lesion that should be avoided, the surgical navigation helps to achieve effective and safe surgery while minimizing the invasiveness of the surgery [1].

The display used for the surgical navigation system is often placed in a nonsterile field from surgeon. This hand-eye coordination problem forces the surgeon to take extra steps to match guidance information on the display with the actual anatomy of the patient [2]. The problem has been discussed as possible cause of the interruption of surgical flow [3]. To overcome this problem, several groups have developed techniques that merge images into real-world views in a more natural and unconstrained

T. Dohi, I. Sakuma, and H. Liao (Eds.): MIAR 2008, LNCS 5128, pp. 367–376, 2008.

manner. Those works involved image overlay that visually merges a computer-generated anatomical model, reconstructed from medical images, with the patient's body [4-6]. Another example is the use of augmented reality visualization with microscopes or endoscopes in image-guided surgery [7-8].

Most of the image overlay system focused on how to overlay pre-/intra- operative images to the patient. Less of them solved the problem of guiding surgical instrument. Some of surgical treatment such as orthopedic surgery requires high-precision accuracy of the position and orientation of the surgical tools insertion. For example, during the surgical implementation of knee joint surgery, surgeon needs to identify both the information of the surgical area and the insertion path for tunneling or drilling. Sasama et al. developed a laser guidance system to monolithic integration with optical tracker [9-10]. The laser beams are projected onto the surgical field so that surgeon can obtain guidance information directly. These systems still have a problem of lack of intuitive visualization of anatomical 3-D information.

To improve the safety and accuracy of surgical treatment, especially for the use of linear surgical tool such as drills and wires, we develop a 3-D autostereoscopic image overlay system that integrated with laser guidance. The fusion of image overlay and the laser guidance enable both visualization of patient and guidance of surgical instrument. Experimental results show that this precision guided system will give a promising support to surgeon for executing the surgical treatment. Our system developed in this study is simple and fast to provide an intra-operative overall information of anatomical structure and enable the surgeon to perform identification of the insertion path of the surgical instrument in intuitive.

2 Materials and Methods

2.1 Laser Guidance System

Laser guidance system includes two laser beam shooters, which project individual laser plane to generate an intersection line in the space (Fig. 1). The laser beam shooters are fixed to a motor on a stand. We use mirrors to reflect the laser beams to the target surgical area. The directions of mirror planes are rotated by motors so that the plane of laser beams can be adjusted according to the position of the target. Two laser planes are projected onto the surgical field, and the projection direction are controlled by navigation system.

The intersection line generated by the laser planes is used to guide insertion path for linear surgical instrument. Fig. 2 shows the procedure of aligning the surgical instrument.

1) Two laser planes are projected onto the surgical area as crossing lines (Fig. 2a). The projection positions are decided by patient registration method that described in subsection 2.4 and 2.5.

2) Move the tip of the surgical instrument to the crossing point (Fig. 2b). The position of the crossing point should be calculated according to the 3-D shape of the anatomical structure.

3) Rotate the surgical instrument around the crossing point and align the insertion path (Fig. 2c). The orientation can be decided by a coaxial point localized at the tail of

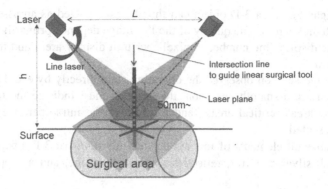

Fig. 1. Laser guidance with intersection line generated by two laser planes

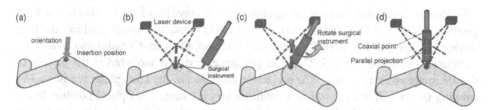

Fig. 2. Procedure of surgical instrument alignment: (a) Target in surgical area; (b) Move the tip of surgical instrument to the insertion point; (c) Rotate surgical instrument and adjust its orientation; (d) Surgical instrument aligned to the target orientation by identifying coaxial point or parallel projection lines

the surgical instrument or parallel projection straight lines on cylindrical surface of the surgical instrument (Fig. 2d).

4) Stabilize the surgical instrument after achieving surgical path by the alignment of the insertion point and orientation.

2.2 IV Autostereoscopic Image Overlay System

We adopt an autostereoscopic image overlay technique that can be integrated into a surgical navigation system by superimposing an actual 3-D image onto the patient using a half-silvered mirror. The autostereoscopic image is generated by using a modified version of integral videography (IV) [11-12], which is an animated extension of the integral photography [13].

The IV display we developed consists of a high-resolution LCD with a micro convex lens array. The computer-generated images of the anatomical object are rendered behind the lens array. The source image shown on the IV display is generated from the 3-D data by high-speed IV rendering. Any kind of 3-D data source can be processed, such as MRI and CT images. Each point shown in a 3-D space is reconstructed at the same position as the actual object by the convergence of rays from the pixels of the element images on the computer display after they pass through the lenses in a micro convex lens array. The surgeon can see any point on the display from various directions, as though it were fixed in 3-D space. Each point appears as a different light source; a 3-D object can thus be constructed as an assembly of reconstructed light sources. The quality of the IV image depends primarily on the pixel density of the display (the number of pixels per unit display area) and the lens pitch of the lens array.

Generally, the surgeon observed the operating field directly by eye during the operation. To ensure a smooth operation, the surgeon must indicate the target object, avoid specific areas (critical areas), and respond to the intra-operative information when it is presented.

The fundamental elements of this system include intuitive 3-D image on the IV display, a half-silvered mirror, reflected spatial 3-D image, and a supporting stage [14].

2.3 System of IV Image Overlay with Laser Guidance

The IV-overlay based surgical navigation system consists of an IV display, a laser guidance device, 3-D data source collection equipment, an optical position tracking device (POLARIS, Northern Digital Inc., Waterloo, Ontario, Canada) and a personal computer, as shown in Fig.3. The laser guidance device is mounted in the bottom of the IV image-overlay device. The projection direction of the laser plane is adjusted by rotating the axis of mirror, which is controlled by a motor. The optical position tracking system is used for both calibration of the laser guidance device and registration of the IV-image to patient. To project the laser beams onto the required position and orientation, we calibrate the original projection and calculate the relationship between the reflection direction of the mirror and the rotation of the motor.

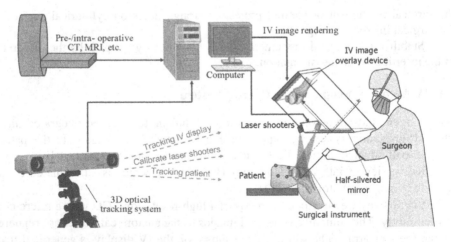

Fig. 3. System configuration of IV image overlay with laser guidance

2.4 Calibration of Laser Guidance Device

The laser guidance system is registered with POLARIS optical tracking device. A set of test laser beams are projected onto a plate at different directions. The 3-D position of the projection laser beams are measured by optical tracking device. The relationship between the projected laser plane and the rotation angle of the mirror can be thus determined. Since the laser guidance devices are fixed in the IV display, which can be tracked by the same optical tracking device, we can calculate the transformation matrix between the original laser plane and the optical tracking device. After finishing patient-image registration described in next section, we drive the motors to rotate the axes of the laser shooter and the mirror to targeted angles. The insertion path of the surgical instrument can be obtained by the intersection line of the two laser beam planes.

2.5 Patient-Image Registration

Patient-image registration can be based on a set of distinct features (geometrical landmarks or natural anatomical landmarks) that can be accurately identified in both spaces. In this study, the fiducial markers used in image registration provide pairs of corresponding 3-D points in the spaces to be registered. Additionally, the same fiducials can be localized in the position sensor space by computing their 3-D coordinates. Once the coordinates of the fiducials in the image space and in the patient coordinate space have been determined, the geometric transformation that associates these two spaces can be derived [15].

The position and orientation of the IV display can also be tracked for image overlay. It is also possible to calculate the relative position of projected IV images and the corresponding organ with these results. The target objects are represented in the form of IVs, which are displayed in real time on the IV display.

3 Experiments and Results

3.1 Laser Guidance Devices

We manufactured a prototype of laser guidance device (Fig. 4). Two lasers and four motors were mounted on the bottom of the IV image overlay device. The orientation of laser beam plane was driven by two motors. The laser shooter was fixed in one of the motors, which can rotate the axis of the projected laser beam. A mirror was fixed to another motor, which could adjust the laser plane to the surgical field (Fig. 4b). The projection laser beams are shown in Fig. 4a. A set of optical tracking markers were attached in the base of the laser guidance device, which was fixed in the IV image overlay device.

3.2 Accuracy Measurement of Laser Guidance

We carried out an experiment to evaluate the accuracy of the laser guidance. In order to achieve a high-precision laser beam projection, we calibrated the laser guidance device by a set of test patterns. The accuracy evaluation experiments were performed based on the calibration and correction results of relationship between the motors and

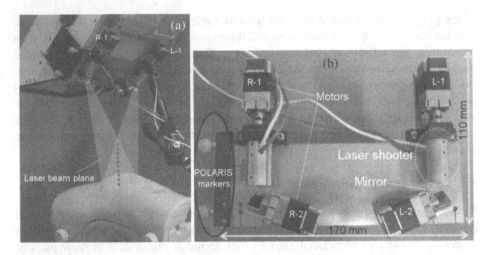

Fig. 4. Laser guidance devices: (a) laser plane intersected into a line; (b) Motors and mirrors for adjustment of the orientation of the projection laser planes

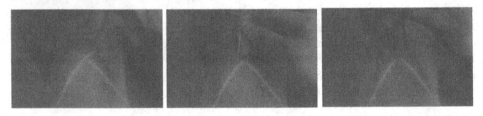

Fig. 5. Alignment of surgical instrument under the guidance of laser beams intersection path: (a) Move the tip of the surgical instrument to the crossing point of laser planes; (b) Adjust the orientation of the surgical instrument; (c) Identify coaxial point and parallel projection lines on the surgical instrument and stabilize the surgical instrument

laser projection planes. We used POLARIS to measure the projected crossing point and the intersection line of the two laser planes. Experimental evaluation of 25 tests showed that the mean value of position error of the insertion point was 2.48 mm and the standard deviation was 1.76 mm, and the mean value of the orientation error of the intersection line was 2.96 degree and the standard deviation was 2.12 degree.

We conducted another set of experiments to assess the feasibility of surgical instrument aligning with an insertion path generated by the laser planes (Fig. 5). Experimental results show that the system could provide the intuitive 3-D information of anatomical structure of the organ and guidance of surgical instrument.

3.3 IV Image Overlay

We manufactured an IV image overlay device with a micro convex lens array, a half-silvered mirror, and a supporting stage (Fig.6a). The primary specifications of the IV display are listed in Table I. The rendering time of IV image depended highly on the complexity of the rendered object. We integrated a Graphic Processing Unit (GPU)-accelerated IV rendering method to realize real-time IV rendering. Despite of the complexity of the data, the developed method enabled an update speed of 14 frames per second for a data of 256×256×256 voxels (Intel Pentium 4, 3.2 GHz CPU). With our optimized algorithm, the IV image could be calculated and displayed in almost real-time.

The IV image could be superimposed onto the patient with fiducial markers based registration. Once all displayed objects have been transformed into the same coordinate space using these transformations, they will appear to the surgeon exactly as if they were in their virtual spatial locations. It took less than 0.2 second to update each IV image. One of the registration results was shown in Fig. 6b.

Table 1. Primary Specifications of IV Display

Size	184.50 mm × 30.6 mm × 139.5 mm
Size of display	129.0mm×96.7mm
Number of pixels	1024 × 768 pixels
Pixel pitch	0.127 mm
Lens pitch	1.001 mm (H), 0.876mm(V); (hexagon)
Lens focal length	3.0 mm
Lens refractive index	Nd = 1.49
Viewing angle	about ± 10°
Weight	700 g

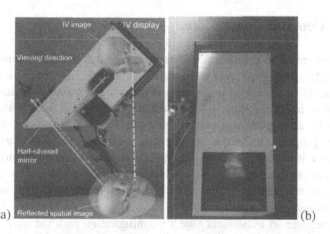

Fig. 6. IV image overlay device: (a) IV image overlay device; (b) Image-overlay result

3.4 Feasibility Study of IV Image Overlay and Laser Guidance System

A volunteer clinical trial was implemented to evaluate the feasibility of the developed system. We performed CT scanning to take photo of in-vivo knee. The volumetric CT images of knee (512×512pixels×347 slices, thickness of 0.5mm) were segmented and the results were rendered and transmitted to IV display. We integrated IV segmentation image in knee surgery and superimposed IV image into the patient in surgical implementation (Fig.7a). The position of the insertion point and the orientation of the intersection line were calculated and the laser planes were adjusted by the rotation of corresponding motors. Fig. 7b showed the procedure of alignment of a surgical instrument with the guidance of lasers, and Fig. 7c showed the image-patient registration results with the laser guidance surgical instrument. These combinations enabled safe, easy, and accurate navigation.

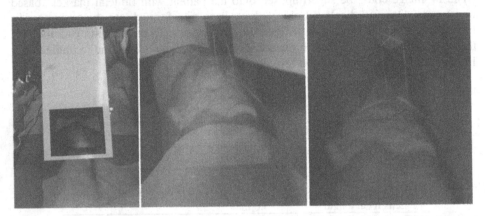

Fig. 7. The laser guidance with autostereoscopic image overlay: (a) Scheme of device and patient with IV image overlay; (b) Alignment of surgical instrument; (c) Image-patient registration results and surgical path guidance of laser beams

4 Discussion and Conclusions

We have demonstrated a fusion autostereoscopic image overlay technique and laser guidance technique for surgical navigation. An actual 3-D image is superimposed onto the patient using a semi-transparent display based on an adaptation of integral videography to image overlay. A laser guidance technique is used to guide the insertion path of linear surgical instrument. The experimental findings demonstrated feasibility of the proposed technique. The accuracy of laser guidance was 2.48 mm on average, which is almost satisfactory for precision-guided knee joint surgery.

Although the orientation evaluation of the laser guidance showed the error was 2.96 degree and the standard deviation was 2.12 degree, improvement of precision of the laser shooter and corresponding motors should obviate this problem. It will then be possible to register an anatomical object's configuration with the intra-operative surgical instrument in high precision with a real-time IV image rendering. For soft tissue or deformable tissue around the bone, the patient-IV image registration should be corrected by sensing intra-operative tissue images and automatically updating the displayed image.

In conclusion, our precision-guided surgical navigation system is possible to superimpose a real 3-D image onto a patient's body for accurate and less-invasive surgery and an intuitive guidance of linear surgical instrument. The experimental results show that the errors were in the range of about 2 mm. Due to the simplicity and accuracy of real-time projected point location by the introduction a display device with higher pixel density and a laser guidance device with higher precision, this system should be of practical use in the precision guidance orthopedic surgery and other medical field.

Acknowledgment

This study was supported in part by the Special Coordination Funds for Promoting Science and Technology commissioned by the Ministry of Education, Culture, Sports, Science and Technology (MEXT) in Japan, Grant for Industrial Technology Research (07C46050) of New Energy and Industrial Technology Development Organization, Japan, and the Communications R & D Promotion Programme (062103006) of the Ministry of Internal Affairs and Communications in Japan.

References

1. Rosen, M., Ponsky, J.: Minimally Invasive Surgery. Endoscopy 33, 358–366 (2001)
2. Breedveld, P., Wentink, M.: Eye-hand coordination in laparoscopy - an overview of experiments and supporting aids. Minim. Invasiv. Ther. 10(3), 155–162 (2001)
3. Breedveld, P., Stassen, H.G., Meijer, D.W., Stassen, L.P.S.: Theoretical background and conceptual solution for depth perception and eye-hand coordination problems in laparoscopic surgery. Minim. Invasiv. Ther. 8, 227–234 (1999)
4. Stetten, G.D., Clib, V.S.: Overlaying Ultrasonographic Images on Direct Vision. J. Ultrasound Med. 20, 235–240 (2001)
5. Rosenthal, M., State, A., Lee, J., Hirota, G., Ackerman, J., Keller, K., Pisano, E.D., Jiroutek, M., Muller, K., Fuchs, H.: Augmented reality guidance for needle biopsies: An initial randomized, controlled trial in phantoms. Medical Image Analysis 6, 313–320 (2002)
6. Fichtinger, G., Deguet, A., Masamune, K., Balogh, E., Fischer, G.S., Mathieu, H., Taylor, R.H., Zinreich, S.J., Fayad, L.M.: Image Overlay Guidance for Needle Insertion in CT Scanner. IEEE Trans. Biomedical Engineering 52(8), 1415–1424 (2005)
7. Edwards, P.J., King, A.P., Maurer Jr., C.R., Cunha, D.A., Hawkes, D.J., Hill, D.L.G., Gaston, R.P., Fenlon, M.R., Jusczyzck, A., Strong, A.J., Chandler, C.L., Gleeson, M.J.: Design and evaluation of a system for microscope-assisted guided interventions (MAGI). IEEE Trans. Med. Imag. 19, 1082–1093 (2000)
8. Shahidi, R., Bax, M.R., Maurer, C.R., Johnson, J.A., Wilkinson, E.P., Wang, B., West, J.B., Citardi, M.J., Manwaring, K.H., Khadem, R.: Implementation, calibration and accuracy testing of an image-enhanced endoscopy system. IEEE Trans. Med. Imag. 21, 1524–1535 (2002)
9. Sasama, T., Sugano, N., Sato, Y., Momoi, Y., Nakajima, Y., Koyama, T., Nakajima, Y., Sakuma, I., Fujie, M., Yonenobu, K., Ochi, T., Tamura, S.: A Novel Laser Guidance System for Alignment of Linear Surgical Tool: Its Principles and Performance Evaluation as a Man-Machine System. In: Dohi, T., Kikinis, R. (eds.) MICCAI 2002. LNCS, vol. 2489, pp. 125–132. Springer, Heidelberg (2002)
10. Nakajima, Y., Yamamoto, H., Sato, Y., Sugano, N., Momoi, Y., Sasama, T., Koyama, T., Tamura, T., Yonenobu, K., Sakuma, I., Yoshikawa, H., Ochi, T., Tamura, S.: Available range analysis of laser guidance system and its application to monolithic integration with optical tracker. In: CARS 2004, pp. 449–454 (2004)

11. Liao, H., Hata, N., Nakajima, S., Iwahara, M., Sakuma, I., Dohi, T.: Surgical Navigation by Autostereoscopic Image Overlay of Integral Videography. IEEE Transactions on Information Technology in Biomedicine 8(2), 114–121 (2004)
12. Liao, H., Iwahara, M., Hata, N., Dohi, T.: High-quality integral videography using a multi-projector. Optics Express 12(6), 1067–1076 (2004)
13. Lippmann, M.G.: Epreuves reversibles donnant la sensation du relief. J. de Phys. 7(4th series), 821–825 (1908)
14. Liao, H., Matsui, K., Dohi, T.: Design and Evaluation of Surgical Navigation for Anterior Cruciate Ligament Reconstruction using Autostereoscopic Image Overlay of Integral Videography. In: 27th Annual International Conference of the IEEE Engineering In Medicine and Biology Society (EMBS) 2005. CD-ROM (September 2005)
15. Liao, H., Inomata, T., Sakuma, I., Dohi, T.: Surgical Navigation of Integral Videography Image Overlay for Open MRI-Guided Glioma Surgery. In: Yang, G.-Z., Jiang, T., Shen, D., Gu, L., Yang, J. (eds.) MIAR 2006. LNCS, vol. 4091, pp. 187–194. Springer, Heidelberg (2006)

Augmented Display of Anatomical Names of Bronchial Branches for Bronchoscopy Assistance

Shunsuke Ota[1], Daisuke Deguchi[2], Takayuki Kitasaka[2,3], Kensaku Mori[1,2],
Yasuhito Suenaga[1,2], Yoshinori Hasegawa[4], Kazuyoshi Imaizumi[4],
Hirotsugu Takabatake[5], Masaki Mori[6], and Hiroshi Natori[7]

[1] Graduate School of Information Science, Nagoya University, Japan
[2] Mext Innovative Research Center for Preventive Medical Engineering,
Nagoya University, Japan
[3] Faculty of Management and Information Science,
Aichi Institute of Technology, Japan
[4] School of Medicine, Nagoya University, Japan
[5] Sapporo Minami Sanjo Hospital, Japan
[6] Sapporo-Kosei General Hospital, Japan
[7] Keiwakai Nishioka Hospital, Japan

Abstract. This paper presents a method for an automated anatomical labeling of bronchial branches (ALBB) for augmented display of its result for bronchoscopy assistance. A method for automated ALBB plays an important role for realizing an augmented display of anatomical names of bronchial branches. The ALBB problem can be considered as a problem that each bronchial branch is classified into the bronchial name to which it belongs. Therefore, the proposed method constructs classifiers that output anatomical names of bronchial branches by employing the machine-learning approach. The proposed method consists of four steps: (a) extraction of bronchial tree structures from 3D CT datasets, (b) construction of classifiers using the multi-class AdaBoost technique, (c) automated classification of bronchial branches by using the constructed classifiers, and (d) an augmented display of anatomical names of bronchial branches. We applied the proposed method to 71 cases of 3D CT datasets. We evaluated the ALBB results by leave-one-out scheme. The experimental results showed that the proposed method could assign correct anatomical names to bronchial branches of 90.1 % up to segmental lobe branches. Also, we confirmed that an augmented display of the ALBB results was quite useful to assist bronchoscopy.

Keywords: bronchus, anatomical labeling, bronchoscopy guidance, virtual bronchoscopy, chest CT image, multi-class AdaBoost.

1 Introduction

Virtual Bronchoscopy System (VBS) becomes a very important tool for a bronchoscopist to make the bronchoscopy much safer and effective[1]. In the respiratory field, a bronchoscope is a quite useful tool for diagnosis of inside the

T. Dohi, I. Sakuma, and H. Liao (Eds.): MIAR 2008, LNCS 5128, pp. 377–384, 2008.
© Springer-Verlag Berlin Heidelberg 2008

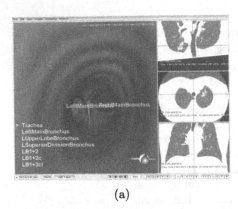
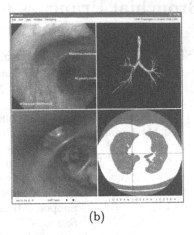

(a)   (b)

Fig. 1. (a) A sequence of the anatomical names of bronchial branches where the bronchoscope should be passed through toward a target location. (b) An example of augmented display of anatomical names of bronchial branches. They are overlaid on the real bronchoscopic view (Top-left)). Outside view of the bronchus is depicted with the trajectory of a bronchoscope on the top-right window. Inside view and slice view are shown in Bottom-left and -right windows, where their observing position is corresponding to that of the bronchoscope.

bronchus. During bronchoscopy, a bronchoscopist inserts a bronchoscope into a bronchus to diagnose its inside with watching a TV monitor. An ultra-thin bronchoscope has enabled him/her to observe thinner bronchi and to perform biopsy against peripheral lung tumors. In the case of peripheral lung tumors, however, he/she may be easily confused and lose the way to the target location, since the bronchus has a very complex tree structure and it is necessary to visit several branches before reaching the desired location. Therefore, the path planning is a crucial and indispensable task to perform bronchoscopy smoothly and safely[2,3]. In the path planning, a bronchoscopist usually generates an optimal path to a target using VB images generated from patient's CT images. Here, the path is represented as a sequence of the anatomical names of bronchial branches where the bronchoscope should visit. Therefore, augmented display of anatomical names of bronchial branches on real bronchoscopic views are quite helpful for a bronchoscopist as shown in Fig. 1

To generate such augmented display, anatomical names of bronchial branches should be labeled before the planning. However, due to the complexity of bronchial tree structure, it is heavily time-consuming to label them manually. Several research groups proposed methods for automated ALBB[4,5]. They performed automated ALBB by comparing a bronchial tree structure with branching-pattern models. Kitaoka et al.[4] prepared one branching-pattern model for ALBB. Then, automated ALBB was performed using a weighted maximum clique search approach. However, their method could not deal with variations of branching patterns. In contrast, Mori et al.[5] utilized several branching-pattern models for each part of the bronchus (right upper lobe, right middle and lower lobes, left upper lobe and left lower lobe). Their models have information about running directions, parent branch names and parent-child relationships. Using several branching models, this method could deal with variations of branching-patterns. However, they considered only variations of branching patterns and did not consider variations of running directions. Since the running directions of bronchial branches can differ greatly among individuals, it is impossible to perform ALBB accurately when running directions of bronchial branches were different from those of their models.

Therefore, we consider the ALBB as a problem that each bronchial branch is classified into its anatomical name. We try to solve this problem by classifiers which learn variations of running directions of bronchial branches as well as branching-patterns. Since the bronchus consists of hundreds of branches with unique anatomical names, our problem is formulated as a multi-class classification problem in which each bronchial branch is to be assigned to each class corresponding to its anatomical name. We utilize multi-class AdaBoost technique to construct classifiers. Multi-class AdaBoost[6,7,8] is a powerful tool for a multi-class classification problem. The proposed method uses the multi-class AdaBoost technique proposed by Li et al.[8].

2 Methods

2.1 Anatomical Labeling of Bronchial Branches

The ALBB problem can be considered as a problem that each bronchial branch is classified into the bronchial name to which it belongs. The bronchus consists of hundreds of bronchial branches having unique anatomical names. Therefore, our problem is formulated as a multi-class classification problem. To solve this problem, the proposed method constructs classifiers by utilizing the multi-class AdaBoost technique, and each classifier is trained by using features of bronchial branches, such as length and running directions of bronchial branches. Automated ALBB consists of five steps: (a) extraction of bronchial tree structures from 3D CT images, (b) normalization of patient's position and orientation, (c) feature calculation of bronchial branches, (d) construction of classifiers using multi-class AdaBoost technique, and (e) automated ALBB by using the constructed classifiers.

(a) Extraction of bronchial tree structure. The first step of the proposed method is to extract the bronchial region and analysis of its tree structure from the 3D CT image. Bronchial regions are extracted by Kitasaka's method [9]. They extract bronchial regions by region growing using branch-by-branch VOI (Volume of Interest) placement technique. This method can detect the bifurcation points of a bronchus during extraction procedure of the bronchial region. The tree structure is obtained by connecting the detected bifurcation points. The proposed method uses the extracted tree structure for automated ALBB and augmented display of anatomical names of bronchial branches on the RB views.

(b) Normalization of patient's position and orientation. Patient's position and orientation may vary among CT images of individuals. Therefore, individual differences may be included in the features calculated in the next step. To reduce individual differences caused by shift of patient's position and orientation, the proposed method introduces two normalization scheme: (1) global normalization and (2) local normalization. Global normalization is performed by equalizing the plane defined by the right and the left main bronchi between individual CT images. The individual differences about the patient's position and orientation will be roughly reduced by applying this normalization. Also, local normalization is obtained by applying the same process against the plane defined by the parent branch and its sibling branch. This normalization aims to reduce variance about a running direction of each branch.

(c) Computation of features for each branch. This step calculates five types of bronchial features: (i) length of a branch, (ii) running direction of a branch, (iii) relative position from the parent branch, (iv) average direction of the child branches, and (v) running direction of sibling branches.

(d) Construction of classifiers using multi-class AdaBoost technique. Before construction of classifiers, the proposed method calculates candidate branch names that should be classified by each classifier. Sets of candidate branch names are grouped by the parent's name of a target branch, and each classifier is trained by a set of feature vector calculated from candidate branches that have candidate branch names. Here, since the complexity of a classification problem may depend on the number of classes or categories that should be classified, we try to reduce the number of candidate branch names by using parent-child relationships. The proposed method lists up this relationships into the "correspondence table". And each classifier is trained to output its bronchial name by using each record on the correspondence table, and then added into the correspondence table. Finally, multi-class AdaBoost technique is utilized in this training process.

(e) Automated ALBB. At first, the proposed method labels the root of the tree structure as "TRACHEA". Next, ALBB is applied for child branches of "TRACHEA". In this step, child branches of "TRACHEA" are labeled by a classifier selected from the correspondence table. A classifier for labeling these branches is obtained by finding a record which has "TRACHEA" as the parent's name. Then child branch names are checked whether the combination of their branch names is appropriate or not. (ex. "RB1" is not a sibling branch of "RB13M" or "RB1B"). These processes are repeated in the width first search way until all branches are labeled.

2.2   Augmented Display of Anatomical Names on RB Views

Finally, we generate augmented display of anatomical names of bronchial branches for bronchoscopists by overlaying ALBB results onto RB views. To overlay anatomical names on RB views, the proposed method calculates branches being observed by a bronchoscope. These branches are defined as the branch where a bronchoscope is currently located (current branch) and child branches of the current branch. The location of a bronchoscope is obtained by Deguchi's method in real time [10].

3 Experiments

We applied the proposed method to 71 cases of 3D CT images. The acquisition parameters of the CT images were 512×512 pixels, 80 – 728 slices, 0.549 – 0.625 mm in pixel spacing, 1.0 – 2.5 mm in slice thickness, and 0.5 mm – 2.5 mm in reconstruction intervals. The following computer was used in the experiments: CPU: Quad-Core Intel Xeon 3.00 GHz $\times$ 2, Memory: 4GByte, OS: Microsoft Windows VistaD First of all, we extracted the bronchial region, the medial line and its tree structure from CT images by Kitasaka's method [9]. Then, we manually corrected missing or incorrect branches. Finally, we obtained 26,873 bronchial branches (2,523 bronchial branches up to segmental lobe branches). In prior to ALBB, all bronchial branches were manually labeled by 3 experienced engineers who had knowledge about bronchoscopy.

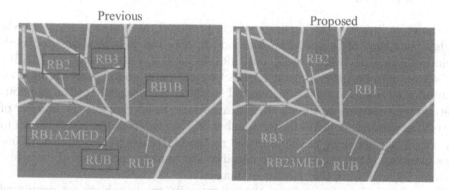

Fig. 2. Examples of ALBB results by the previous [5] and the proposed methods. Boxes show mis-labeled branches by the methods.

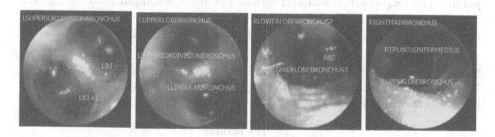

Fig. 3. Examples of augmented display of anatomical names of bronchial branches. Anatomical name of an observing branch was displayed on the left top of each image. Also, anatomical names of child branches of an observing branch were displayed close to their bronchial branches.

To evaluate the performance of the proposed method, we utilized the leave-one-out scheme. In the experiments, the accuracy of ALBB was measured by $\frac{N_a}{N_s} \times 100\,\%$, where N_a is the number of correctly labeled branches up to segmental lobe branches, and N_s is the total number of branches up to segmental lobe branches. The experimental results showed that the accuracy of the proposed method was 90.1 %, while that of the previous method [5] was 76.8 %. The average computation time of the classifier construction was 1.49 seconds. Figure 2 shows results of ALBB by the previous [5] and the proposed methods . In this figure, boxes shows mis-labeled branch obtained by the methods. Table 1 shows the accuracy of ALBB in each lobe, such as Right Upper, Right Middle and Lower, Left Upper, Left Lower Lobes, and the others (Trachea, Right main bronchus, Left main bronchus).

Also, Fig. 3 shows examples of augmented display of anatomical names of bronchial branches on our guidance system. Our guidance system could display anatomical names of an observing branch and its child branches. Augmented display of them could enable a bronchoscopist to recognize the current position and insertion direction visually.

4   Discussion

As shown in Table 1, the accuracy of the proposed method was about 13.3 % higher than that of the previous method [5]. The previous method used multiple branching pattern models, and suitable models were selected for ALBB. This procedure becomes difficult to select appropriate model when the number of branching pattern models increase. Therefore, the accuracy of the previous method may decrease as the number of images increased, because the number of branching patterns depends on the number of images. From the result shown in the Fig. 4, the accuracy of the proposed method increases as the number of images increases. This is because the classifier learns more variations of bronchial features by increasing the number of images.

To evaluate the usefulness of the parent-child relationships, we compared the proposed method with the method which constructs classifiers without the parent-child relationships. In this case, the accuracy of ALBB without the parent-child relationships was 47.2 %, and the average computation time of the classifier construction was 108.1 seconds. From this result, the parent-child relationships can significantly increase the accuracy of ALBB and reduce the

Table 1. Accuracy of the previous [5] and the proposed methods in each lobe (TR: Trachea, LM: Left main bronchus, RM: Right main bronchus, RU: Right upper lobe, RL: Right middle and lower lobe, LU: Left upper lobe and LL: Left lower lobe).

	The accuracy of ALBB[%]					
	TR, RM, LM	RU	RL	LU	LL	Total
Previous method[5]	100.0	70.1	70.8	87.9	71.0	76.8
Proposed method	100.0	84.7	88.5	97.6	85.8	90.1

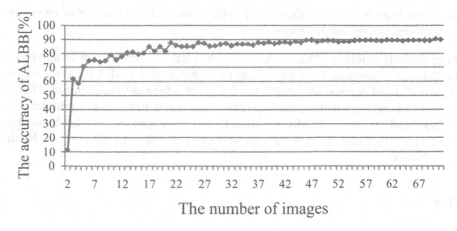

Fig. 4. The accuracy of ALBB when the number of samples was increasing

computation time for constructing classifiers. However, since the classifier for child branches is selected by the parent branch information, the results of ALBB for descendant branches depends on the result of ALBB for a parent branch. Therefore, this may greatly deteriorate the accuracy of the proposed method. In future work, it is necessary to develop a mechanisms to check whether the parent branch name has been correctly assigned.

In this experiment, the proposed method was evaluated by only 71 images. This may be insufficient number of images for training classifiers by multi-class AdaBoost technique. Therefore, we have to evaluate the proposed method by increasing the number of images more than hundreds. In addition, most of images used in this paper includes nodules close to bronchial branches. Since the positions of the bronchial branches are distorted by nodules, bronchial features calculated by the proposed method were greatly affected by these nodules. To evaluate the influence of the nodules, we have to compare the accuracy of the proposed method by using images which does not have nodules.

5   Conclusions

This paper presented a method for automated ALBB for bronchoscopy guidance system. The proposed method constructed classifiers that output anatomical names of bronchial branches by employing the machine-learning approach. Multi-class AdaBoost technique was utilized for construction of classifiers. We applied the proposed method to 71 images, and it was evaluated by leave-one-out scheme. Experimental results showed that the proposed method could assign correct anatomical names to bronchial branches of 90.1% up to segmental lobe branches. Also, we confirmed presentation of anatomical names of bronchial branches on real bronchoscopic views was quite useful to assist the bronchoscopy. Future work includes: (1) development of the method for checking whether the parent branch name has been correctly assigned, (2) application to large number of cases, and (3) experiments on normal cases.

Acknowledgements. This work was supported in part by the Grant-In-Aid for Scientific Research from the Ministry of Education (MEXT), the program of formation of innovation center for fusion of advanced technologies "Establishment of early preventing medical treatment based on medical-engineering for analysis and diagnosis" funded by MEXT, and the Japan Society for Promotion of Science, the Grant-In-Aid for Cancer Research from the Ministry of Health and Welfare.

References

1. Rogalla, P., van Scheltinga, J.T., Hamm, B., et al.: Virtual endoscopy and related 3D techniques. Springer, Berlin (2001)
2. Paik, D.S., Beaulien, C.F., Jeffrey, R.B., et al.: Automated flight path planning for virtual endoscopy. Med. Phys. 25(5), 629–637 (1998)
3. Kiraly, A.P., Helferty, J.P., et al.: Three-Dimensional Path Planning for Virtal Bronchoscopy. IEEE Transaction of Medical Imaging 23, 1365–1379 (2004)
4. Kitaoka, H., Park, Y., Tschirren, J., et al.: Automated nomenclature labeling of the bronchial tree in 3D-CT lung images. In: Dohi, T., Kikinis, R. (eds.) MICCAI 2002. LNCS, vol. 2489, pp. 1–11. Springer, Heidelberg (2002)
5. Mori, K., Ema, S., Kitasaka, T., et al.: A method for automated nomenclature of bronchial branches extracted CT images. In: CARS 2005, 19th International Congress and Exhibition. International Congress Series, vol. 1281, pp. 86–91 (2005)
6. Schapire, R.E.: Using output codes to boost multiclass learning problems. In: Machine Learning: Proceedings of the Fourteenth International Conference, pp. 313–321 (1997)
7. Guruswami, V., Sahai, A.: Multiclass Learning, Boosting, and Error-Correcting Codes. In: Proceedings of the Twelfth annual Conference on Computational Learning Theory, pp. 145–155. ACM Press, New York
8. Li, L.: Multiclass Boosting with Repartitioning. In: Proceedings of the 23rd International Conference on Machine Learning, pp. 569–576 (2006)
9. Kitasaka, T., Mori, K., Hasegawa, J., Toriwaki, J.: A Method for Extraction of Bronchus Regions from 3D Chest X-ray CT Images by Analyzing Structural Features of the Bronchus. FORMA 17(4), 321–338 (2002)
10. Deguchi, D., Ishitani, K., Kitasaka, T., et al.: A method for bronchoscope tracking using position sensor without fiducial markers. In: Proceedings of SPIE, vol. 6511, pp. 65110N-1-12 (2007)

Non-metal Slice Image Overlay Display System Used Inside the Open Type MRI

Ken Masamune[1], Ikuma Sato[2], Hongen Liao[3], and Takeyoshi Dohi[1]

[1] Deptatment of Mechano Informatics, Graduate School of Information Science,
The University of Tokyo
[2] Graduate School of Advanced Science and Technology, Tokyo Denki University
[3] Graduate School of Engineering, The University of Tokyo,
7-3-1 Hongo, Bunkyo-ku, Tokyo, 113-8656, Japan
{masa, ikuma_is, takdohi}@atre.t.u-tokyo.ac.jp,
liao@bmpe.t.u-tokyo.ac.jp

Abstract. MRI is now utilized not only for diagnosis but also for intraoperative surgical treatment. In the MRI environment, the surgeon imagines the position of target region by observing pre-acquired images and patient body during the operation, therefore the spatial position of the diseased part depends on the surgeon's knowledge and experience. Thus information from the MRI image is not fully utilized. In order to solve this problem, we developed the prototypes of slice image overlay system for open-type MRI, which comprises the MRI compatible display device, image communication, registration system and visualization software, which is adopted to clinical 0.2T Open MRI. Phantom experiments were performed and the TRE of the overlay device was less than 1.0mm at the center of the display.

1 Introduction

In recent years, MRI imaging system is not utilized only for diagnosis but also for intra-operative surgical treatment, and surgeons put their hands to perform the surgical procedure in the narrow gantry space. In the MRI environment, the surgeon imagines the position of target region by observing pre-acquired images and patient body during the operation, therefore the spatial position of the diseased part depends on the surgeon's knowledge and experience. In this sense, the information from the MRI image is not fully utilized though the image data is digital and quantitative. In order to solve this problem, we introduced the Augmented Reality concept to develop a slice image overlay system for open-type MRI, which comprises the MRI compatible display device, image communication and visualization software, which is adopted to clinical 0.2T Open MRI.

The concept of the image overlay is not a new idea [1-6] and many researchers are/were involved to develop the image overlay system for medical use. Among them, the distinguished researches are conducted by the groups of G. Stetten's[4] and us[1], which tries to combine the imaging system (ultrasound imaging and X-ray CT respectively) and the overlaid image simultaneously on the patient, i.e. the surgeon observes

T. Dohi, I. Sakuma, and H. Liao (Eds.): MIAR 2008, LNCS 5128, pp. 385–392, 2008.

the patient and the image floating inside the body on real-time. The principle of the image integration is shown in Fig. 1. The plane position of reflection of the display screen depends on the geometrically relationship between the position of the screen and half mirror, therefore the integrated image does not shift if the viewpoint changes.

In this paper, we present the image overlay device under the MRI imaging system. As is well known, there is a strong magnetic field in the MR environment and conventional displays are not available especially inside the MRI gantry, and our research purpose is to develop the MRI compatible display and the overlay device, and build up the registration system to perform the image-overlay inside the MRI gantry. 'MRI compatible' means that the device will not disturb the image acquisition, and vice versa at the same time. In chapter 2, we described the design of MRI compatible display, and the registration algorithm in 2.2. The quantitative evaluations and their results are shown in chapter 3 including the experiment of the image registration error and head phantom. Discussions are written in chapter 4 and the conclusion in chapter 5.

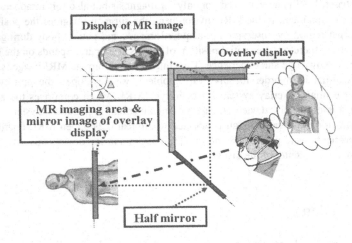

Fig. 1. Principle of image integration

2 Material and Methods

2.1 MRI Compatible Display

MRI compatibility is well described in [3]. Basically the electric devices produce the noise/artifact on the MRI image. Fischer et al. tried to use normal LCD display covered with electro-magnetic shields to use in the MRI room[2], however this method will not be adopted to use inside the MRI gantry because of the image distortions caused by the noise from magnetism of the display itself. In this research, to use the display device in the MRI gantry, an image-guide fiber (the bundle of optical fibers) is used to transfer the image from an LCD projector to a screen via lens system and a half-mirror is attached to the screen to create overlay images. The number of the image-guide fiber is approx. 50000 pixels in a circle, and the image resolution of 1mm/pixel is obtained on the screen. The display device is composed of engineering

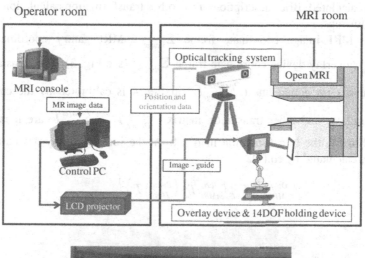

Operator room   MRI room

MRI console

MR image data

Position and orientation data

Optical tracking system

Open MRI

Control PC

Image - guide

LCD projector

Overlay device & 14DOF holding device

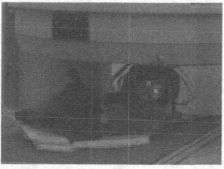

Fig. 2. Top) MRI compatible display with image guide fiber and the projector Bottom) The display device installed inside the open-MRI gantry

plastics, acrylic sheets, which are made of all non-metal materials and non-ferromagnetic materials. The weight of the device is below 2kg, and a cylindrical rod is attached for easy handling. As a preliminary testing of MRI compatibility, S/N and the deformation of MRI images are evaluated with 0.2T MRI. The decrease of S/N of the image was 4.7% with no deformations. Fig. 2 shows the system integration and the overview located in the MRI gantry.

2.2 Image Registration

To place the slice image at the correct position from the MRI data, the registration between the overlay device and MRI image is required. To obtain the relationship between MRI image (in the virtual space) and the real device, the translation from MRI image to the Open MRI gantry should be firstly calibrated. The overlay device has four spherical markers for its position tracking, and MRI gantry has also a rigid marker on the upper side wall of the MRI gantry. A 3D position measurement system Polaris™ (NDI Inc., Canada) is used to detect each position and then the transform matrix is calculated. Brief description of the other transformation calculation is shown in the followings.

Define MRI image coordinate frame Σ_{image} , MRI gantry coordinate frame $\Sigma_{MRIgantry}$, overlay device coordinate frame Σ_{device} (see Fig. 3). The translation formation matrix on dotted line ($^{OpenMRI}_{MRimage}T$) in Fig. 4 is calibrated by the customized calibration box, and other translation matrix $^{Polaris}_{Device}T$, $^{Polaris}_{OpenMRI}T$ are measured by Polaris. Finally, the transformation matrix from the image overlay device and MRI image are calculated by eq.(1).

$$^{OpenMRI}_{MRimage}T \cdot {}^{Polaris}_{OpenMRI}T \cdot \left({}^{Polaris}_{Device}T \right)^{-1} \tag{1}$$

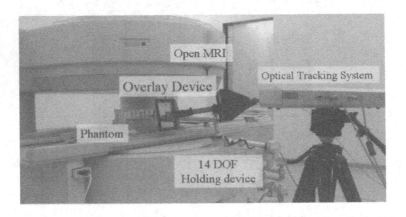

Fig. 3. System Overview with registration system

With these matrix equations, the device's image and MRI image is registered and we can provide the slice image floating inside the patient's body with the same size and position.

3   Evaluation Experiments and Results

3.1   Registration Error

Image registration errors are evaluated. We prepared a lattice phantom which has a 10mm x 10mm grid filled with water. By using this phantom, the image distortion derived by the device is measured. For TRE (= Target Registration Error) evaluation, 6 points are chosen on the edge of the lattice phantom (see in Fig. 5 Right), and the distance between these points and these points on the overlaid image are measured from the camera image processing, which distortion is pre-calibrated. The distance from each point and the center of the display is listed in Table 1. It is expected that the image distortion is distributed in a concentric fashion, and the best result of the

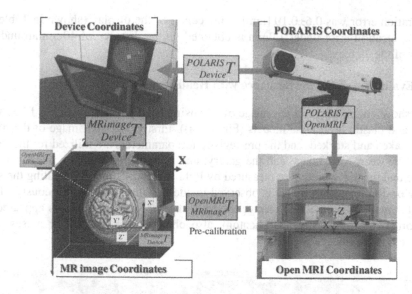

Fig. 4. Coordinate relationships between each modality

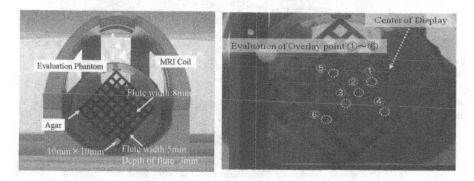

Fig. 5. Evaluation phantom and the evaluation experiment

Table 1. Evaluation result of the location errors

Location	Distance from the center (mm)	Location error (mm)
Point①	12.9	0.6 ±0.10
Point②	29.9	0.9 ±0.18
Point③	44.4	0.9 ±0.18
Point④	43.1	0.8 ±0.18
Point⑤	43.7	1.0 ±0.10
Point⑥	63.7	1.9 ±0.18

registration error was 0.6±0.10 [mm] at the center of the display (shown in Table 1), and the location error under 1.0mm is obtained on the distance of 40mm around the center of the display.

3.2 Evaluation of the Performance with Head Phantom

Fig.6 shows the example of the image overly using head phantom which is filled with water and plastic head bone models (Fig. 6, (a)). Firstly 3D MRI image of the phantom is taken and stacked, and the pre-registration parameters are utilized for the registration between MRI image and the gantry, and the position tracking marker on the device and the MRI gantry are measured by Polaris on real-time. By creating the slice image on ROI, overlaid image is observed inside the phantom simultaneously. If the operator moves the device to change the ROI, the slice image, which is appeared on the correct position inside the phantom, also changes. No artifacts or noises were observed on the images.

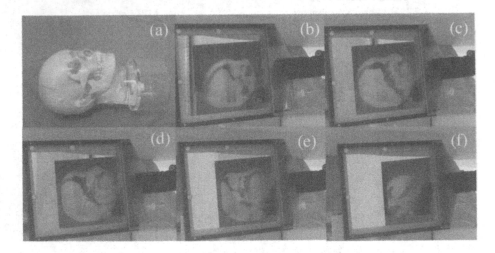

Fig. 6. Demonstration phantom experiments with different position

4 Discussion

In this prototype system, we used the pre-acquired 3D MRI image data to create the slice image for the overlay, thus if the patient moves during the operation or the patient's organ is deformed, the overlay image provides incorrect information. It takes over a few minutes to obtain the 3D MRI data (it depends on the protocol). To create the real-time overlay system, we're waiting for many researches of fast-MR imaging, which has now 1 to 2 Hz updating of the slice image with better image quality. Our next system will include this real time imaging onto the system. And more, if we use the pre-acquired 3D image, the patient should not move during through whole operation. By applying the fast imaging for this overlay system, we will observe the real-time deformation with correct information and the surgeon will perform more safe and precise surgical treatment.

MRI image quality depends on the strength of the magnetic field. For interventional MRI, 0.1 to 1.0 T open-type MRI are commonly used and our device was evaluated under the 0.1 T and 0.3T MRI for open-type MRI guided intervention, and basically it's very difficult to obtain the clear image. In case of stronger magnetic field, our device will work correctly with no artifacts because this device is non-metal materials and using no electricity in principle. Thus, we can also use the display device for visual stimulation in the functional MRI researches, e.g. brain research.

In our MRI compatible display, the display image resolution depends on the number of image-guide's fibers. 50000 fibers are appeared on the circle of ϕ=180mm, so the resolution of 0.7 mm/pixel is obtained, however, there are black contour lines between each pixel on the display because the image guide fibers are bundled in hexagonal close-packed structure.

Toward clinical application, we should re-design the device to be light-weighted for easy handling. In the clinical setting, the surgeon will hold the device in his left/right hand to adjust the device, and fix its position by MRI compatible stabilizer arm device. About sterilization of the device, this is just the device for the observation, so the sterilized plastic cover sheets will be used like the surgical microscope. The total weight of the prototype was below 2 kg and slightly it was difficult to handle this device in the narrow gantry space. We designed the size of the display to provide 200mm square image to see wide ROI, however, in case of minimally invasive surgery, we often concentrate on very small ROI and the small display is acceptable. Thus, we're considering downsizing the display and the device in the next development.

5 Conclusion

We developed the non-ferromagnetic / non-metal image overly display device, and surgeons and staffs are able to look at the patient's body and the internal MRI image simultaneously which is floating inside his body at the same position with the same size. Thus, without looking away from the region of interest, surgeon can operate the surgical procedures with the MRI image information on time of image update.

Our system is adapted to clinical 0.2T Open MRI, and the phantom experiments were performed and the TRE of the overlay device was less than 1.0mm at the center of the display. We conclude that this technology will create a new surgical environment in near future.

This research is partly supported by Grant in Aid for scientific research of JSPS (#18680042).

References

[1] Masamune, K., et al.: An Image Overlay System with Enhanced Reality for Percutaneous Therapy Performed Inside CT Scanner. In: Dohi, T., Kikinis, R. (eds.) MICCAI 2002. LNCS, vol. 2489, pp. 77–84(part 2). Springer, Heidelberg (2002)

[2] Fischer, G.S., Deguet, A., Csoma, C., Taylor, R.H., Fayad, L., Carrino, J.A., Zinreich, S.J., Fichtinger, G.: MRI image overlay: Application to arthrography needle insertion. Computer Aided Surgery 12(1), 2–14 (2007)

[3] Tsekos, N.V., Khanicheh, A., Christoforou, E., Mavroidis, C.: Magnetic Resonance Compatible Robotic and Mechatronics Systems for Image-Guided Interventions and Rehabilitation: A Review Study. Annu. Rev. Biomed. Eng. 9(14), 1–14 (2007)

[4] Stetten, G., et al.: Tomographic Reflection to Merge Ultrasound Images with direct Vision. In: IEEE Proc. AIPR 2000, Washington, D.C, pp. 200–205 (2000)

[5] Sauer, F., et al.: A Head-Mounted Display System for Augmented Reality Image Guidance: Towards Clinical Evaluation for iMRI-guided Neurosurgery. In: Niessen, W.J., Viergever, M.A. (eds.) MICCAI 2001. LNCS, vol. 2208, pp. 707–716. Springer, Heidelberg (2001)

[6] Edwards, P.J., et al.: Design and evaluation of a system for microscope-assisted guided interventions (MAGI). IEEE Transactions On Medical Imaging 19(11), 1082–1093 (2000)

Extracting Curve Skeletons from Gray Value Images for Virtual Endoscopy*

Christian Bauer and Horst Bischof

Institute for Computer Graphics and Vision, Graz University of Technology, Austria
{cbauer, bischof}@icg.tu-graz.ac.at

Abstract. The extraction of curve skeletons from tubular networks is a necessary prerequisite for virtual endoscopy applications. We present an approach for curve skeleton extraction directly from gray value images that supersedes the need to deal with segmentations and skeletonizations. The approach uses properties of the Gradient Vector Flow to derive a tube-likeliness measure and a medialness measure. Their combination allows the detection of tubular structures and an extraction of their medial curves that stays centered also in cases where the structures are not tubular such as junctions or severe stenoses. We present results on clinical datasets and compare them to curve skeletons derived with different skeletonization approaches from high quality segmentations. Our approach achieves a high centerline accuracy and is computationally efficient by making use of a GPU based implementation of the Gradient Vector Flow.

1 Introduction

Modern volumetric imaging techniques provide detailed information about tubular structures such as colon, blood vessels, or the bronchial tree. To make use of this information virtual endoscopy (VE) systems can be used. These systems have become powerful tools for aiding procedures such as diagnosis, preoperative planning, or intraoperative support. To achieve this, VE combines methods of medical image understanding with virtual reality methods and typically involves three tasks: 1) Identification/segmentation of the interesting structures in the volumetric dataset. 2) Extraction of the associated curve skeleton (CS) representing the flight paths through the tubular networks. 3) Visualization of the interesting structures from points on the given flight paths using isosurface or other volume rendering techniques.

The first two tasks are usually treated separately - segmentation with a consecutive skeletonization. There are robust general purpose methods for extraction of CSs from discrete objects that can be used application independent [1,2,3,4]; however, the segmentation methods are typically application dependent, require manual initialization, or adaption of parameters. Methods that extract centerlines directly from gray value images on the other hand are rare and either

---

* This work was supported by the Austrian Science Fund (FWF) under the doctoral program Confluence of Vision and Graphics W1209.

T. Dohi, I. Sakuma, and H. Liao (Eds.): MIAR 2008, LNCS 5128, pp. 393–402, 2008.

require specification of start- and endpoints of the flight path [5,6] - for highly branched tubular structures such as the bronchial tree this is difficult - or they are based on tube detection approaches [7,8,9]. These methods have problems to extract valid centerlinepaths in proximity of junctions or diseases like stenosis and require additional postprocessing steps that do not guarantee centered paths [10,8,11].

In a previous work we used the Gradient Vector Flow (GVF) [13] for identification of tubular objects as a replacement for the multi-scale gradient vector computation used by most tube detection filters [12]. In combination with Frangi's vesselness measure [9] the overall approach allows detection of tubular objects (more precisely their centerlines) independent of the tubes size and contrast and the method shows a high robustness against image noise and disturbances outside the tubular objects. But similar to other tube detection filters the method does not produce valid centerline paths in the proximity of junctions or diseases like stenosis where the objects are not tubular. However, the GVF shows another property that can be used to solve this problem and that has been used for extraction of CSs from binary segmentations by the skeletonization approach of Hassouna and Farag [2]. In contrast to skeletonization approaches that are based on the distance transformation the magnitude of the GVF is always guaranteed to vanish at the medial curves independent of the object's shape. This enables the extraction of the centerlines also in case of junctions or plate like structures.

In this work, we present a system for extraction of complete CSs from tubular networks directly from gray value images. This supersedes the need to deal with two problems - segmentation and skeletonization. We propose to use the GVF's properties in two ways: first, for detection of tubular objects and thus selection of the interesting structures. Second, for extraction of the complete medial curves that stay centered also in case of junctions or diseases. This approach combines the advantages of tube detection filters - their robustness against leakage and their ability to detect small low contrast structures - with the advantage of Hassouna and Farag's skeletonization approach - its ability to extract centered lines also in areas where the objects are not tubular. The proposed approach may be used in several application areas and not just VE applications, but, as it extracts centered paths, it is especially suited for VE applications. It is further computationally efficient - as it uses the GVF as a core component similar to Hassouna and Farag's skeletonization approach - and may perform fully automatic for some application domains since it performs a bottom up detection of tubular objects for identification of the interesting structures.

2   Methodology

The basic idea of our approach is outlined in Fig. 1 for some simple 3D tubular objects. The approach consists of three processing steps: 1) Performing the GVF on the gray value image. 2) Identification of tubular objects. 3) Extraction of the medial curves that are associated with tubular objects (thus not only the

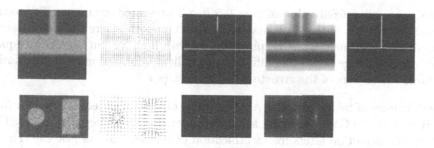

Fig. 1. Illustration of the basic idea on 2D cross section profiles of some 3D structures. Top row: cross section T-junction of a tubular object; bottom row: tube and plate like structures. From left to right: original dataset, GVF, derived tube-likeliness, derived medialness (after appropriate weighting for visualization purposes), extracted CS.

tubular part is extracted, but also areas of stenoses/aneurisms or junctions are handled).

Gradient Vector Flow: The first step of the processing pipeline is performing the GVF on the gray value image. This allows an edge-preserving diffusion of gradient information from the boundaries towards the centers of the interesting structures.

Depending on the application domain the initial gradient information is obtained differently: $F = \nabla(G_\sigma \star I)$ for structures surrounded by darker tissue (e.g. angiography images), $F = -\nabla(G_\sigma \star I)$ for structures surrounded by brighter tissue (e.g. airways), $F = -\nabla|\nabla(G_\sigma \star I)|$ for structures surrounded by arbitrary step edges (e.g. blood vessels containing calcifications), whereby I is the original image and G_σ is a Gaussian filter kernel with a given variance (we used a variance of one voxel in all presented experiments). In contrast to other tube detection filters the gradient information is obtained only on a small scale that only accounts for image noise. We do not require multiple scales which may result in an undesired diffusion of nearby structures into one another on larger scales. This would influence the detection of tubular objects and the accuracy of the associated centerlines [12].

The given initial gradient information is normalized to account for varying contrast situations, $F^n(\mathbf{x}) = F(\mathbf{x})/|F(\mathbf{x})| * (min(|F(\mathbf{x})|, F_{max})/F_{max})$ where $\mathbf{x} = (x, y, z)$, and used to initialize the GVF. The GVF as proposed by Xu and Prince [13] is defined as the vector field $V(\mathbf{x})$ that minimizes:

$$E(V) = \iiint_\Omega \mu|\nabla V(\mathbf{x})|^2 + |F^n(\mathbf{x})|^2|V(\mathbf{x}) - F^n(\mathbf{x})|^2 d\mathbf{x}, \qquad (1)$$

where μ is a regularization parameter that usually has to be adapted according to the amount of noise. We use the normalized gradient vector information F^n to account for varying noise levels (σ) and contrast levels (F_{max}) as these parameters are more intuitive to set than the GVF's regularization parameter.

Thus, we used a fixed value of $\mu = 0.5$ in all presented examples. The variational formulation of the GVF makes the result smooth where the initial vector magnitudes are small, while keeping vectors with high magnitude nearly equal. This allows an edge-preserving diffusion of gradient information from boundaries towards the centers of the structures of interest (see Fig. 1).

Identification of tubular objects: At the centers of tubular objects the vector field derived from the GVF shows the same characteristic properties that are used by other tube detection filters for identification of tubular objects (see Fig. 1): All vectors point directly towards the centerline of the tubular object; they show a large variance in two dimensions and a low variance in the third dimension. Therefore, the GVF can be used a replacement for the multi-scale gradient vector computation performed by other tube detection filters [12].

To derive a tube-likeliness from these vectors $V^n(\mathbf{x}) = V(\mathbf{x})/|V(\mathbf{x})|$ the Hessian matrix $H(\mathbf{x}) = \nabla V^n(\mathbf{x})$ with its eigenvalues $|\lambda_1| \leq |\lambda_2| \leq |\lambda_3|$ can be used. Currently we are using Frangi's vesselness measure [9] to derive the final tube-likeliness from these eigenvalues since it is simple and well known:

$$T(\mathbf{x}) = \begin{cases} 0 & \text{if } \lambda_2 > 0 \text{ or } \lambda_3 > 0 \\ \left(1 - exp\left(-\frac{R_A^2}{2\alpha^2}\right)\right)exp\left(-\frac{R_B^2}{2\beta^2}\right)\left(1 - exp\left(-\frac{S^2}{2c^2}\right)\right) & \text{otherwise} \end{cases}$$

$$(2)$$

with $R_A = |\lambda_1|/\sqrt{|\lambda_2||\lambda_3|}$ indicating blob-like structures, $R_B = |\lambda_2|/|\lambda_3|$ to distinguish between plate-like and line-like structures, and $S = \sqrt{\lambda_1^2 + \lambda_2^2 + \lambda_3^2}$ for suppression of random noise effects. The parameters α, β, and c allow to control the sensitivity of the filter to the measures R_A, R_B, and S, respectively. In combination with our approach the third term of Frangi's vesselness measure that controls the noise-sensitivity becomes obsolete since noise is already suppressed. Also for the other parameters Frangi's suggested default values are used: $\alpha = 0.5$, $\beta = 0.5$, and $c = 100$.

The overall combination of the GVF with Frangi's vesselness measure allows detection of tubular objects (more precisely their centerlines), whereby the response is independent of the tubes size and contrast (see Fig. 1). But similar to other tube detection filters it does not produce valid centerlines where the objects are not tubular such as in areas of junctions or diseases like stenoses where the cross section profile is more plate-like.

Medial curve extraction: As outlined in the introduction, the magnitude of the GVF vanishes at medial curves also for non-tubular objects and this property can be used to extract the complete medial curves of identified tubular objects also in areas where the tubes do not show a circular cross-section.

The magnitude of the GVF vanishes towards the centers of the objects but it not necessarily becomes zero. As a measure of medialness we use $M(\mathbf{x}) = 1 - |V(\mathbf{x})|$. Fig. 1 shows the derived medialness after an appropriate weigthing (this weighting is only used for visualization but not for computation). In the so derived medialness map medial curves form height-ridges that can be extracted. We use a height ridge traversal procedure for this purpose for two main reasons:

first, it is computationally highly efficient (see Sec. 3). Second, it allows immediate extraction of a higher-level representation that describes the complete CS including the centerlines, junction points, and connectivity information between the single tubular objects.

Given the medialness map M and a starting point x_0 on a height-ridge the complete associated medial curve can be extracted using a procedure similar to the method suggested by Aylward and Bullit [7]. This procedure needs an estimate of the ridge orientation $t(x)$; we obtain this information from the Hessian matrix as the eigenvector associated with its smallest eigenvalue. Thus, given a starting point x_0 the heigh-ridge is traversed into both directions $t(x_0)$ and $-t(x_0)$. For a current point on the height ridge x_i all local neighbors x_i^n with $\overrightarrow{x_i x_i^n} \cdot t_i > 0$ are considered and the neighbor with the highest medialness is chosen as the next point x_{i+1} on the medial curve. The tangent direction $t(x_{i+1})$ is set to $t(x_{i+1}) = \text{sign}(\overrightarrow{x_i x_{i+1}} \cdot t(x_{i+1})) t(x_{i+1})$ to maintain the correct direction during traversal and the procedure is repeated until a stopping criterion is met. The procedure it stopped when the medialness falls below a given threshold m_{min} (an endpoint of the medial curve is found; we used $m_{min} = 0.1$ in all presented experiments) or an already traversed point is found (a junction of two medial curves is found). This way the complete medial curves are extracted.

Combination: The final step is to combine the results of the last two steps: we use the tube-likeliness for identification of the interesting structures and the medial curve extraction to obtain the complete centerlines associated with the tubular structures.

This requires specification of starting points for the height-ridge traversal procedure. As we know that the tube-likeliness increases for tubular structures and that the response falls off in proximity of junctions, we can conclude that every tubular object contains at least one local maximum in the tube-likeliness map. Thus all local maxima in the tube-likeliness map with a value $T(x) > T_{min} = 0.5 * \max_{y \in \Omega} T(y)$ are considered as starting points for the height-ridge traversal (for robustness reasons these starting points are processed in descending order of their associated tube-likeliness). However, as the tube detection filter may produce some short spurious responses due to noise one further condition is necessary; the direct neighbors of the candidate starting points along the height-ridge also have to be tubular $(T(x) > T_{min})$. This strategy discards short spurious responses and is comparable with pruning strategies used with other skeletonization approaches [1,4] or tube extraction methods [10].

Applying this procedure allows a bottom up detection of the complete medial curves associated with tubular objects that is robust to local variations along the tube such as junctions, stenoses, or aneurisms. As the height-ridge traversal also provides connectivity information between the single medial curves, the complete CSs of the tubular networks are also known immediately and in some application domains the structure of interest can be identified as the largest connected component (concerning its centerline length).

3   Evaluation

In this section we present results achieved on clinical datasets and compare them quantitatively and qualitatively to other methods with similar objectives. We will show two things: first, our approach is able to extract medial curves that stay centered also in complicated cases where pure tube detection filters have problems; we do this by comparing our approach to results achieved with another approach that extracts medial curves directly from the gray value images [8,10]. Second, the accuracy of the extracted centerlines is comparable to those achieved with pure skeletonization approaches from accurate segmentations; we do this by comparing the results of our approach to the skeletons extracted with three different skeletonization approaches [2,4,1] from known gold standards (available segmentations of the interesting structures).

Datasets and methods: The three clinical datasets we used for evaluation show a bronchial tree (see Fig. 2), a contrast CT of an aorta containing a severe stenosis due to calcification (see Fig. 3), and a CT angiography image of the brain (see Fig. 4). High quality segmentations of the bronchial tree and the aorta were available; the segmentation of the aorta follows the interior of the aorta excluding the calcifications. For the CTA of the brain only a low quality segmentation based on thresholding was available.

The approaches we used for comparison are three sophisticated skeletonization approaches (using binary segmentations) that were presented for VE applications and one method that derives the medial curves directly from the gray

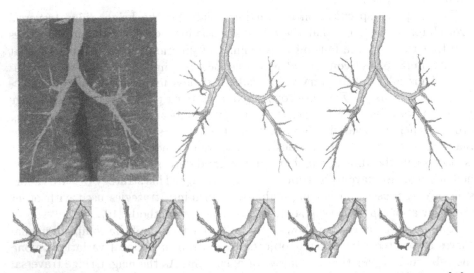

Fig. 2. Airway tree and resulting CSs. Top row (overview): volume rendering of the original dataset, CS of the proposed approach and Hassouna's approach. Bottom row (subregion around a junction): CS of the proposed approach, Krissian's approach, Hassouna's approach, Bouix's approach, and Palagyi's approach (green: proposed approach; red: other approaches).

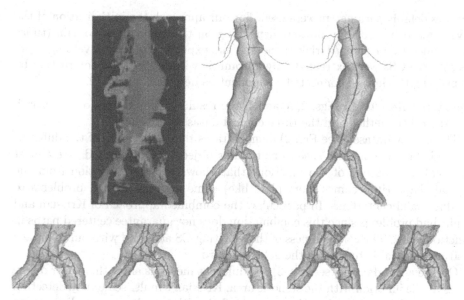

Fig. 3. Contrast CT dataset of the aorta containing a severe stenosis due to calcification. Top row (overview): volume rendering of the original dataset, CS of the proposed approach and Hassouna's approach. Bottom row (subregion around the stenosis): CS of the the proposed approach, Krissian's approach, Hassouna's approach, Bouix's approach, and Palagyi's approach (green: proposed approach; red: other approaches).

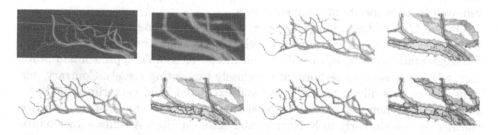

Fig. 4. CT angiography dataset of the brain and resulting CSs. Shown are a sub-branch of the dataset and a subregion with some closely adjacent vessels. From left to right, from top to bottom: MIP of the original dataset, CS of the proposed approach, Krissian's approach, and Hassouna's approach (green: proposed approach; red: other approaches).

value image. The skeletonization approaches are that of Hassouna et al. [2,3], Bouix et al. [4], and Palagyi et al. [1]. Hassouna's approach also uses the GVF similarly to our approach; the other two methods were specifically developed for tubular objects. As a representative example of a method that tries to extract centerlines directly from gray value images we decided to use a combination of the methods of Krissian et al. [8] (for a bottom up detection of tubular structures) and Bullitt et al. [10] (for grouping the single tubular objects into tree structures and an extraction of the complete CS). For all approaches the

authors default parameters were used. For our approach the initialization of the
GVF had to be set appropriately depending on the application domain (tubes
surrounded by brighter/darker tissue and the expected contrast level F_{max}; see
Sec. 2); the CSs were extracted fully automatic without any user interaction by
identifying the largest connected component as described in Sec. 2.

Qualitative Results: In Figs. 2, 3, and 4, the results achieved with our approach
and the other methods on the three clinical datasets are shown.

The airway dataset (see Fig. 2) demonstrates that the results of the different
methods for the standard case - one tubular object - of all methods are almost
identical. But at one of the junctions that shows a larger variation from the
typical shape (it becomes more plate like) some approaches had problems to
produce valid centerlines. In particular, the combined approach of Krissian and
Bullit had problems since this combination does not guarantee centered paths in
junction areas. The completeness of the resulting CS achieved with our approach
is also comparable to that of the gold standard.

On the aorta dataset (see Fig. 3) the different methods show the major differences at the junction with the stenotic area. Krissian's multi-scale tube detection
filter was influenced by the calcification and thus the resulting centerline moved
far away from the desired position. Our approach was able to extract a medial
curve that stayed centered in proximity of the stenosis with a quality comparable
to that of the skeletonization approaches. The approaches of Bouix and Palagyi
showed some sensitivity to surface noise and produced additional centerlines; the
authors themselves mention this behaviour and these spurious branches can be
removed by appropriate pruning strategies.

On the CTA of the brain (see Fig. 4) closely tangenting vessels with diffuse
boundaries and thin low contrast vessels are typically the difficult situations
for segmentation methods/tube detection filters. Krissian's approach had problems to extract valid centerlines for the closely tangenting vessels. Contrary, our
approach successfully separated them and extracted valid centerlines for these
structures. Further, our approach was also able to extract most of the thin low
contrast vessels similarly to Krissian's tube detetion filter. As only a low quality
segmentation was available none of the skeletonization approaches was able to
extract valid centerlines for the tangenting vessels; therefore we show only the
result of one of the skeletonization methods.

Quantitative Results: The quantitative comparison of the centerline accuracy
is based on the average centerline distances between the different methods. To
make the CSs comparable, the skeletons obtained with the methods of Bouix
and Palagyi were pruned and only branches detected by all methods (the segme-
nation methods and the tube detection filter methods) were considered. Table 1
summarizes the average centerline distances between the different methods for
the two datasets with the high-quality segmentations. All the methods are quite
comparable (except the results achieved with the combined approach of Krissian and Bullitt). Most notably is the small difference between our proposed
method and Hassouna's approach on the airway tree, but this may be explained
since both methods are based on the GVF. As these results show, the achieved

Table 1. Average centerline distances (in voxels) between the CSs extracted with different approaches from the bronchial tree and the aorta dataset

	Bronchial Tree					Aorta				
	M1	M2	M3	M4	M5	M1	M2	M3	M4	M5
proposed (M1)	–	0.24	0.41	0.40	0.58	–	0.66	0.62	0.79	1.49
Hassouna (M2)	0.22	–	0.37	0.34	0.72	0.63	–	0.60	0.72	1.14
Bouix (M3)	0.47	0.36	–	0.45	0.67	0.59	0.63	–	0.78	1.58
Palagyi (M4)	0.44	0.33	0.44	–	0.70	0.78	0.75	0.80	–	1.53
Krissian (M5)	0.59	0.53	0.57	0.66	–	1.61	1.17	1.70	1.60	–

centerline accuracy of our proposed method is comparable to the variation found between different skeletonization approaches; and this although all the skeletonization approaches use the same binary segmentations while our method does not know this gold standard. This proofs that our approach is able to extract CSs of comparable quality directly from the gray value images.

Implementational and computational effort: Our current implementation is based mainly on standard ITK-Filters[1] and a GPU based implementation of the GVF using the CUDA Framwork[2] as the main computational effort is due to the GVF. This allows an efficient computation of the GVF (500 iterations): $150 \times 110 \times 60$ voxels in ~ 3 seconds; $256 \times 256 \times 256$ voxels in ~ 15 seconds; $380 \times 210 \times 425$ voxels in ~ 30 seconds on an NVIDIA GeForce 8800 GTX. The second non-standard component is the height-ridge traversal procedure (see Sec. 2) that is computationally highly efficient. Even for large datasets containing many tubular objects the computation times are below one second. Thus, using a GPU based implementation of the GVF, the whole processing pipeline can be computed on a standard workstation within times comparable to some pure skeletonization approaches [2,4], exclusive of the additional computation times these methods require for the segmentation step.

4   Conclusion

In this work we presented an approach for extraction of CSs directly from gray value images. The approach combines the advantages of a bottom up tube detection filter with the GVF's ability for extraction of medial curves also in cases where the objects are not tubular. This combination enables robustness against local disturbances such as stenoses/aneurisms along the tubes and an extraction of medial curves also in these areas. We demonstrated the applicability of our approach on various clinical datasets and showed that the accuracy of the resulting centerline is comparable to that achieved with state of the art skeletonization approaches that are all based on the same known segmentations. Thus, the final CSs extracted with our approach are directly applicable for VE applications and

---

[1] www.itk.org

[2] www.nvidia.com/object/cuda_home.html

other application areas that require CS extraction and this supersedes the need to deal with segmentations and skeletonizations.

Acknowledgements. The authors thank Univ.Doz.Dr. Erich Sorantin from the Dep. of Radiology, Medical University Graz, Austria, and Prof.Dr.-Ing. Georgios Sakas for providing the clinical datasets.

References

1. Palagyi, K., Sorantin, E., Balogh, E., Kuba, A., Halmai, C., Erdohelyi, B., Hausegger, K.: A sequential 3D thinning algorithm and its medical applications. In: Insana, M.F., Leahy, R.M. (eds.) IPMI 2001. LNCS, vol. 2082, pp. 409–415. Springer, Heidelberg (2001)
2. Hassouna, M.S., Farag, A.A.: On the extraction of curve skeletons using gradient vector flow. In: Proc. of ICCV, pp. 1–8 (2007)
3. Hassouna, M.S., Farag, A.A., Falk, R.: Differential fly-throughs (DFT): A general framework for computing flight paths. In: Duncan, J.S., Gerig, G. (eds.) MICCAI 2005. LNCS, vol. 3750, pp. 654–661. Springer, Heidelberg (2005)
4. Bouix, S., Siddiqi, K., Tannenbaum, A.: Flux driven automatic centerline extraction. MIA 9(3), 209–221 (2005)
5. Deschamps, T., Cohen, L.D.: Fast extraction of minimal paths in 3d images and applications to virtual endoscopy. MIA 5(4), 281–299 (2001)
6. Wink, O., Niessen, W., Viergever, M.: Multiscale vessel tracking. IEEE TMI 21(2)23(1), 130–133 (2004)
7. Aylward, S., Bullit, E.: Initialization, noise, singularities, and scale in height ridge traversal for tubular object centerline extraction. IEEE TMI 21(2), 61–75 (2002)
8. Krissian, K., Malandain, G., Ayache, N., Vaillant, R., Trousset, Y.: Model-based detection of tubular structures in 3D images. CVIU 2(80), 130–171 (2000)
9. Frangi, A.F., Niessen, W.J., Vincken, K.L., Viergever, M.A.: Multiscale vessel enhancement filtering. In: Wells, W.M., Colchester, A.C.F., Delp, S.L. (eds.) MICCAI 1998. LNCS, vol. 1496, pp. 130–137. Springer, Heidelberg (1998)
10. Bullitt, E., Aylward, S., Smith, K., Jukherji, S., Jiroutek, M., Muller, K.: Symbolic description of intracerebral vessels segmented from magnetic resonance angiograms and evaluation by comparision with x-ray angiograms. MIA 5(2), 157–169 (2001)
11. Szymczak, A., Stillman, A., Tannenbaum, A., Mischaikow, K.: Coronary vessel trees from 3d imagery: A topological approach. MIA 10(4), 548–559 (2006)
12. Bauer, C., Bischof, H.: A novel approach for detection of tubular objects and its application to medical image analysis. In: Proc. of DAGM 2008 (in print) (2008)
13. Xu, C., Prince, J.L.: Snakes, shapes, and gradient vector flow. IEEE TMI 7(3), 359–369 (1998)

Automatic Hepatic Vessel Segmentation Using Graphics Hardware

Marius Erdt[1], Matthias Raspe[2], and Michael Suehling[3]

[1] Fraunhofer Institute for Computer Graphics, Cognitive Computing & Medical
Imaging, Fraunhoferstrasse 5, 64283 Darmstadt, Germany
`marius.erdt@igd.fhg.de`
[2] University of Koblenz-Landau, Institute of Computational Visualistics,
Universitaetsstrasse 1, 56070 Koblenz, Germany
[3] Siemens Medical Solutions, Computed Tomography: Physics & Applications,
Siemensstrasse 1, 91301 Forchheim, Germany

Abstract. The accurate segmentation of liver vessels is an important
prerequisite for creating oncologic surgery planning tools as well as medical visualization applications. In this paper, a fully automatic approach
is presented to quickly enhance and extract the vascular system of the
liver from CT datasets. Our framework consists of three basic modules:
vessel enhancement on the graphics processing unit (GPU), automatic
vessel segmentation in the enhanced images and an option to verify and
refine the obtained results. Tests on 20 clinical datasets of varying contrast quality and acquisition phase were carried out to evaluate the robustness of the automatic segmentation. In addition the presented GPU
based method was tested against a CPU implementation to demonstrate
the performance gain of using modern graphics hardware. Automatic
segmentation using graphics hardware allows reliable and fast extraction
of the hepatic vascular system and therefore has the potential to save
time for oncologic surgery planning.

Keywords: Segmentation, Automation, Computed Tomography, Graphics Hardware, Hepatic Vessels.

1 Introduction

Shape and location of the intrahepatic vessels are of significant importance to
liver surgery. Modern minimal invasive operation methods like laser surgery as
well as established surgical intervention techniques require the detection of vessels with a diameter down to 2 mm to decide whether an operation can be
realised or not.

In order to develop oncologic operation planning tools it is necessary to segment the vessel systems of the liver in a pre-computing step. Therefore, contrast
agents are injected in the bloodstream to raise the opacity of those structures and
make them appear bright in the CT scan. However, the distribution of the agent
and hence the quality of the contrast between the vessels and the liver-tissue
depends on the point of time the scan is started. This leads to heavily varying

T. Dohi, I. Sakuma, and H. Liao (Eds.): MIAR 2008, LNCS 5128, pp. 403–412, 2008.

results regarding the amount of contrast in the image. Usually filter based methods are used to enhance the quality of CT images since they can be applied as soon as the image comes out of the machine and require no user interaction. In [1] gaussian/median filters are used to intensify the liver vessels. However, those filters are insufficient to enhance low contrasted CT images since image details and therefore small vessels may get lost. A common approach is to model the vessels locally as tube like objects and applying hessian based eigenanalysis to find those structures in the images [2,3,4,5,6]. Such methods have proven to yield good results on the extraction of vessel systems like pulmonary vessels as well as coronary and retinal arteries. However, often several parameters need to be set that do not have a direct geometrical meaning and have to be statistically determined by testing a large amount of representative datasets. Our filter is based on a reduction of the parameter space by creating a vesselness function that is directly calculated from a pre-defined vessel model, thus supporting a fully automatic solution.

There are few fully automatic approaches for vessel segmentation from hessian based filter outputs. Often the result is thresholded based on either semi-automatically or statistically found values. Selle et al. [1] use an automatic and iterative algorithm after applying their gaussian and laplace like filters. However, hessian based filter outputs fundamentally differ from the results of pure denoising algorithms. Our method is therefore based on two principles: We first calculate a threshold based on a pre-defined ideal vessel model. Then an iterative region growing is used directly on the filter output to ensure that only tube like structures are segmented.

As described earlier, clinical datasets often considerably vary in their contrast quality which can make it impossible to segment the whole vessel tree without any artefacts attached. Therefore we implemented a real time preview function that allows the user to visually verify and refine the segmentation before rendering the result.

Recent advances in the development of graphics processors (GPUs) have increased their programmability and performance, making them interesting for non-graphical applications especially in the field of medical imaging. Owens et al. [7] give an exhaustive overview of current "General Purpose GPU" research and applications. Especially filtering processes are highly suited for a GPU implementation since GPUs are by their architecture massively parallel processors, as shown for example in Langs et al. [8]. In order to evaluate the benefit of using graphics hardware we present a CPU-GPU performance comparison of components of our filter implementation.

In what follows, we outline our approach towards segmenting liver vessels from CT datasets. Section 2 shows the methods used to enhance and automatically extract the vessels as well as the previewing option to verify and manually select a segmentation in low contrast CT images. Section 3 shows the results regarding performance on CPU and GPU as well as robustness of the extraction process on clinical datasets. In 4 we discuss the obtained results and give an outlook of future work on the proposed approach.

2   Methods

2.1   Tube Detection

First, the vessels in the CT images have to be enhanced in order to handle low contrast datasets. For this purpose, a hessian based filter is developed since this kind of filters have proven to yield good results in terms of 3D vessel detection. Following [2] we compose the filter $h(\boldsymbol{r})$ as a linear combination of second order derivatives of a gaussian $g(\boldsymbol{r})$ $(\boldsymbol{r} = (x, y, z))$:

$$h(\boldsymbol{r}) = \alpha_1 g_{xx}(\boldsymbol{r}) + \alpha_2 g_{xy}(\boldsymbol{r}) + \alpha_3 g_{xz}(\boldsymbol{r}) + \alpha_4 g_{yy}(\boldsymbol{r}) + \alpha_5 g_{yz}(\boldsymbol{r}) + \alpha_6 g_{zz}(\boldsymbol{r}), \quad (1)$$

i.e. the filter consists of 6 basis filters given by $h_1 = g_{xx}, .., h_6 = g_{zz}$.

The goal is now to tune the filter to a certain vessel model in order to design a vesselness function that can be applied without setting any parameters in advance. Therefore we model the vessel $v(\boldsymbol{r})$ locally by a cylinder along the x-axis with a radial Gaussian intensity profile:

$$v(\boldsymbol{r}) = b + (a - b)e^{-\frac{y^2+z^2}{2\sigma_v^2}}, \quad (2)$$

with a and b denoting the intensity at the vessel center and boundary respectively. The standard deviation σ_v is chosen to be the same as the standard deviation of the gaussian basis filters $h_1, .., h_6$. The coefficients α_n can now be determined analytically solving the optimization problem given by the maximization of the convolution of filter and vessel signal:

$$S = v * h = \int_{\Re^3} v(\boldsymbol{r})h(\boldsymbol{r})d\boldsymbol{r}, \quad (3)$$

The solution of S using the mathematical framework of Lagrange multipliers yields:

$$h(\boldsymbol{r}) = c \cdot \left(\frac{2}{3}g_{xx}(\boldsymbol{r}) - g_{yy}(\boldsymbol{r}) - g_{zz}(\boldsymbol{r})\right), \quad (4)$$

where $c = \sqrt{\frac{3}{5\pi^{\frac{3}{2}}}} \cdot \sqrt{\sigma_v}$.

To attain a maximum response, the filter has to be oriented along the vessel. This direction can be obtained by eigenvalue analysis of the Hessian H since the eigenvector corresponding to the largest eigenvalue $\lambda_1 = \max(\lambda_1, \lambda_2, \lambda_3)$ points in direction of the biggest local change of grey values (i.e. from vessel center to the vessel boundary). Applied to (4) the optimal filter output can be computed as:

$$S_{opt} = v * h_{rot} = \frac{2}{3}\lambda_1 - \lambda_2 - \lambda_3. \quad (5)$$

In order to avoid the detection of very bright, plate-like structures, i.e., regions where the cross-sectional intensity decreases rapidly in one direction but remains almost constant in the orthogonal one, we multiply (5) by an isotropy factor

$$\kappa = 1 - \frac{||\lambda_2| - |\lambda_3||}{|\lambda_2| + |\lambda_3|} \qquad \in [0, 1]. \quad (6)$$

The factor κ approaches 1 if $|\lambda_2| \approx |\lambda_3|$, i.e. the intensity decreases uniformly with increasing radial distance from the center, which is typically the case for vessels.

The filter output is maximal if the size of the filter mask matches the vessel thickness (i.e. have same standard deviations). Multiscale results are therefore obtained by selecting the maximum response over the range of all scales. In our tests 4 different ($\sigma_v = 1$–4) scales turned out to be sufficient for covering most liver vessels. Fig. 1(a) and (b) show the result of the 3D filtering procedure.

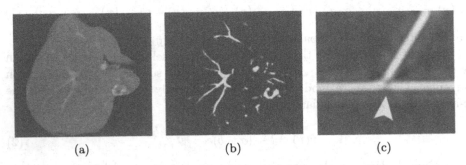

(a)   (b)   (c)

Fig. 1. Contrasted CT dataset of the liver. (a) Original. (b) Filter result. (c) Lower filter response on branches due to deviation from the tube-shaped vessel model (synthetic dataset).

2.2 GPU Implementation

As mentioned in the introduction, current commodity graphics hardware is able to outperform software implementations by several orders of magnitude due to their parallel architecture. In order to investigate how advanced filtering of volume data can be accelerated by hardware we have implemented the filtering steps described above in shader programs. These small programs are executed for every primitive (vertex, geometry, or fragment), depending on the type of program. In our framework, these shaders perform computations on special 2D textures to exploit the two-dimensional memory layout of commodity graphics hardware also for volumetric data. To utilize also the vector-processing capabilities (SIMD) we employ an additional packing scheme that combines four subsequent volume slices in one RGBA texture slice (i.e., tile in our representation).

Although our framework is designed for building complete workflows to process medical volume data while visualizing the (intermediate) results, we have implemented the aforementioned computations in one shader. This fragment program is executed for every voxel and writes the results into an equally sized texture. Depending on the available hardware multiple execution units (pipelines) perform the computations in parallel. However, using the GPU requires to transfer the data to the video memory and, if successive computations are not also performed in hardware, load the results back to the host. In table 1 we have therefore listed the timings for computations and transfer seperately. Although current CPUs provide facilities for parallel computation like SIMD units or multiple cores as well, their design is not as data-processing oriented as graphics hardware. In addition, the price/performance ratio for GPU-based implementations is clearly superior to multi-CPU systems.

The algorithm first fetches the voxels from the texture depending on the current neighborhood size. Then, all partial derivatives are computed according to equation (1) by convolving the voxels with 1D gaussian kernels. In order to compute the filter response, the eigenvalues are determined by using the closed solution for symmetric 3×3 matrices. After the last computations according to the equations above the results are finally written into the target memory.

2.3   Vessel Segmentation

The enhanced vessels are now extracted by applying an automatic region growing algorithm directly on the filter output. The idea behind this is to guarantee that all segmented vessels are connected to each other. Furthermore no post processing is required to remove outlying artefacts that usually appear on tissue borders with high gradients. To operate on the filter output only implicates problems when the vessel splits into two or more branches. In those areas the vessel deviates from the ideal tube-like model and forms a blob-like structure (compare Fig. 1(c)). A possibility to alleviate that problem is to adapt the vesselness function to detect blob-like structures as well as tubes [9]. However, we found that such an approach amplifies the false positive rate of the segmentation procedure in noisy regions with small vessels too heavily. Therefore we rely on the described tube vesselness function alone. As a consequence, the region growing thresholds have to be automatically determined in a way that all vessels and branches are sufficiently segmented while artefacts should be avoided as much as possible.

Fig. 2(a) shows the automatic region growing algorithm used to segment the vessels. First, the volume is divided into layers and seed points are automatically placed on local maxima of the filter output in order to evenly distribute the seeds on the data. Then, the thresholds are initialized with the response value for the ideal vessel model defined in (2). That response can be computed analytically as

$$v * h = (a - b)\kappa\sqrt{\frac{6}{5}}\pi^{\frac{3}{4}}\sigma_h^{\frac{3}{2}},\tag{7}$$

where σ_h denotes the standard deviation of the filter analysis window.

Since real vessels will deviate from the ideal model to a certain degree, the thresholds are iteratively refined. For this task, the original unfiltered data is comprised, because it is not feasible to decide from the filter output alone whether any detected structure is a real vessel or just appeared due to local noise. The reason for this lies in the aim of the Hessian based filters to detect tubular structures. Therefore the filter output will show many small tubular patterns, that cannot be directly classified as vessels. As a result, the region growing shows no clearly identifiable leaking from the vessels into the background like it is given on an ordinary dataset.

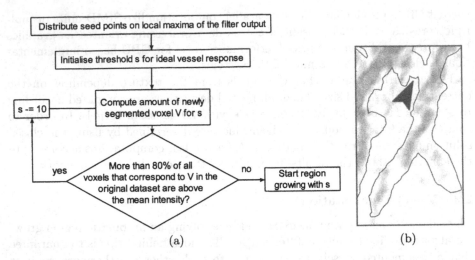

Fig. 2. (a) Automatic region growing algorithm on the filter output. (b) Continous segmentation on a low contrast dataset. A connection between two adjacent vessels needs to be refined by manual interaction (arrow).

The iterative refinement of the region growing thresholds using the original data works as follows: For the given threshold the mean value of the pixels in the original data corresponding to the detected pixels in the filter output is computed. This value is compared to the mean intensity of the dataset. If 80% of the pixels are above that value the threshold is lowered and the procedure is applied anew. Otherwise the iteration stops and the current threshold is taken as the final threshold. This automatic approach allows the continous segmentation of vessels that are disconnected in the original dataset while preventing the segmentation of noisy structures. However in the case of very low contrasted datasets, unwanted connections between vessels may appear Fig. 2(b).

2.4   Real Time Preview of Parameter Variations

As an enhancement of the automatic approach of the last section our framework gives the opportunity of a manual refinement of the segmentation result by implicitly adjusting the underlying parameters. Especially for people who do not have a computer science background, it is favorable to have a simple and intuitive dialog that gives the user the opportunity to manipulate the segmentation result without the need to manually adjust any parameters. By introducing a parameter free vesselness function in section 2.1 the threshold of the region growing is the only variable value in the segmentation process. In order to give the user a direct feedback of adjusting the threshold a real time preview of pre-computed segmentations is provided.

Starting with the automatically determined threshold, the region growing is applied with slightly varying values leading to different segmentation results. The

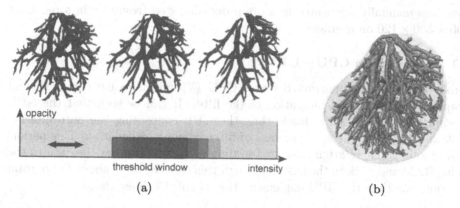

Fig. 3. Real time preview of manual parameter refinement. (a) A dynamic transfer function is used to visually seperate the pre-computed segmentation results. (b) The desired view is selected by the user and then rendered as a 3D mesh.

computed results are all stored in a single tagged volume separated by different values. This procedure can already be partly realized during the refinement process of 2.3 by storing the segmentation results of each iteration. The tagged volume is then visualized by direct volume rendering. In order to display all segmentations separately a dynamic transfer function is applied which only maps values to an opacity > 0 that correspond to the current threshold. Because the manipulation of the transfer function does not require to change or reload the dataset representation in memory it is very fast and therefore a real time preview of the different segmentation results is possible. Fig. 3(a) shows the results of adjusting the thresholds by moving a slider for the 3D case. After selecting the desired view the segmentation can be rendered as a 3D mesh using the marching cubes algorithm (Fig. 3(b)).

3   Results

We applied the segmentation method to 20 clinical CT datasets (14 for portal-venous phase, 6 for arterial phase) with an in-plane-resolution of 512^2 (0.613 to 0.84 mm voxel size) and an axial spacing of 1.0 to 2.5 mm. For the tests the

Table 1. Comparison of CPU and GPU performance. The first two columns show the computation time of the filter response in seconds on an AMD 1.8 GHz CPU using a $7 \times 7 \times 7$ kernel. The last two columns present the results of the GPU implementation performed on an Nvidia Geforce 8800 GTS with 640 MB of VRAM.

Dataset	$278 \times 271 \times 139$	$278 \times 308 \times 99$	$278 \times 271 \times 139$	$278 \times 308 \times 99$
Partial derivative ($\times 6$)	3.27(19.62)	2.72(16.32)	0.23(1.38)	0.19(1.14)
Filter response	11.93	9.87	0.11	0.09
Transfer to/from VRAM	$\times$	$\times$	0.28/0.20	0.21/0.16
Total	31.55	26.19	1.97	1.59

liver was manually segmented in a pre-processing step (resulting in a region of $300 \times 300 \times 120$ on average).

3.1   Comparison CPU – GPU

Table 1 shows a comparison between CPU (VisualStudio 6.0 compiler) and graphics hardware implementation of the filter. It can be seen that the GPU is approximately 15 times faster than the CPU concerning the pure filtering task and 100 times faster in the case of filter response calculation. This performance gain is partly attenuated by the time needed to transfer the data to the video RAM and back to the host. Although this transfer takes about 1/4 of total computation time the GPU implementation is still 15 times ahead.

3.2   Segmentation

A region growing (manual settings of seeds and thresholds) running on the unfiltered datasets was used for a visual comparison with the automatic approach. Hereby, the parameters of the region growing were chosen to prevent a leaking to the liver tissue while segmenting as much vessels as possible at the same time. Fig. 4(a)-(d) shows an exemplary result for the portal venous phase. With the

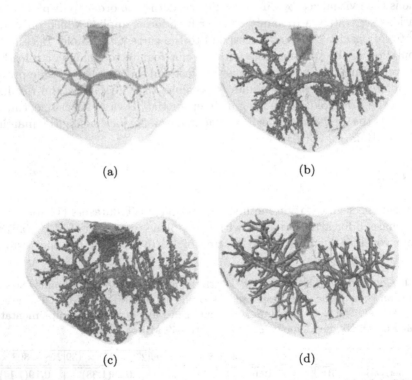

(a)   (b)

(c)   (d)

Fig. 4. Comparison of a manual region growing segmentation with the automatic method (portal venous phase). (a) Volume rendering of the original dataset. (b) and (c) Rendered masks of region growing with different thresholds. (d) Our approach.

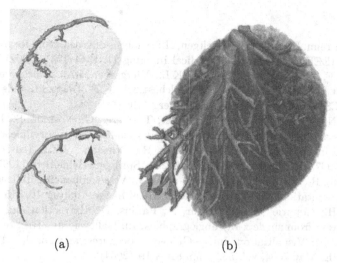

(a)   (b)

Fig. 5. (a) Arterial phase: manual region growing (top) and automatic segmentation with an artefact attached (bottom, arrow). (b) Illustration of an operation planning prototype using the proposed approach.

proposed approach more and better defined vessels can be segmented compared to the manual region growing. In fig. 5(a) an artefact appeared, because the automatic threshold was slightly too low. In such a case the preview function described in section 2.4 has to be used to refine the result. In order to detect falsely segmented structures, our operation planning prototype is providing a visual comparison with Maximum Intensity Projection, transparence and transfer function refinement. Fig. 5(b) illustrates a tumor resection scenario build with the proposed methods.

4   Discussion

We proposed an automatic hepatic vessel enhancement and segmentation approach together with a user friendly real time preview function to manually refine the resulting masks. A comparison with a manual region growing showed the potential of the method to save surgery planning time while providing accurate segmentations at the same time. An implementation on the GPU showed that a hardware implementation is able to perform the filter operations approximately 15 times faster, even for larger neighborhoods. The overall performance could be increased by the same factor.

Future work includes the isolation of portal and hepatic veins. For that task, knowledge about the tree structure of the vascular systems has to be incorporated. In addition, this procedure is promising to further reduce artefacts on low contrasted images. Also, we will further investigate on extending the use of graphics hardware to the other steps of the procedure.

References

1. Selle, D., Preim, B., Schenk, A., Peitgen, H.: Analysis of vasculature for liver surgical planning. IEEE Transactions on Medical Imaging 21, 1344–1357 (2002)
2. Frangi, A.F., Niessen, W.J., Vincken, K.L., Viergever, M.A.: Multiscale vessel enhancement filtering. In: Wells, W.M., Colchester, A.C.F., Delp, S.L. (eds.) MICCAI 1998. LNCS, vol. 1496. Springer, Heidelberg (1998)
3. Sato, Y., Nakajima, S., Atsumi, H., Koller, T., Gerig, G., Yoshida, S., Kikinis, R.: 3d multi-scale line filter for segmentation and visualization of curvilinear structures in medical images. In: Troccaz, J., Mösges, R., Grimson, W.E.L. (eds.) CVRMed-MRCAS 1997. LNCS, vol. 1205, pp. 213–222. Springer, Heidelberg (1997)
4. Manniesing, R., Viergever, M.A., Niessen, W.J.: Vessel enhancing diffusion: A scale space representation of vessel structures. Medical Image Analysis 10, 815–825 (2006)
5. Koehler, H., Couprie, M., Bouattour, S., Paulus, D.: Extraction and analysis of coronary tree from single x-ray angiographies. In: Galloway Jr., R.L. (ed.) Medical Imaging 2004: Visualization, Image-Guided Procedures, and Display. Proceedings of the SPIE, May 2004, vol. 5367, pp. 810–819 (2004)
6. Langs, G., Radeva, P., Rotger, D.: Explorative building of 3d vessel tree models. In: Digital Imaging in Media and Education. 28th annual workshop of the Austrian Association for Pattern Recognition (OAGM/AAPR) (2004)
7. Owens, J.D., Luebke, D., Govindaraju, N., Harris, M., Krueger, J., Lefohn, A.E., Purcell, T.J.: A Survey of General-Purpose Computation on Graphics Hardware. Computer Graphics Forum 26(1), 80–113 (2007)
8. Langs, A., Biedermann, M.: Filtering Video Volumes Using the Graphics Hardware. In: Ersbøll, B.K., Pedersen, K.S. (eds.) SCIA 2007. LNCS, vol. 4522, pp. 878–887. Springer, Heidelberg (2007)
9. Zhou, C., Chan, H.-P., Hadjiiski, L.M., Patel, S., Cascade, P.N., Sahiner, B., Wei, J., Ge, J., Kazerooni, E.A.: Automatic pulmonary vessel segmentation in 3D computed tomographic pulmonary angiographic (CTPA) images. In: Reinhardt, J.M., Pluim, J.P.W. (eds.) Medical Imaging 2006: Image Processing., March 2006, vol. 6144, pp. 1524–1530 (2006)

Learning Longitudinal Deformations for Adaptive Segmentation of Lung Fields from Serial Chest Radiographs*

Yonghong Shi[1] and Dinggang Shen[2]

[1] Digital Medical Research Center, Fudan University, Shanghai, China 200032
Yonghong.Shi@fudan.edu.cn
[2] Department of Radiology and Biomedical Research Imaging Center
University of North Carolina, Chapel Hill, NC 27510
dgshen@med.unc.edu

Abstract. We previously developed a deformable model for segmenting lung fields in serial chest radiographs by using both population-based and patient-specific shape statistics, and obtained higher accuracy compared to other methods. However, this method uses an *ad hoc* way to evenly partition the boundary of lung fields into some short segments, in order to capture the patient-specific shape statistics from a small number of samples by principal component analysis (PCA). This *ad hoc* partition can lead to a segment including points with different amounts of longitudinal deformations, thus rendering it difficult to capture principal variations from a small number of samples using PCA. In this paper, we propose a learning technique to adaptively partition the boundary of lung fields into short segments according to the longitudinal deformations learned for each boundary point. Therefore, all points in the same short segment own similar longitudinal deformations and thus small variations within all longitudinal samples of a patient, which enables effective capture of patient-specific shape statistics by PCA. Experimental results show the improved performance of the proposed method in segmenting the lung fields from serial chest radiographs.

Keywords: Statistical model, Active shape model, Hierarchical principal component analysis, Scale space analysis.

1 Introduction

Segmentation of lung fields in chest radiographs has been an active topic of research for over several decades, since chest radiograph is a popular diagnosis model to observe the dynamical behavior of the heart. However, the low signal-to-noise ratio (SNR) and the multiplicative nature of the noise (speckle) corrupting the chest radiograph make the segmentation of lung fields difficult [1-3]. We previously developed

* This work is supported by Science and Technology Commission of Shanghai Municipality of China (Grant number: 06dz22103).

T. Dohi, I. Sakuma, and H. Liao (Eds.): MIAR 2008, LNCS 5128, pp. 413–420, 2008.

an algorithm of segmenting lung fields in serial chest radiographs by using both population-based and patient-specific shape statistics, and obtained higher accuracy compared to other methods [4]. However, this algorithm uses an *ad hoc* way to evenly partition the boundary of lung fields into some short segments, in order to capture the patient-specific shape statistics from a small number of samples by using hierarchical principal component analysis (*hierarchical PCA*) [5]. In particular, the boundary of lung fields is evenly partitioned into a number of short segments and then PCA is performed for each segment, as well as for the set of middle points of all segments. This *ad hoc* partition can lead to a segment including points with different amounts of longitudinal deformations, thus rendering it difficult to capture principal variations from a small number of samples using PCA.

It would be very attractive to develop an optimal partition technique to replace the *ad hoc* partition in our algorithm, thus the variation in each short segment can be assumed to be linear and thus can be better captured by PCA. In this paper, we develop a learning technique to adaptively partition the boundary of lung fields into short segments according to the longitudinal deformations learned for each boundary point. Therefore, all points in the same short segment own similar longitudinal deformations and thus small variations within all longitudinal samples of a patient, which enables effective capture of patient-specific shape statistics by PCA. Experimental results show the improved performance of the proposed method in segmenting the lung fields from serial chest radiographs.

This paper is organized as follows. In Section 2, we first summarize the whole framework of our previous segmentation algorithm, and then describe a technique to learn longitudinal deformations from online acquired longitudinal samples and use them to adaptively partition the boundary of lung fields by using a scale space analysis method. The performance of this improved lung field segmentation method is demonstrated in Section 3. This paper concludes in Section 4.

2   Method

2.1   Summary of Our Previous Segmentation Algorithm

For segmenting lung fields from serial clinical chest radiographs, we have developed a deformable segmentation model using both population-based and patient-specific shape statistics [4]. This model demonstrated better accuracy in segmenting serial chest radiographs, compared to other model-based segmentation methods. There are two novelties in this algorithm. *First*, a more distinctive local descriptor, referred to as scale invariant feature transform (SIFT) [6], is used to characterize the image features in the vicinity of each pixel, thus allowing the deformable model to accurately match correspondences in the image. *Second*, two types of shape statistics are used to guide the deformable model. In particular, for segmenting the *initial* time-point images, the population-based shape statistics is mainly used to guide the deformable model. As more subsequent longitudinal images are acquired from the same patient, the patient-specific shape statistics is collected from the previous segmentation results, and used to guide the deformable model. This patient-specific shape statistics is updated each time when a new segmentation result is obtained, and the updated patient-specific shape statistics is further used to refine the segmentation of all available time-point images. When a sufficient number of longitudinal images are acquired and segmented from the same patient, the patient-specific shape statistics is considered sufficient to completely capture the variability of lung fields in the specific patient, without the need of using population-based shape statistics for the segmentation of future time-point images. Experimental results confirm that the use of this patient-specific shape statistics yields more robust and accurate segmentation of lung fields for serial chest radiographs.

However, to capture patient-specific shape statistics from a small number of longitudinal samples, the boundary of lung fields is currently partitioned into short segments using an *ad hoc* way. This *ad hoc* partition can lead to a segment including points with different amounts of longitudinal deformations, thus rendering it difficult to capture principal variations from a small number of samples using PCA. To overcome this limitation, we develop a learning technique to adaptively partition the boundary of lung fields into short segments according to the learned longitudinal deformations for each boundary point. This results in each short segment having similar longitudinal deformations, thus enabling the effective capture of patient-specific shape statistics by PCA. The details of our proposed technique are provided in the next subsection.

2.2   Adaptive Boundary Partition Using the Learned Longitudinal Deformations

To demonstrate the importance of learning the longitudinal deformations to guide the adaptive partition of lung field boundary, we *first* summarize our previous *ad hoc* partition method and point out its limitations by giving a visual example. Then, we will provide the details of our learning-based method for achieving adaptive partition of lung field boundary according to the learned longitudinal deformations.

Ad hoc boundary partition for capturing patient-specific shape statistics

At time-point t, we have t-1 previously segmented images and a current time-point image I_t. We can use the t-1 segmentation results from the images $I_1,...,I_{t-1}$, as the training samples, to capture the patient-specific shape statistics. For effectively capturing the shape statistics from a small number of longitudinal samples of the same patient, we adopt a hierarchical representation of shape statistics, namely *Hierarchical PCA*. In particular, we partition the contours along the boundaries of lung fields into G overlapping segments, each of which consists of g contour points. The top level of the contours consists of G middle points of G segments, reflecting the spatial relationships between different segments, while the bottom level has G segments, each with g contour points to capture local shape changes. If g is comparable with the number of longitudinal samples, *i.e.*, t-1, statistical variation of each segment might be well captured by this number of samples. Thus, by computing the local shape statistics for each segment and also the global shape statistics for the G middle points of G segments, we might be able to capture both local and global shape variation information from the longitudinal samples using $G+1$ PCA models.

Fig. 1(a) shows an example of evenly partitioning the boundaries of lung fields into 9 segments by our previous method. Also, the longitudinal variation of each boundary point is visualized by an ellipse that indicates both the directions and the amounts of

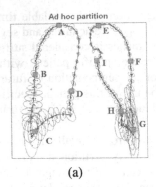 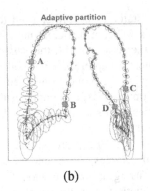

(a)	(b)

Fig. 1. Illustration of the importance of performing adaptive boundary partition, to allow each segment to have the points with similar longitudinal deformations

longitudinal deformations. It can be observed that there exist large longitudinal deformations for the bottom parts of lungs. The locations of points C and G are not reasonably placed in partition of boundaries of lung fields into nine segments. In particular, the segments CD and FG include points with different longitudinal deformations, which make it difficult to capture the statistical variations from a small number of samples by PCA. On the other hand, by using the learning technique developed in this paper, we can obtain optimal partition of boundaries according to the learned longitudinal deformations. For example, four segments are partitioned in Fig. 1(b), each having points with similar longitudinal deformations.

Adaptive **partition for capturing patient-specific shape statistics**
To adaptively partition the boundaries of lung fields into a number of short segments, we first learn the statistical variations for each point in the boundaries. We particularly use a PCA to capture the longitudinal deformation for each point from all available longitudinal samples of a specific patient. For example, for a patient image shown in Fig. 2(a), longitudinal deformation for each point is shown by a corresponding ellipse in Fig. 2(b). The long and short axes of the ellipse represent the major and the secondary directions of longitudinal deformation, and the size of ellipse represents the amount of longitudinal deformation. Figs. 2(c) and (d) show respectively the amounts of principal longitudinal deformation for each boundary point on the boundaries of right and left lungs. This information can be used as a reasonable foundation for adaptive partition of boundaries of lung fields.

However, the curves of principal longitudinal deformation (Figs. 2(c) and 2(d)) have many local details, as also shown in Figs. 3(b) and (d) by blue dashed curves. For determining the best partition positions, a scale space analysis technique, which can decide the parts to be smoothed out and the amount of smoothing, is used to approximate each curve by smoothing out only small details [7]. In this way, the approximated curve represents the global shape of a given curve. For example, as shown in Figs. 3(b) and (d), with the increase of scale, the curvature of the approximated curve becomes more even and constant, as demonstrated by pink, light blue, red and

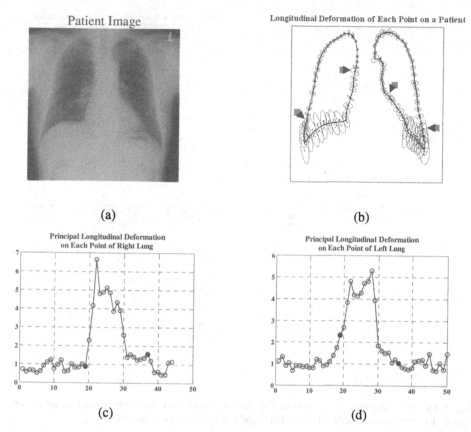

Fig. 2. Demonstration of longitudinal deformation of each point on the boundaries of right and left lungs of a patient

green curves, respectively. Then, the inflection points, i.e., the zero-crossings of second derivatives of the curve, can be used to judge the best partition positions of optimal subparts of the curve. When we plot the inflection points at every scale on the scale space, we can obtain so-called the finger print patterns. For example, in Figs. 3(a) and (c), different colors correspond to different scales, and as the scale increases from pink to light blue, red and green, the number of the inflection points decreases. Note, the scale space is spanned by the original position and the scale, for easy comparison across results from different scales.

It is known that the inflection points disappear only when two or more inflection points meet together in the scale space. Therefore, the finger print pattern closes upward as shown in Figs. 3(a) and (c). We define a shape segment as a part of a given contour between two inflection points which meet together when they disappear. As the scale increases, the number of shape segments decreases, and finally no shape segment remains. In Figs. 3(b) and (d), green curves correspond to the largest scale we used, and the green triangles indicate the inflection points which partition the curve into segments, i.e., with stronger and weaker longitudinal deformations. Finally, when we map these inflection points to the original contours of lung fields, we can

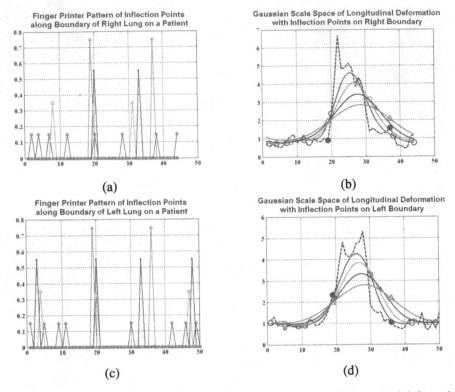

Fig. 3. Detecting the inflection points on the scale space of the leaned longitudinal deformation curves, for optimal boundary partition. *This figure is best viewed with color.*

acquire the optimal partition positions as blue triangles in Fig. 2(b). The advantage of using this adaptive partition technique for better capturing the patient-specific shape statistics is demonstrated in the experiments below.

3 Experiments

Various experiments are performed to evaluate the performance of our improved algorithm in segmenting the serial frontal chest radiographs of 39 patients. Most of these 39 patients have up to 17 monthly scanned images, each with 256x256 pixels. The lung fields of all these serial images have been manually delineated by a human observer, thus these manual segmentation results can be used as a golden standard to evaluate the segmentation results obtained by our method and all other methods in [4]. Two quantitative measures are used to evaluate the performance of the segmentation algorithm, i.e., the average overlay percentage and the average contour distance between automated segmentation result and manual segmentation result [4].

In order to objectively evaluate the performance of our algorithm, we compare the following five segmentation methods. *Method 1* is our complete method, which uses SIFT features, population-based shape statistics, and patient-specific shape statistics captured by *Adaptive* boundary partition. *Method 2* uses *ad hoc* boundary partition to replace *Adaptive* boundary partition in *Method 1* to capture patient-specific shape statistics. *Method 3* is similar to *Method 2,* except that *Method 3* uses *global PCA,* without partition on the patient lung field boundaries, to directly estimate patient-specific shape statistics. In addition, the *ASM SIFT,* which is our method without using patient-specific shape statistics, and the *ASM Intensity,* which is the standard ASM algorithm [3, 4], are also compared in this paper.

The average overlay percentages and the average contour distances of all the five methods are shown in Table 1 and Table 2, respectively. It can be observed that the average overlay percentage of *Method 1* (95.0%), *Method 2* (94.9%) and *Method 3* (94.8%) that use patient-specific shape statistics are much higher than that of *ASM SIFT* (91.0%) and *ASM Intensity* (87.3%). Similar conclusion can be drawn for the average contour distance in Table 2. All of these results indicate that the methods using the patient-specific shape statistics (*Methods 1~3*) outperform those without using patient-specific shape statistics (*ASM SIFT* and *ASM Intensity*). On the other hand, the use of SIFT features improves the segmentation performance, e.g., *ASM SIFT* is better than *ASM Intensity*.

Furthermore, by comparing the results obtained by *Methods 1-3* in Tables 1 and 2, it can be observed that the use of boundary partition (*Method 1-2*) performs better than no partition on patient's lung field boundaries (*Method 3*), when used to capture

Table 1. Average overlay percentage between manual segmentation and automated segmentation by five methods on the serial chest radiographs database of *39 patient.s* (%)

Algorithm	Mean ± std	Minimum	Median	Maximum
Method 1 (Adaptive boundary partition)	95.0±1.2	90.3	95.2	97.0
Method 2 (Ad hoc boundary partition)	94.9±1.3	88.4	95.0	97.0
Method 3 (No boundary partition)	94.8±1.4	88.2	95.1	96.9
ASM SIFT	91.0±1.7	85.0	91.4	94.8
ASM Intensity	87.3±4.9	76.9	89.2	93.7

Table 2. Average contour distance between manual segmentation and automated segmentation by five methods on the serial chest radiographs database of *39 patients.* (Unit in pixel)

Algorithm	Mean ± std	Minimum	Median	Maximum
Method 1 (Adaptive boundary partition)	1.05±0.26	0.58	1.01	2.12
Method 2 (Ad hoc boundary partition)	1.10±0.31	0.62	1.06	2.72
Method 2 (No boundary partition)	1.10±0.30	0.62	1.07	2.75
ASM SIFT	2.06±0.46	1.06	1.97	3.76
ASM Intensity	3.07±1.35	1.32	2.45	6.05

the patient-specific shape statistics from a small number of longitudinal samples of the same patient.

Finally, the use of adaptive partition (*Method 1*) produces better segmentation results than the use of ad hoc partition (*Method 2*). For example, the average overlay percentage is increased from 94.9% to 95.0%, and standard deviation is reduced from 1.3% to 1.2%. In the meanwhile, the minimum overlay percentage is increased from 88.4% to 90.3%. Similarly, we can see the average contour distance is decreased from 1.10 to 1.05 pixels, and the standard deviation is decreased from 0.31 to 0.26 pixel. In the meanwhile, the minimum, median, maximum contour distances are all greatly decreased by using adaptive boundary partition.

4 Conclusion

We have developed an improved method for segmenting boundaries of lung fields from serial chest radiographs. The better performance is achieved by the improved collection of patient-specific shape statistics using adaptive boundary partition according to the learned longitudinal boundary deformations. In the current paper, only the amount of principal longitudinal deformation is used to guide the boundary partition. In the future, we will include both the direction and the amount of principal longitudinal deformations to guide the partition of lung field boundaries. This can potentially make each resulting segment have not only similar amount of longitudinal deformation but also similar direction of longitudinal deformation, thus enabling better capture of patient-specific shape statistics for guiding the lung field segmentation.

References

1. van Ginneken, B., ter Haar Romeny, B.M., Viergever, M.A.: Computer-Aided Diagnosis in Chest Radiography: a Survey. IEEE Trans. On Medical Imaging 20(12), 1228–1241 (2001)
2. van Ginneken, B., Stegmann, M.B., Loog, M.: Segmentation of Anatomical Structures in Chest Radiographs using supervised methods: a Comparative Study on a Public Database. Medical Image Analysis 10, 19–40 (2006)
3. Cootes, T.F., Taylor, C.J.: Statistical Models of appearance for Computer Vision. Technical Report, Wolfson Image Analysis Unit, University of Manchester (2001)
4. Shi, Y., Qi, F., Xue, Z., Chen, L., Ito, K., Matsuo, H., Shen, D.: Segmenting Lung Fields in Serial Chest Radiographs Using Both Population-based and Patient-specific Shape Statistics. In: Larsen, R., Nielsen, M., Sporring, J. (eds.) MICCAI 2006. LNCS, vol. 4190, pp. 83–91. Springer, Heidelberg (2006)
5. Davatzikos, C., Tao, X., Shen, D.: Hierarchical Active Shape Models Using the Wavelet Transform. IEEE Trans on Medical Imaging 22(3), 414–423 (2003)
6. Lowe, D.G.: Distinctive Image Features from Scale-Invariant Keypoints. International Journal of Computer Vision 60(2), 91–110 (2004)
7. Hontani, H., Deguchi, K.: Primitive Curve Generation Based on Multiscale Contour Figure Approximation. In: Proceeding of 15th International Conference on Pattern Recognition, vol. 2, pp. 887–890 (2000)

Automatic Extraction of Proximal Femur Contours from Calibrated X-Ray Images Using 3D Statistical Models

Xiao Dong and Guoyan Zheng

MEM Research Center, University of Bern, CH-3014, Switzerland
guoyan.zheng@ieee.org

Abstract. Automatic identification and extraction of bone contours from x-ray images is the first essential task for further medical image analysis. In this paper we propose a 3D statistical model based framework for the proximal femur contour extraction from calibrated x-ray images. The initialization is solved by an *Estimation of Bayesian Network Algorithm* to fit a multiple component geometrical model to the x-ray data. The contour extraction is accomplished by a non-rigid 2D/3D registration between a 3D statistical model and the x-ray images, in which bone contours are extracted by a graphical model based Bayesian inference. Our experimental results demonstrate its performance and efficacy even when part of the images are occluded.

Keywords: statistical models, segmentation, fluoroscopy, Bayesian network.

1 Motivation

Accurate extraction of bone contours from x-ray images is an important component for computer analysis of medical images for diagnosis [1][2][3], planning [4][5][6] or 3D reconstruction of anatomic structures [7][8][9][10]. X-ray images may vary a lot in brightness and contrast as well as in the imaged region of anatomy. Therefore conventional segmentation techniques [1][5][6] can not offer a satisfactory solution and model based segmentation is usually implemented to obtain robust and accurate results [11][12][13][3][7].

In [14][3][15][12], 2D statistical models, active shape model (ASM) or active appearance model (AAM), are constructed from a training image set under the assumption that the images are taken from a certain view direction. 2D statistical models can encode both the shape and texture information learnt from training data set, which is helpful in improving robustness and accuracy in noisy images. Due to the limited convergence region, 2D statistical model asks for a proper initialization. Fully automatic initialization can be accomplished by the generalized Hough transformation [12], neural nets [13] or evolutionary algorithms [15][14]. But both the initialization and segmentation performance rely on whether the view direction assumption can be fulfilled.

3D statistical models are also used for 2D segmentation and 3D reconstruction from calibrated 2D x-ray images [7][8][9][10]. One of the main advantages is that it can be used for segmenting an image taken from an arbitrary view direction. The initialization of the 3D model is usually manually defined [7][9]. Due to the dense mesh of the 3D

T. Dohi, I. Sakuma, and H. Liao (Eds.): MIAR 2008, LNCS 5128, pp. 421–429, 2008.

statistical model, fully automated solutions based on evolutionary algorithm is computational expensive [17].

Bayesian network based approaches [18][19][20] has been used to identify or track objects. The Bayesian network embeds the object information in a graphical model, where the constraints among subparts of the object are represented as *potentials* among nodes and the local image information correspondent to each subpart as *observation* of the node. Bayesian network is also exploited to find deformable shapes [21][22]. Belief propagation is usually used to perform approximate inference on the graph to find an MAP estimation.

We propose a 3D statistical model based fully automatic proximal femur bone contour segmentation for calibrated x-ray images. The initialization is accomplished by an Estimation of Bayesian Network Algorithm on a simplified multiple component model instead of the triangulated surface mesh of the 3D model, which reduces the computational complexity. The statistical model based contour extraction is achieved by a Bayesian inference on a Bayesian network, which encodes both the shape and texture information of the model and therefore enhances the robustness and accuracy of the contour extraction.

2 Methods

2.1 Image Acquisition

In our work calibrated x-ray images from C-arm are used. Due to the limited imaging volume of C-arm, we ask for four images for the proximal femur from different view directions, of which two images focus on the proximal femoral head and the other two focus on the femoral shaft. The calibrated x-ray image set is represented by $\mathbf{I}$.

2.2 3D Statistical Model of the Proximal Femur

A *Principle Component Analysis* (PCA) based 3D statistical model $\mathcal{M}$ with 4098 vertices of the proximal femur is constructed from a collection of 13 CT data of the proximal femur as shown in Fig. 1(a). An instance generated from the statistical model with parameter set $\mathbf{Q} = \{\alpha, \beta_0, \beta_1, \ldots, \beta_{11}\}$ can be described as

$$\mathcal{M} : \mathbf{S}(\mathbf{Q}) = \alpha(\mathbf{S}_0 + \sum_{i=0}^{11} \beta_i \lambda_i^{\frac{1}{2}} \mathbf{P}_i) \tag{1}$$

where $\mathbf{S}_0$ is the mean model, α is the scaling factor, λ_i and $\mathbf{P}_i$ are the ith eigenvalue and the the correspondent eigenvectror of the correlation matrix of the training data set.

2.3 Automated Initialization of the 3D Statistical Model

To find the initial rigid transformation $\mathbf{T}_0$ and parameter set $\mathbf{Q}_0$ to align the model instance $\mathbf{S}(\mathbf{Q}_0)$ with the observed x-ray images, we model the proximal femur by a multiple component geometrical model consisting of three components: head, neck and shaft, which are described by a sphere, a trunked cone and a cylinder with parameter set $\mathbf{X}_{geo} = \{\mathbf{X}_H, \mathbf{X}_N, \mathbf{X}_S\}$ respectively as shown in Fig. 1(b).

A graphical model is then constructed for the geometrical model as shown in Fig. 1(c). The constraints among components are encoded in the conditional distributions among nodes [18][20]. $\pi(X_S), \pi(X_N), \pi(X_H)$ are the prior information for the shaft, neck and head. The conditional distributions $p(X_N|X_S), p(X_H|X_N)$ are set so that the geometrical model can represent a meaningful anatomical structure of the proximal femur. A combination of particle filter and probability logic sampling, which can also be regarded as an Estimation of Bayesian Network Algorithm (EBNA), is implemented (see details in [23]) to find an instance of the geometrical model $\mathbf{X}_{geo}^0$ which fits the x-ray images as shown in Fig. 1(d).

From the mean shape of the 3D statistical model S_0, the model vertices can be classified into three regions, femoral head, neck and shaft. The femoral head center and radius, axes of femoral neck and shaft can be determined in the model coordinate space by a 3D sphere fitting to the femoral head region and cylinder fittings to the femoral neck and shaft regions. The initial rigid transformation $\mathbf{T}_0$ and parameter set $\mathbf{Q}_0 = \{\alpha_0, 0, \ldots, 0\}$ can then be computed to fit the statistical model(the scaled mean shape) to the geometrical model as shown in Fig. 1(e).

2.4 3D Statistical Model Based Contour Extraction

After the initialization of the statistical model, the contour extraction is accomplished by a joint registration and segmentation as summarized in Algorithm 1.

---

1. *Simulated x-ray and silhouette extraction*

Given the current instanced statistical model $\mathcal{M} : S(\mathbf{Q}^n)$ and the transformation $\mathbf{T}^n$, project the aligned statistical model on each of the K x-ray image planes using the projection geometry of each x-ray image. From the simulated x-ray images the silhouettes $\{\mathbf{C}_{model}^{k,n}\}_{k=0,\ldots,K-1}$ are extracted[9].

2. *2D template based segmentation*

On each x-ray image, taking the correspondent silhouette of the projected statistical model $\mathbf{C}_{model}^{k,n}$ as a template, a Bayesian network based shape matching is implemented to search for the bone contour $\mathbf{C}_{image}^{k,n}$.

3. *Nonrigid 2D/3D registration*

A 2D/3D nonrigid registration is carried out to fit the extracted bone contours $\{\mathbf{C}_{image}^{k,n}\}_{k=0,\ldots,K-1}$ and the statistical model $\mathcal{M}$, which results in an updated model instance $\mathcal{M} : S(\mathbf{Q}^{n+1})$ and rigid transformation $\mathbf{T}^{n+1}$

4. Go to 1, until the procedure converges.

Algorithm 1. 3D statistical model based contour segmentation

2D template based segmentation using belief propagation. From the silhouette of the projected 3D statistical model, we sample M points(nodes) tracing along the contour as the shape prior. Each point is described by a parameter set $q_i = \{\mathbf{x}_i, \mathbf{g}_i, flag_i\}$, $i = 1, \ldots, M$, where $\mathbf{x}_i = (x_i, y_i)$ is the position of ith point in the image coordinate system, $\mathbf{g}_i = (g_{xi}, g_{yi})$ is the gradient vector of the x-ray image, $flag_i = 1$ if the current node belongs to the femur head projection silhouette and $flag_i = 0$ otherwise. The

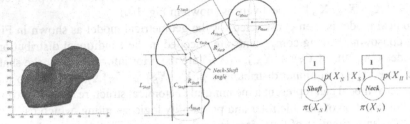

(a) PCA based 3D statisti-   (b) Multiple component geo-   (c) Graphical model for the
cal model   metrical model   multiple component geometrical
                                                              model

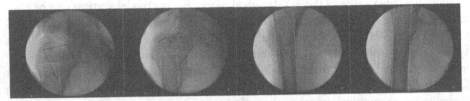

(d) Fitting the geometrical 3D model with x-ray images

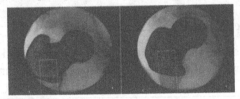

(e) Fitting the statistical model with the geometrical model

Fig. 1. Automatic initialization of the 3D statistical model

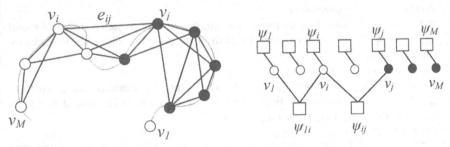

(a) Graphical model for the contour extraction,   (b) Factor graph for the graphical model for
filled dots: head nodes, circles: non-head nodes   the contour extraction

Fig. 2. Bayesian network for the template based contour extraction

configuration of our model can then be written as $\mathbf{Q}_{model} = \{\mathbf{q}_i\}_{i=1,...,M}$, where $\mathbf{g}_i$ is set as the normal vector of the template curve at position $\mathbf{x}_i$. The configuration of a candidate contour can be written as $\mathbf{Q}_{cand} = \{\mathbf{q}'_i\}_{i=1,...,M}$.

We then establish a partially connected graph with M vertices as: $\mathbf{G}(\mathbf{V}, \mathbf{E})$, $\mathbf{V} = \{v_i,\}_{i=1,\ldots,M}$, $\mathbf{E} = \{e_{ij}\}_{i,j=1,\ldots,M}$, where $e_{ij} = 1$ for $(a)(|i-j| <= N_{Shaft}) \cap (i \neq j) \cap (flag_i = 0) \cap (flag_j = 0)$, $(b)(flag_i = 0) \cap (flag_j = 1)$, $(c)(|i-j| <= N_{Head}) \cap (flag_i = 1) \cap (flag_j = 1)$ as shown in Fig. 2(a). N_{Head} and N_{Shaft} determine the number of connected neighbors for the head nodes and the non-head nodes respectively. Larger N_{Head} and N_{Shaft} will keep the rigidity of the shape but will fail to track deviation from the template. The reason that all the head nodes are connected with the non-head nodes is that we need the non-head nodes(which are supposed to be relatively easier to be located than the head nodes) to guide the localization of the head nodes. The correspondent factor graph is shown in Fig. 2(b).

Given the template $\mathbf{Q}_{model} = \{\mathbf{q}_i\}_{i=1,\ldots,M}$, the joint probability distribution of the factor graph with an candidate configuration $\mathbf{Q}_{cand} = \{\mathbf{q}_i'\}_{i=1,\ldots,M}$ is then given by

$$p(\mathbf{Q}_{cand}) = \frac{1}{Z} \prod_i \psi_i(\mathbf{q}_i') \prod_{e_{ij}=1} \psi_{ij}(\mathbf{q}_i', \mathbf{q}_j') \qquad (2)$$

where $\psi_i(\mathbf{q}_i') = dot(\mathbf{g}_i, \mathbf{g}_i')$, which means to penalize candidates with weak gradient amplitude and inconsistent gradient direction with the model.

$\psi_{ij}(\mathbf{q}_i', \mathbf{q}_j') = e^{-(\mu \frac{(\mathbf{x}_i' - \mathbf{x}_j') \cdot (\mathbf{x}_i - \mathbf{x}_j)}{\|\mathbf{x}_i' - \mathbf{x}_j'\| \|\mathbf{x}_i - \mathbf{x}_j\|} + \nu \frac{\|\|\mathbf{x}_i' - \mathbf{x}_j'\| - \|\mathbf{x}_i - \mathbf{x}_j\|\|}{\|\mathbf{x}_i - \mathbf{x}_j\|})}$, which is set so that the global shape of the model will be kept by penalizing the deviation of the angle and distance between vertices from our model.

Under these definitions, a bone contour that keeps the global shape of our model and at the same time locates itself to the strong edge positions can be obtained by a *Maximal Likelihood*(ML) estimation as

$$C_{image}^* = \max_{\mathbf{Q}_{cand}=\{\mathbf{q}_i'\}} \prod_i \psi_i(\mathbf{q}_i') \prod_{e_{ij}=1} \psi_{ij}(\mathbf{q}_i', \mathbf{q}_j') \qquad (3)$$

In our approach, the candidate positions for each node of the bone contour are sampled along the normal direction of the model and standard loopy belief propagation [21] is used to approximate the ML estimation as shown in Fig. 3(a).

2D/3D nonrigid registration. Our statistical model can then fit to the extracted bone contours $\{C_{image}^{k,n}\}$ using a 2D/3D nonrigid registration procedure [8]. For

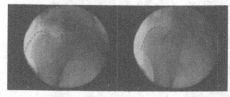 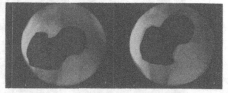

(a) Bayesian network based 2D segmentation, where circles show the projected silhouettes and dots show the extracted contours

(b) 2D/3D nonrigid registration to fit the 3D statistical model to the extracted bone contours

Fig. 3. Bayesian network for the template based contour extraction

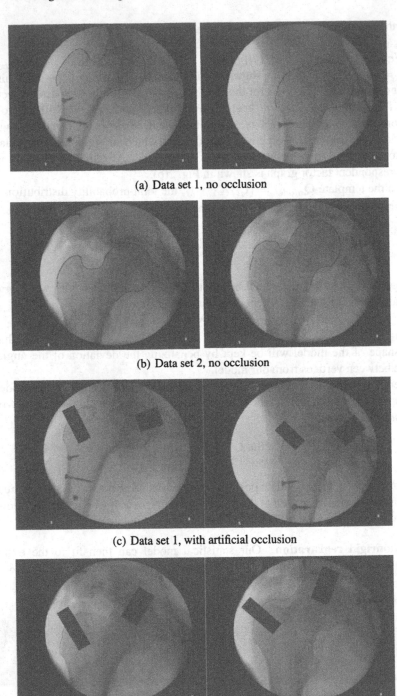

(a) Data set 1, no occlusion

(b) Data set 2, no occlusion

(c) Data set 1, with artificial occlusion

(d) Data set 2, with artificial occlusion

Fig. 4. Results of automatic proximal femur bone contour extraction on clinical data

each point P_l on the extracted bone contour, the correspondence between its back-projection line $BP(P_l)$ and a vertex $v_{corr(P_l)}$ on the current instanced statistical model $\mathcal{M} : S(Q^n)$ can be established using the current rigid transformation $\mathbf{T}^n$. Projecting $v_{corr(P_l)}$ onto $BP(P_l)$ will generate a correspondent 3D point pair $(v_{corr(P_l)}, Proj(v_{corr(P_l)}, BP(P_l)))$. A rigid transformation $\mathbf{T}^{n+1}_{update}$ can be calculated to align the current statistical model $\mathcal{M} : S(Q^n)$ to the extracted contours by minimizing the distances between all 3D point pairs. The rigid transformation can then be updated as $\mathbf{T}^{n+1} = \mathbf{T}^{n+1}_{update} \mathbf{T}^n$. The residual error between those correspondent point pairs can be further reduced by generating a new instance $\mathcal{M} : S(Q^{n+1})$ using an statiatically regularized instantiation [16]. An example of the nonrigid registration is shown in Fig. 3(b).

3 Experimental Results

We verified our approach on two set of clinical data, each data set includes four calibrated x-ray images of the proximal femur. We first run our algorithm on the original data set with parameters set as $M = 35, N_{Head} = 4, N_{Shaft} = 3, \mu = 2, \nu = 1$ and the results are shown in Fig. 4(a) and 4(b). To further verify its performance against occlusion, we added artificial occlusion with different sizes to the x-ray images. The contour extraction results with $M = 35, N_{Head} = 5, N_{Shaft} = 6, \mu = 2, \nu = 1$ are shown in Fig. 4(c) and 4(d). It can be observed that due to the existence of occlusion, we have to select larger N_{Head} and N_{Shaft} to hold the global shape of the contour, which on the other hand leads to a failure in tracking local deviation between the real contour and the template in the femur neck area as shown in Fig. 4(c) and 4(d)

4 Conclusions

We introduced a 3D statistical model based fully automatic bone contour extraction framework from calibrated x-ray images. The automatic initialization is achieved by fitting a simplified multiple component geometrical 3D model to the observed x-ray images. The 3D model based initialization algorithm does not ask for strict view direction assumption compared with 2D model based initialization. The 3D statistical model based bone contour extraction is solved as a simultaneous 2D/3D registration and segmentation. The model based segmentation is accomplished by a Bayesian inference procedure which in principle can overperform ASM/AAM based algorithms by simultaneously optimize both the global shape constraints and the local image feature information. Our experimetal results demonstrate its performance and efficacy even when part of the images are occluded.

References

1. Chen, Y., et al.: Automatic Extraction of Femur Contours from Hip X-ray Images. In: Liu, Y., Jiang, T., Zhang, C. (eds.) CVBIA 2005. LNCS, vol. 3765, pp. 200–209. Springer, Heidelberg (2005)

2. de Luis-Garcia, R., et al.: A Fully Automatic Algorithm for Contour Detection of Bones in Hand Radiographs Using Active Contours. In: ICIP 2003, Part. III, pp. 421–424 (2003)
3. Roberts, M.G., et al.: Automatic segmentation of lumbar vertebrae on digitised radiographs using linked active appearance models. In: MIUA 2006, Part. I, pp. 120–124 (2006)
4. Gottschling, H., et al.: Intraoperative, Fluoroscopy-based Planning for Complex Osteotomies of the Proximal Femur. The International Journal of Medical Robotics & Computer Assisted Srugery 1(3), 67–73 (2005)
5. Bartolini, F., et al.: Model-based Extraction of Femoral Medulla Ducts from Radiographic Images. Image and Vision Computing 22, 173–182 (2004)
6. Tian, T.P., et al.: Computing Neck-Shaft Angle of Femur for X-ray Fracture Detection. In: Petkov, N., Westenberg, M.A. (eds.) CAIP 2003. LNCS, vol. 2756, pp. 82–89. Springer, Heidelberg (2003)
7. Benameur, S., et al.: 3D/2D Registration and Segmentation of Scoliotic Vertebrae Using Statistical Models. Computerized Medical Imaging and Graphics 27(5), 321–337 (2003)
8. Zheng, G., Nolte, L.-P.: Surface Reconstruction of Bone from X-ray Images and Point Distribution Model Incorporating a Novel Method for 2D-3D Correspondence. In: CVPR 2006, Part II, pp. 2237–2244 (2006)
9. Lamecker, H., et al.: Atlas-based 3D-Shape Reconstruction from X-ray Images. In: ICPR 2006, Part I, pp. 371–374 (2006)
10. Tang, T.S., Ellis, R.E.: 2D/3D Deformable Registration Using a Hybrid Atlas. In: Duncan, J.S., Gerig, G. (eds.) MICCAI 2005, Part II. LNCS, vol. 3750, pp. 223–230. Springer, Heidelberg (2005)
11. Behiels, G., et al.: Active Shape Model-based Segmentation of Digital X-ray Images. In: Taylor, C., Colchester, A. (eds.) MICCAI 1999. LNCS, vol. 1679, pp. 128–137. Springer, Heidelberg (1999)
12. Howe, B., et al.: Hierarchical Segmentation of Cervical and Lumbar Vertebrae Using a Customised Generalized Hough Transform and Extensions to Active Appearance Models. In: Proc. IEEE 6th SSIAI, March 2004, pp. 182–186 (2004)
13. Langs, G., et al.: Determining Position and Fine Shape Detail in Radiological Anatomy. In: Michaelis, B., Krell, G. (eds.) DAGM 2003. LNCS, vol. 2781, pp. 532–539. Springer, Heidelberg (2003)
14. Seise, M., et al.: Probabilistic Segmentation of the Knee Joint from X-ray Images. In: MIUA 2006, pp. 110–114 (2006)
15. de Bruijne, M., Nielsen, M.: Image Segmentation by Shape Particle Filtering. In: ICPR 2004, Part. III (2004)
16. Zheng, G., et al.: Use of a Dense Surface Point Distribution Model in a Three-Stage Anatomical Shape Reconstruction from Sparse Information for Computer Assisted Orthopaedic Surgery: A Preliminary Study. In: Narayanan, P.J., Nayar, S.K., Shum, H.-Y. (eds.) ACCV 2006, Part II. LNCS, vol. 3852, pp. 52–60. Springer, Heidelberg (2006)
17. Ma, B., Ellis, R.E.: Surface-based Registration with a Particle Filter. In: Barillot, C., Haynor, D.R., Hellier, P. (eds.) MICCAI 2004, Part I. LNCS, vol. 3216, pp. 566–573. Springer, Heidelberg (2004)
18. Lee, M.W., Cohen, I.: Human Upper Body Pose Estimation in Static Images. In: Pajdla, T., Matas, J(G.) (eds.) ECCV 2004, Part II. LNCS, vol. 3022, pp. 126–138. Springer, Heidelberg (2004)
19. Sigal, L., et al.: Tracking loose-limbed people. In: CVPR 2004, Part. 1, pp. 421–428 (2004)
20. Wu, Y., et al.: Tracking articulated body by dynamic Markov network. In: ICCV 2003, vol. 1, pp. 1094–1101 (2003)
21. Coughlan, J., Ferreira, S.: Finding deformable shapes using loopy belief propagation. In: Heyden, A., Sparr, G., Nielsen, M., Johansen, P. (eds.) ECCV 2002. LNCS, vol. 2350, pp. 453–468. Springer, Heidelberg (2002)

22. Rangarajan, A., et al.: A Bayesian Network Framework for Relational Shape Matching. In: ICCV 2003, pp. 671–678 (2003)
23. Dong, X., Zheng, G.: Fully Automatic Determination of Morphological Parameters of Proximal Femur from Calibrated Fluoroscopic Images Through Particle Filtering. In: Campilho, A., Kamel, M. (eds.) ICIAR 2006. LNCS, vol. 4142, pp. 535–546. Springer, Heidelberg (2006)

Anisotropic Haralick Edge Detection Scheme with Application to Vessel Segmentation

Ali Gooya[1], Takeyoshi Dohi[2], Ichiro Sakuma[1], and Hongen Liao[1,3]

[1] Graduate School of Engineering, The University of Tokyo, The University of Tokyo
[2] Graduate School of Informaiton Science and Technology, The University of Tokyo
[3] Translational Systems Biology and Medicine Initiative, The University of Tokyo
{gooya,ichiro,liao}@bmpe.t.u-tokyo.ac.jp
7-3-1, Hongo, Bunkyo, Tokyo, 113-8656

Abstract. In this paper, detection of edges in oriented fields is addressed. Haralick edge detection is an accurate scheme for estimation of the edge in a Euclidean space. However, in some applications such as edge detection for vessel segmentation because of the intrinsic orientation of structures, accuracy is only demanded in a particular subspace. This is specially usefull when a curve evolution is chosen for segmentation since gradients in parallel to vessel orientation stops evolution. Haralick edge detection is generalized on a Riemannian space using the inner product of the vectors under a space metric tensor. This eliminates the spurious gradients and preserves the accuracy on the vessel border. Examples are given and the comparison is made with the state-of-the-art flux maximizing flow indicating that significant improvements in terms of leakage minimization and thiner vessel delineation is achievable using our methodology.

1 Introduction

Magnetic Resonance Angiography (MRA) is increasingly used to provide volumetric information of vascular system. Accurate assessment of MRA images requires that the vessel structures to be extracted from MRA data sets. Currently, a number of techniques have been developed for vessel segmentation based on the advanced level set evolutionary methods. Lorigo *et al* [1] has proposed CURVES using image gradient strength information, and the surface minimum curvature as the smoothing term. Also capillary active contours is invented by Yan *et al.* [2], a method that is based on the capillary force acting on the free fluid surface through a capillary tube. A local variance maximizer edge detection method is proposed in [13], where the detected edge field is used for computation of a multi-scale flux image, and segmentation is achieved based on the technique described in flux maximizing flow proposed by Vasilevsky [3].

Despite of relative success from some of these methods, segmentation of long thin structures is still considered as a delicate task. Most of these techniques are edge detection based and therefore, their success mainly depends on the accuracy of the detected edges. Typical gradient patterns in non-contrast agent vascular

T. Dohi, I. Sakuma, and H. Liao (Eds.): MIAR 2008, LNCS 5128, pp. 430–438, 2008.

imaging techniques, are not step-like but indicate smooth graduations. Haralick
edge detection [10] is a well known scheme that defines the edge as a point where
the gradient magnitude is maximized along side the image gradient orientation.
The main concern here is that if the gradient has a noisy direction the estimation
will produce inappropriate results. As we will see the original Haralick edge
detection is not appropriate to segment thin vessels that are highly vulnerable
against the noise. The reason is that Haralick edge detector has a isotropic
behaviour, and is equally sensitive to gradients in all orientations. Therefore,
those noisy image gradients which are in parallel to the vessel orientation luck the
contour and prevent further propagation. In fact, the inherited Haralick accuracy
is only needed across the planes normal to vessel. This can be interpreted as a
general form of Haralick edge detection in oriented fields. We will implement this
scheme on a Riemannian space where the norm of the vector is defined using a
metric tensor. An appropriate form of such a tensor will be given and illustrated
using an example.

1.1 Related Work

Our method is inspired by the work of Gazit *et al.*[4] for segmentation of thin
structures, a combinational method, using Haralick edge detector and Chan-Vese
minimal variance functional and geodesic active contours [5]. Our methodology
is different from that model, since we propose a novel Haralick like edge detection
that utilizes structural information for edge detection, and does not depend on
GAC and Chan-Vese model. In another related work to our algorithm, a level set
method is introduced by Vasilevsky [3] that integrates the directions of gradient
vectors into the evolution equation so that the gradient flux through the evolving
curve is maximized (here after called FLUX). A multi-scale method is used to
compute the divergence by estimation the outward flux of the gradient vectors
on multiple hemo-centric spherics and choosing the maximum response over the
scales. We show that leakage is likely to happen using FLUX and usually the
estimated edges are not accurate, while using our method the risk of the leakage
is minimized and better segmentation is achieved in lower contrast vessels.

2 Haralick Edge Detection

Zero crossing of Laplacian was proposed by "Marr-Hildreth" in [12] as an edge
detector, later Haralick [10] only considered the direction along the gradient and
then it was used by Canny [11] as a 2D edge detector. More precisely, Haralick
edge detector finds the image locations where $|\nabla I|$ has a local maximum along
the gradient. In other word, edge is defined as a point where the directional
derivative of $|\nabla I|$ along side $\boldsymbol{\xi} = \frac{\nabla I}{|\nabla I|}$, i.e, $I_{\xi\xi}$ is zero:

$$\nabla |\nabla I|.\boldsymbol{\xi} = 0 \tag{1}$$

This means that the inside the object $\nabla|\nabla I|.\boldsymbol{\xi}$ is negative and the outside posi-
tive. Haralick observed that, using only the gradient direction component of the

Laplacian, gives better edges. In [4], it is shown that $I_{\xi\xi} = \Delta I - I_{\eta\eta}$ and this corresponds to two independent energy functionals on the Euclidean space, one is maximizing the inward flux on the surface of the evolving front [3], and the other one minimizes the variability of the grey levels inside the front. In this paper, an energy functional is proposed which is directly inspired by negativity of $\nabla|\nabla I|.\xi$ inside the object.

3   Formation of Energy Functional

Assume for a given open region D, the evolving surface is represented as the zero level of the level set function $\phi(x)$ where $\phi(x) < 0$ for inside of the object, and $\phi(x) > 0$ for outside. $H(x)$ is representing Heaviside function such that $H(x) = 1$ if $x \geq 0$ otherwise $H(x) = 0$. Also $\delta(x) = \frac{d}{dx}H(x)$ is the Dirac delta function. Further, assume that M is the Riemannian manifold defined on D and endowed by the metric $g = \{g_{i,j}\}$ [6].

4   Riemannian Haralick Edge Detection

The generalization of Haralick edge deteection into a Riemannian space is straight forward using the fact that on the Euclidean space $\nabla|\nabla I|.\xi < 0$ inside the object. We should maximize this value on the manifold M where ever $\phi(x) < 0$. Considering the fact that dot product under the space metric is now defined as: $< x, y >_g = x^t.g.y$ and taking care of all the quantities involved in terms of the metric g such energy functional can be written as:

$$E = \int_M H(-\phi)\nabla_g^t \| \nabla_g I \|_g . g . \frac{\nabla_g I}{\| \nabla_g I \|_g} \tag{2}$$

where ∇_g and $\| \cdot \|_g$ denotes the gradient and the norm on the manifold. Minimization of this regional functional implies negative riemannian interpretation of dot product operator employed in 1 inside the object. Using co-area formula equation (2) can be written as:

$$\int_D H(-\phi)\nabla_g^t \| \nabla_g I \|_g . g . \frac{\nabla_g I}{\| \nabla_g I \|_g} |g|^{1/2} dx \tag{3}$$

in which $|g|$ denotes the determinant of the metric. Using the fact that $\nabla_g I = g^{-1}\nabla I$, one can write: $\| \nabla_g I \|_g = \| \nabla I \|_{g^{-1}}$. Therefore (3) can be simplified as:

$$E = \int_D H(-\phi)\nabla^t \| \nabla I \|_{g^{-1}} . g^{-1} . \frac{\nabla I}{\| \nabla I \|_{g^{-1}}} |g|^{1/2} dx \tag{4}$$

It is easy to see that the Euler-Lagrangian minimizing equation of (4) is as follows:

$$\frac{\partial \phi}{\partial t} = \delta(\phi)\nabla^t \| \nabla I \|_{g^{-1}} . g^{-1} . \frac{\nabla I}{\| \nabla I \|_{g^{-1}}} |g|^{1/2} \tag{5}$$

This can be written as:

$$\frac{\partial \phi}{\partial t} = \delta(\phi)[div(|g|^{1/2}g^{-1}\nabla I) - \| \nabla I \|_{g^{-1}} \ div(\frac{|g|^{1/2}g^{-1}\nabla I}{\| \nabla I \|_{g^{-1}}})] \tag{6}$$

Let us have a closer look at different terms of (6). The first term in computes the Laplacian of the projected image gradient and it has high responses if ∇I has large components in parallel to main eigen vector of g^{-1}. This is an important property which is especially usefull in design of the g, the metric tensor. The second term is *geodesic* mean curvature of the image isolevels, and has a similar role as topological complexity minimizer, i.e., $I_{\eta\eta}$ in the Euclidean version. We observe that for $g = I_d$, (the identity matrix), equation (6) reduces to $\partial\phi/\partial t = \Delta I - I_{\eta\eta}$. This means that in Euclidean case the contour stops in the Haralick edge point. However, generalization using the metric tensor g allows a selective behaviour of the edge detection mechanism. All we have to do is to design an appropriate tensor that eliminates the gradient vectors that are in parallel with main orientation of the local structure.

5   Design of the Metric Tensor

In this paper, we utilize the structural tensor to define our metric tensor. The structure tensor of the image can be obtained using the following convolution[9]:

$$T(x) = w(x) * \nabla I \nabla^t I \tag{7}$$

Where $w(x)$ is a Gaussian with a standard deviation σ. Let $0 \leq \lambda_1 < \lambda_2 < \lambda_3$ and $C_i = e_i e_i^t, i = 1, 2, 3$ be the eigen values and their corresponding eigen components of the structure matrix T.

As mentioned in the previous section the tensor g^{-1} should maintain its main components in support of ∇I if it is normal to the local orientation, and in other way, the gradients that are in parallel to local orientation should be eliminated. In this paper we consider a simple form for g^{-1}:

$$g^{-1} = \epsilon C_1 + C_2 + C_3 \tag{8}$$

Where $0 \leq \epsilon \leq 1$ is a user selected parameter controlling the anisotropic behaviour of the tensor and must be a very small value if a totally anisotropic metric is desired. Under this definition $|g|^{1/2}$ is a constant which can be ignored from the evolution equation (6).

6   Multi-scale Computation

Multi-scale implementation of (6) can be achieved in a similar way as described in [3]. That means $div(v)$ terms are computed as the outward flux of the v on hemo-centric spheres with different radius $r_k = r_0 e^{k.dr}, k = 0, \ldots, q - 1$, and then maximum is chosen over the range of scales:

$$div(\boldsymbol{v}) = \sup_r \{1/N \sum_q \boldsymbol{v}(r\boldsymbol{n}_q).\boldsymbol{n}_q\} \qquad (9)$$

Where $\boldsymbol{n}_q$ is unit outward normal vector on the sphere surface. In our implementation N, the number of the sampling points on the sphere is fixed to 24, minimum radius $r_0 = 0.5$ voxel, q was set to 2 and entries of $\boldsymbol{v}$ and $\boldsymbol{n}$ with non-integer index, are interpolated linearly.

7   Implementation

In order to have a working contour evolution a few issues must be considered. Since we segment vessels that appear brighter than background, to allow proper vessel edge detection we only allow negative values on the second term in (6). This eliminates the edges resulting from objects with opposite brightness polarity. The second issue concerns weighting of this term. As indicated in [4], the (geodesic) image curvature term has a regional energy functional with interpretation as topological complexity of the grey levels, hence it can be independently scaled.

Also a regularized version of delta function,δ_ε is utilized with the same definition as in [8], we used $\varepsilon = 0.5$. Finally smoothness is achieved using minimal surface principle curvature introduced in [1]. Therefore using the tensor metric defined in (8), vessel segmentation evolution is as follows:

$$\frac{\partial \phi}{\partial t} = \delta_\varepsilon(\phi)[\nabla.(g^{-1}\nabla I) - \rho. \parallel \nabla I \parallel_{g^{-1}} S(\nabla.(\frac{g^{-1}\nabla I}{\parallel \nabla I \parallel_{g^{-1}}})) + \alpha \hat{k}] \qquad (10)$$

Where $S(x) = x$ if $x < 0$ otherwise 0. During our experiments we observed that the best performance in terms of contour propagation and leakage minimization, is obtained for $0.8 \leq \rho \leq 0.95$. Setting $w = 1$ is too conservative and stops the propagation in thinner vessels. The program is implemented using *Insight Toolkit* and mex library funcitons are called from MATLAB on a Linux system.

8   Synthetic Data Experiment

The maximum intensity projection of a synthetic image is shown in Fig.1.a. We embed a few gap-like signal drop effect along side the model and the target volume is *assumed* to be a straight rod. A Gaussian noise was generated and added with the image. Segmentation using FLUX is achieved by setting: $g^{-1} = I_d$, $\rho = 0$ in (10). A few leakage can be observed in the segmented model shown in (b). Setting $g^{-1} \neq I_d$ has resulted a better recovery of the shape, because some noisy gradient vectors have been suppressed by projection through g^{-1} in (c). Euclidean Haralick model (d) is insufficient for segmentation since it

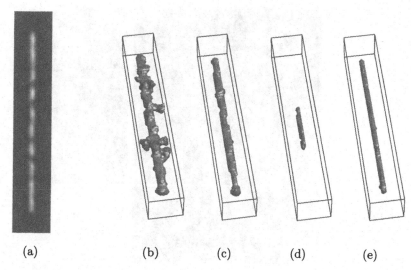

(a)	(b)	(c)	(d)	(e)

Fig. 1. Segmentation of the a noisy data set, (a) Maximum projection image, segmentations obtained from: (b) FLUX ($g^{-1} = I_d$, $\rho = 0$), (c)Anisotropic FLUX ($\rho = 0$), (d)Euclidean Haralick ($g^{-1} = I_d$), (e)Anisotropic Haralick schemes

has detected the embedded gaps and contour has been trapped between those gaps. However, the Riemannian Haralick model has successfully passed over the signal droppings and the target has been successfully segmented. This is because the edges from those gaps has been suppressed by projection with g^{-1}, and meanwhile in contrary to (c), a tighter edges have been obtained across the model, which is also more closer to the actual edge points of the model.

9   Vessel Segmentation

The efficiency of the proposed edge detection scheme was tested on real data sets obtained using 3T TOF-MRA protocol. A typical example is given in this sectionn. The original data set was filtered using a Gaussian smoothing filter with $\sigma = 1$ voxel, and the segmentation was applied on a selected ROI. Fig.2 indicates the maximum intensity projection image from a three different orientation after smoothing. In these experiments, for obtaining a smooth segmenting surface we set $\alpha = 0.3$. This was particularly important for FLUX since without curvature term a significant surface irregularity was obtained.

The segmentation results of the flux maximizing flow is shown in the Fig.3.(a). This has been obtained after 1000 iterations of (10) by setting $g^{-1} = I_d$ and $\rho = 0$. As it can be observed segmented vessels appears wider than MIP. This can be associated with edge localization error of the original "Marr-Hildreth" method. It is also observe that some of thin vessels have been missed. We verified that, these thin vessels can be discovered by less amounts of α. But in that case, irregularity and leakage was rapidly increasing, which made the visualization

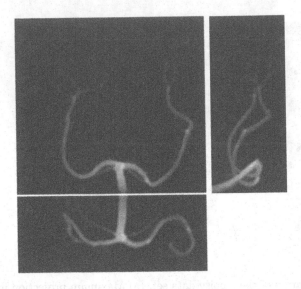

Fig. 2. MIP images of a 150×140×60 of 3T TOF-MRA data set used for segmentation

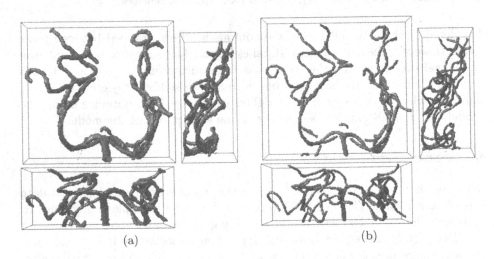

(a)   (b)

Fig. 3. Segmentation using: (a) FLUX, (b) Riemannian Haralick edge detection

difficult. Therefore a compromised result is shown here which consists of most of the vessels with acceptable smooth surface.

In contrary, using g^{-1} as defined in (8) $\alpha = 0.3$ and $\rho = .8$, segmented vessels in Fig.3.(b) appear thinner and render better detail in complex morphological areas. This is because it is based on the Haralick edge detection scheme with higher precision for edge identification, which allows the method to capture finer details.

10 Discussion

In this paper a new Riemannian Haralick like edge detection scheme was proposed. The method generalizes the standard Haralick edge detection scheme to a Riemannian manifold, where the dot product of two vectors is defined under a specific metric tensor. Into our knowledge, this extention is new and has not been addressed yet. Our curve evolution method is based on a regional energy functional defined on the manifold. The tensor metric has a simple form that eliminates noisy gradient vectors. This can be extended to more sophisticated cases in future studies. A comparison with standard FLUX method, revealed that the method is able to segment more detailed structures and finer elements. Validation and comparion using other kind of data sets remains as our future research activities.

Acknowledgement

This study was supported in part by the Special Coordination Funds for Promoting Science and Technology in Japan, and Grant for Industrial Technology Research (07C46050), New Energy and Industrial Technology Development Organization, Japan (both to H. Liao), the Grant-in-Aid for Scientific Research (17100008) of the Japan Society for the Promotion of Science (to T. Dohi).

References

1. Lorgio, L.M., Faugeras, O.D., Grimson, W.E.L., Kerivan, R., Kikinis, R., Nabavai, A., Westin, C.F.: CURVES: Curve evolution for vessel segmentation. Medical Image Analysis 5, 195–206 (2001)
2. Yan, P., Kassim, A.A.: Segmentation of volumetric MRA images by using capillary active contour. Medical Image Analysis 10(3), 317–329 (2006)
3. Vasilevsky, A., Siddiqi, K.: Flux maximizing geometric flows. IEEE Trans. Pat. Anal. Mach. Intel. 24(12), 1565–1578 (2002)
4. Gazit, M.H., Kimmel, R., Peled, N., Goldsher, D.: Segmentation of thin structures in volumetric medical images. IEEE Trans. Image Proc. 15(2), 354–363 (2006)
5. Caselles, V., Kimmel, R., Sapiro, G.: Geodesic Active Contours. Int. Journal of Computer Vision 22(1), 61–79 (1997)
6. Shah, J.: Riemannian Drums, Anisotropic Curve Evolution and Segmentation. In: Nielsen, M., Johansen, P., Fogh Olsen, O., Weickert, J. (eds.) Scale-Space 1999. LNCS, vol. 1682, pp. 129–140. Springer, Heidelberg (1999)
7. Zaho, H.K., Chan, T., Merriman, B., Osher, S.: A variational level set approach to multiphase motion. Journal of Computational Physics 127, 179–195 (1996)
8. Chan, T.F., Vese, A.: Active contours without edges. IEEE Trans. Imag. Proc. 10, 266–277 (2001)
9. Agam, G., Armato, S., Wu, C.: Vessel Tree Reconstruction in Thoracic CT Scans With Application to Nodule Detection. IEEE Trans. Imag. Proc. 24(4), 486–499 (2005)
10. Haralick, R.: Digital step edge from zero crossing of second directional derivatives. IEEE Trans. Patt. Rec. Mach. Vis. 1(1), 58–68 (1984)

11. John Canny, F.: A Computational Approach to Edge Detection. IEEE Trans. Patt. Rec. Mach. Vis. 8, 679–698 (1986)
12. Marr, D., Hildreth, E.: Theory of Edge Detection, A Computational Approach to Edge Detection. Proc. Roy. Soc. Lond. B 207, 187–217 (1980)
13. Law, M.W.K., CHung, A.C.S.: Weighted local variance-based edge detection and its application to vascular segmentation in Magnetic Resonance Angiography. IEEE Trans. Imag. Proc. 26(9), 1224–1241 (2007)

Author Index

Ademoglu, Ahmet   108
Akbari, Hamed   142
Atallah, Louis   270
Azuma, Takashi   300

Bainbridge, Daniel   1
Bauer, Christian   393
Bello, Fernando   202
Benali, Habib   124
Bischof, Horst   393

Camici, Paolo G.   193
Cao, Xianbin   31
Casula, Roberto   202
Chang, Stephen   320
Cheng, Kan   150
Chiba, Toshio   251, 260, 300, 329
Chui, Chee-Kong   320
Chung, Adrian   21
Chung, Adrian J.   193
Chung, Moo K.   177
Colliot, Olivier   124

Dalton, Kim M.   177
Darzi, Ara W.   270
Davidson, Richard J.   177
Deguchi, Daisuke   377
Dohi, Takeyoshi   210, 260, 329,
  349, 367, 385, 430
Dong, Xiao   421
Du, Peng   168
Dubois, Bruno   124
Duru, Adil Deniz   108

Edwards, Philip   202
Emery, Roger J.   270
Erdt, Marius   403

Feng, Jun   31, 168
Figl, Michael   202
Fujie, Masakatsu G.   50, 311
Fujisaki, Masayuki   300
Fuwa, Teruhiko   70

Gallinari, Patrick   124
García, Jaime   185

Gill, Inderbir S.   359
González Ballester, Miguel Á.   160, 185
Gooya, Ali   430
Gu, Lixu   150, 339
Guiraudon, Gérard M.   1

Hahn-Barma, Valérie   124
Hamed, Abbi   220
Hanafusa, Akihiko   70
Hanak, David   279
Hasegawa, Yoshinori   377
Hashizume, Makoto   50, 359
Hattori, Asaki   70
Hawkes, David   202
He, Qizhen   31
Heng, Pheng Ann   116
Herlambang, Nicholas   349
Hoshi, Takeharu   50
Hu, Mingxing   202
Huang, Chung-Hsien   289

Ikeda, Tomozumi   70
Imaizumi, Kazuyoshi   377
Ip, Horace H.S.   31, 168
Ishihara, Hirotaka   367
Ishii, Tetsuko   300
Ishiyama, Akihiko   300

Jiang, Jiefeng   133
Jiang, Tianzi   133
Jones, Douglas L.   1

Kagiyama, Yoshiyuki   40
Katsuike, Yasumasa   300
Kawamura, Kazuya   50, 311
Kinkingnéhun, Serge   124
Kitasaka, Takayuki   377
Kitazumi, Gontaro   300
Kobayashi, Etsuko   329
Kobayashi, Yo   50, 311
Koizumi, Norihiro   231
Kojima, Kazuyuki   142
Kosugi, Yukio   142
Kozic, Nina   160
Kwok, Ka-Wai   21

Lamperth, Michael   220
Lee, Deukhee   231
Lee, Jiann-Der   289
Lee, Shin-Tseng   289
Leff, Daniel R.   270
Lehéricy, Stéphane   124
Leong, Florence   320
Leong, Julian J.H.   270
Li, Kuncheng   133
Li, Wei   150
Liao, Hongen   210, 260, 329,
    349, 367, 385, 430
Lin, Chung-Wei   289
Lin, Lei   133
Linte, Cristian A.   1
Liu, Huafeng   60

Magnin, Benoit   124
Mahadevan, Arul   359
Marescaux, Jacques   241
Masamune, Ken   210, 260, 349, 367, 385
Matsumiya, Kiyoshi   210, 260, 349
Matsumoto, Yoichiro   231
Mendoza-Burgos, Luis   241
Mesrob, Lilia   124
Miki, Tsuneharu   359
Mitsuishi, Mamoru   231
Miyamoto, Yoshitaka   300
Miyoshi, Toshinobu   300
Mochizuki, Takashi   329
Moore, John   1
Mori, Kensaku   377
Mori, Masaki   377
Mutter, Didier   241
Mylonas, George P.   21, 270

Nacewicz, Brendon M.   177
Naganawa, Akihiro   251
Nakamoto, Masahiko   40, 359
Nakamura, Tetsuya   251
Nakayama, Noriyoshi   300
Natori, Hiroshi   377
Nicolau, Stephane A.   241
Nolte, Lutz P.   160

Oka, Kiyoshi   251
Okazaki, Makoto   300
Onishi, Akinori   50
Ota, Kohei   231
Ota, Shunsuke   377
Otomaru, Itaru   40

Pedro, Ose   202
Penney, Graeme   202
Peterhans, Matthias   185
Peters, Terry M.   1
Pollak, Seth   177
Poo, Aun Neow   320

Qi, Wenyuan   339

Raspe, Matthias   403
Reyes, Mauricio   160
Rueckert, Daniel   202

Sakuma, Ichiro   320, 329, 367, 430
Sarazin, Marie   124
Sato, Ikuma   210, 385
Sato, Yoshinobu   40, 359
Shen, Dinggang   413
Shi, Feng   133
Shi, Pengcheng   60, 98
Shi, Yonghong   413
Soler, Luc   241
Song, Zhijian   81
Styner, Martin   185
Suehling, Michael   403
Suenaga, Yasuhito   377
Sugano, Nobuhiko   40
Sugawara, Motoki   70
Suzuki, Naoki   70

Tada, Yukio   40
Takabatake, Hirotsugu   377
Takacs, Barnabas   279
Takamoto, Shinichi   300
Takao, Masaki   40
Talib, Haydar   185
Tanaka, Naofumi   142
Tannast, Moritz   160
Tran, Huy Hoang   367
Tse, Zion Tsz Ho   220
Tsin, Wong Tien   116
Tsuzuki, Masayoshi   329

Ukimura, Osamu   359

Voshburg, Kirby G.   279
Vrtovec, Tomaž   89

Wang, Liansheng   116
Wang, Linwei   60, 98
Wang, Manning   81
Wang, Shubing   177

Wong, Kelvin   12
Wong, Ken C.L.   60, 98
Wong, Stephen   12
Wu, Chien-Tsai   289
Wu, Jianghua   150

Xia, James   31
Xu, Jianrong   150, 339
Xue, Zhong   12

Yamanaka, Noriaki   210, 260
Yamashita, Hiromasa   251, 260, 300
Yang, Guang-Zhong   21, 193, 270

Yang, Liangjing   320
Yoshikawa, Hideki   40
Yoshinaka, Kiyoshi   231
Yoshizawa, Shin   231
Young, Ian   220
Yu, Chunshui   133

Zhang, Dong Ping   202
Zhang, Heye   60, 98
Zhang, Yuanchao   133
Zheng, Guoyan   421
Zhou, Yuan   133
Zuo, Siyang   210

Lecture Notes in Computer Science

Sublibrary 6: Image Processing, Computer Vision, Pattern Recognition, and Graphics

For information about Vols. 1– 3951
please contact your bookseller or Springer

Vol. 5128: T. Dohi, I. Sakuma, H. Liao (Eds.), Medical Imaging and Augmented Reality. XVI, 441 pages. 2008.

Vol. 5116: E.A. Krupinski (Ed.), Digital Mammography. XXVII, 769 pages. 2008.

Vol. 5112: A. Campilho, M. Kamel (Eds.), Image Analysis and Recognition. XXII, 1126 pages. 2008.

Vol. 5099: A. Elmoataz, O. Lezoray, F. Nouboud, D. Mammass (Eds.), Image and Signal Processing. XVI, 625 pages. 2008.

Vol. 5098: F.J. Perales, R.B. Fisher (Eds.), Articulated Motion and Deformable Objects. XIV, 458 pages. 2008.

Vol. 5096: G. Rigoll (Ed.), Pattern Recognition. XIII, 538 pages. 2008.

Vol. 4992: D. Coeurjolly, I. Sivignon, L. Tougne, F. Dupont (Eds.), Discrete Geometry for Computer Imagery. XIII, 554 pages. 2008.

Vol. 4987: X. Gao, H. Müller, M.J. Loomes, R. Comley, S. Luo (Eds.), Medical Imaging and Informatics. XV, 388 pages. 2008.

Vol. 4958: V.E. Brimkov, R.P. Barneva, H.A. Hauptman (Eds.), Combinatorial Image Analysis. XVI, 446 pages. 2008.

Vol. 4931: G. Sommer, R. Klette (Eds.), Robot Vision. XI, 468 pages. 2008.

Vol. 4901: D. Zhang (Ed.), Medical Biometrics. XII, 324 pages. 2007.

Vol. 4889: A. Pasko, V. Adzhiev, P. Comninos (Eds.), Heterogeneous Objects Modelling and Applications. VII, 285 pages. 2008.

Vol. 4844: Y. Yagi, S.B. Kang, I.S. Kweon, H. Zha (Eds.), Computer Vision – ACCV 2007, Part II. XXVIII, 915 pages. 2007.

Vol. 4843: Y. Yagi, S.B. Kang, I.S. Kweon, H. Zha (Eds.), Computer Vision – ACCV 2007, Part I. XXVIII, 969 pages. 2007.

Vol. 4842: G. Bebis, R. Boyle, B. Parvin, D. Koracin, N. Paragios, S.-M. Tanveer, T. Ju, Z. Liu, S. Coquillart, C. Cruz-Neira, T. Müller, T. Malzbender (Eds.), Advances in Visual Computing, Part II. XXXIII, 827 pages. 2007.

Vol. 4841: G. Bebis, R. Boyle, B. Parvin, D. Koracin, N. Paragios, S.-M. Tanveer, T. Ju, Z. Liu, S. Coquillart, C. Cruz-Neira, T. Müller, T. Malzbender (Eds.), Advances in Visual Computing, Part I. XXXIII, 831 pages. 2007.

Vol. 4815: A. Ghosh, R.K. De, S.K. Pal (Eds.), Pattern Recognition and Machine Intelligence. XIX, 677 pages. 2007.

Vol. 4814: A. Elgammal, B. Rosenhahn, R. Klette (Eds.), Human Motion – Understanding, Modeling, Capture and Animation. X, 329 pages. 2007.

Vol. 4792: N. Ayache, S. Ourselin, A. Maeder (Eds.), Medical Image Computing and Computer-Assisted Intervention – MICCAI 2007, Part II. XLVI, 988 pages. 2007.

Vol. 4791: N. Ayache, S. Ourselin, A. Maeder (Eds.), Medical Image Computing and Computer-Assisted Intervention – MICCAI 2007, Part I. XLVI, 1012 pages. 2007.

Vol. 4781: G. Qiu, C. Leung, X.-Y. Xue, R. Laurini (Eds.), Advances in Visual Information Systems. XIII, 582 pages. 2007.

Vol. 4778: S.K. Zhou, W. Zhao, X. Tang, S. Gong (Eds.), Analysis and Modeling of Faces and Gestures. X, 305 pages. 2007.

Vol. 4768: D. Doermann, S. Jaeger (Eds.), Arabic and Chinese Handwriting Recognition. VIII, 279 pages. 2008.

Vol. 4756: L. Rueda, D. Mery, J. Kittler (Eds.), Progress in Pattern Recognition, Image Analysis and Applications. XXI, 989 pages. 2007.

Vol. 4738: A.C.R. Paiva, R. Prada, R.W. Picard (Eds.), Affective Computing and Intelligent Interaction. XVIII, 781 pages. 2007.

Vol. 4729: F. Mele, G. Ramella, S. Santillo, F. Ventriglia (Eds.), Advances in Brain, Vision, and Artificial Intelligence. XVI, 618 pages. 2007.

Vol. 4713: F.A. Hamprecht, C. Schnörr, B. Jähne (Eds.), Pattern Recognition. XIII, 560 pages. 2007.

Vol. 4679: A.L. Yuille, S.-C. Zhu, D. Cremers, Y. Wang (Eds.), Energy Minimization Methods in Computer Vision and Pattern Recognition. XII, 494 pages. 2007.

Vol. 4678: J. Blanc-Talon, W. Philips, D. Popescu, P. Scheunders (Eds.), Advanced Concepts for Intelligent Vision Systems. XXIII, 1100 pages. 2007.

Vol. 4673: W.G. Kropatsch, M. Kampel, A. Hanbury (Eds.), Computer Analysis of Images and Patterns. XX, 1006 pages. 2007.

Vol. 4642: S.-W. Lee, S.Z. Li (Eds.), Advances in Biometrics. XX, 1216 pages. 2007.

Vol. 4633: M. Kamel, A. Campilho (Eds.), Image Analysis and Recognition. XII, 1312 pages. 2007.

Vol. 4625: R. Stiefelhagen, R. Bowers, J. Fiscus (Eds.), Multimodal Technologies for Perception of Humans. XIII, 556 pages. 2008.

Vol. 4584: N. Karssemeijer, B. Lelieveldt (Eds.), Information Processing in Medical Imaging. XX, 777 pages. 2007.

Vol. 4569: A. Butz, B. Fisher, A. Krüger, P. Olivier, S. Owada (Eds.), Smart Graphics. IX, 237 pages. 2007.

Vol. 4538: F. Escolano, M. Vento (Eds.), Graph-Based Representations in Pattern Recognition. XII, 416 pages. 2007.

Vol. 4522: B.K. Ersbøll, K.S. Pedersen (Eds.), Image Analysis. XVIII, 989 pages. 2007.

Vol. 4485: F. Sgallari, A. Murli, N. Paragios (Eds.), Scale Space and Variational Methods in Computer Vision. XV, 931 pages. 2007.

Vol. 4478: J. Martí, J.M. Benedí, A.M. Mendonça, J. Serrat (Eds.), Pattern Recognition and Image Analysis, Part II. XXVII, 657 pages. 2007.

Vol. 4477: J. Martí, J.M. Benedí, A.M. Mendonça, J. Serrat (Eds.), Pattern Recognition and Image Analysis, Part I. XXVII, 625 pages. 2007.

Vol. 4472: M. Haindl, J. Kittler, F. Roli (Eds.), Multiple Classifier Systems. XI, 524 pages. 2007.

Vol. 4466: F.B. Sachse, G. Seemann (Eds.), Functional Imaging and Modeling of the Heart. XV, 486 pages. 2007.

Vol. 4418: A. Gagalowicz, W. Philips (Eds.), Computer Vision/Computer Graphics Collaboration Techniques. XV, 620 pages. 2007.

Vol. 4417: A. Kerren, A. Ebert, J. Meyer (Eds.), Human-Centered Visualization Environments. XIX, 403 pages. 2007.

Vol. 4391: Y. Stylianou, M. Faundez-Zanuy, A. Esposito (Eds.), Progress in Nonlinear Speech Processing. XII, 269 pages. 2007.

Vol. 4370: P.P. Lévy, B. Le Grand, F. Poulet, M. Soto, L. Darago, L. Toubiana, J.-F. Vibert (Eds.), Pixelization Paradigm. XV, 279 pages. 2007.

Vol. 4358: R. Vidal, A. Heyden, Y. Ma (Eds.), Dynamical Vision. IX, 329 pages. 2007.

Vol. 4338: P.K. Kalra, S. Peleg (Eds.), Computer Vision, Graphics and Image Processing. XV, 965 pages. 2006.

Vol. 4319: L.-W. Chang, W.-N. Lie (Eds.), Advances in Image and Video Technology. XXVI, 1347 pages. 2006.

Vol. 4292: G. Bebis, R. Boyle, B. Parvin, D. Koracin, P. Remagnino, A. Nefian, G. Meenakshisundaram, V. Pascucci, J. Zara, J. Molineros, H. Theisel, T. Malzbender (Eds.), Advances in Visual Computing, Part II. XXXII, 906 pages. 2006.

Vol. 4291: G. Bebis, R. Boyle, B. Parvin, D. Koracin, P. Remagnino, A. Nefian, G. Meenakshisundaram, V. Pascucci, J. Zara, J. Molineros, H. Theisel, T. Malzbender (Eds.), Advances in Visual Computing, Part I. XXXI, 916 pages. 2006.

Vol. 4245: A. Kuba, L.G. Nyúl, K. Palágyi (Eds.), Discrete Geometry for Computer Imagery. XIII, 688 pages. 2006.

Vol. 4241: R.R. Beichel, M. Sonka (Eds.), Computer Vision Approaches to Medical Image Analysis. XI, 262 pages. 2006.

Vol. 4225: J.F. Martínez-Trinidad, J.A. Carrasco Ochoa, J. Kittler (Eds.), Progress in Pattern Recognition, Image Analysis and Applications. XIX, 995 pages. 2006.

Vol. 4191: R. Larsen, M. Nielsen, J. Sporring (Eds.), Medical Image Computing and Computer-Assisted Intervention – MICCAI 2006, Part II. XXXVIII, 981 pages. 2006.

Vol. 4190: R. Larsen, M. Nielsen, J. Sporring (Eds.), Medical Image Computing and Computer-Assisted Intervention – MICCAI 2006, Part I. XXXVVIII, 949 pages. 2006.

Vol. 4179: J. Blanc-Talon, W. Philips, D. Popescu, P. Scheunders (Eds.), Advanced Concepts for Intelligent Vision Systems. XXIV, 1224 pages. 2006.

Vol. 4174: K. Franke, K.-R. Müller, B. Nickolay, R. Schäfer (Eds.), Pattern Recognition. XX, 773 pages. 2006.

Vol. 4170: J. Ponce, M. Hebert, C. Schmid, A. Zisserman (Eds.), Toward Category-Level Object Recognition. XI, 618 pages. 2006.

Vol. 4153: N. Zheng, X. Jiang, X. Lan (Eds.), Advances in Machine Vision, Image Processing, and Pattern Analysis. XIII, 506 pages. 2006.

Vol. 4142: A. Campilho, M. Kamel (Eds.), Image Analysis and Recognition, Part II. XXVII, 923 pages. 2006.

Vol. 4141: A. Campilho, M. Kamel (Eds.), Image Analysis and Recognition, Part I. XXVIII, 939 pages. 2006.

Vol. 4122: R. Stiefelhagen, J.S. Garofolo (Eds.), Multimodal Technologies for Perception of Humans. XII, 360 pages. 2007.

Vol. 4109: D.-Y. Yeung, J.T. Kwok, A. Fred, F. Roli, D. de Ridder (Eds.), Structural, Syntactic, and Statistical Pattern Recognition. XXI, 939 pages. 2006.

Vol. 4091: G.-Z. Yang, T. Jiang, D. Shen, L. Gu, J. Yang (Eds.), Medical Imaging and Augmented Reality. XIII, 399 pages. 2006.

Vol. 4073: A. Butz, B. Fisher, A. Krüger, P. Olivier (Eds.), Smart Graphics. XI, 263 pages. 2006.

Vol. 4069: F.J. Perales, R.B. Fisher (Eds.), Articulated Motion and Deformable Objects. XV, 526 pages. 2006.

Vol. 4057: J.P.W. Pluim, B. Likar, F.A. Gerritsen (Eds.), Biomedical Image Registration. XII, 324 pages. 2006.

Vol. 4046: S.M. Astley, M. Brady, C. Rose, R. Zwiggelaar (Eds.), Digital Mammography. XVI, 654 pages. 2006.

Vol. 4040: R. Reulke, U. Eckardt, B. Flach, U. Knauer, K. Polthier (Eds.), Combinatorial Image Analysis. XII, 482 pages. 2006.

Vol. 4035: T. Nishita, Q. Peng, H.-P. Seidel (Eds.), Advances in Computer Graphics. XX, 771 pages. 2006.

Vol. 3979: T.S. Huang, N. Sebe, M. Lew, V. Pavlović, M. Kölsch, A. Galata, B. Kisačanin (Eds.), Computer Vision in Human-Computer Interaction. XII, 121 pages. 2006.

Vol. 3954: A. Leonardis, H. Bischof, A. Pinz (Eds.), Computer Vision – ECCV 2006, Part IV. XVII, 613 pages. 2006.

Vol. 3953: A. Leonardis, H. Bischof, A. Pinz (Eds.), Computer Vision – ECCV 2006, Part III. XVII, 649 pages. 2006.

Vol. 3952: A. Leonardis, H. Bischof, A. Pinz (Eds.), Computer Vision – ECCV 2006, Part II. XVII, 661 pages. 2006.